JOY BAUER'S SUPERFOOD!

150 RECIPES *for* ETERNAL YOUTH

JOY BAUER

Abrams, New York

*To my family . . . superfood tastes even better
with a super-family to share it with.*

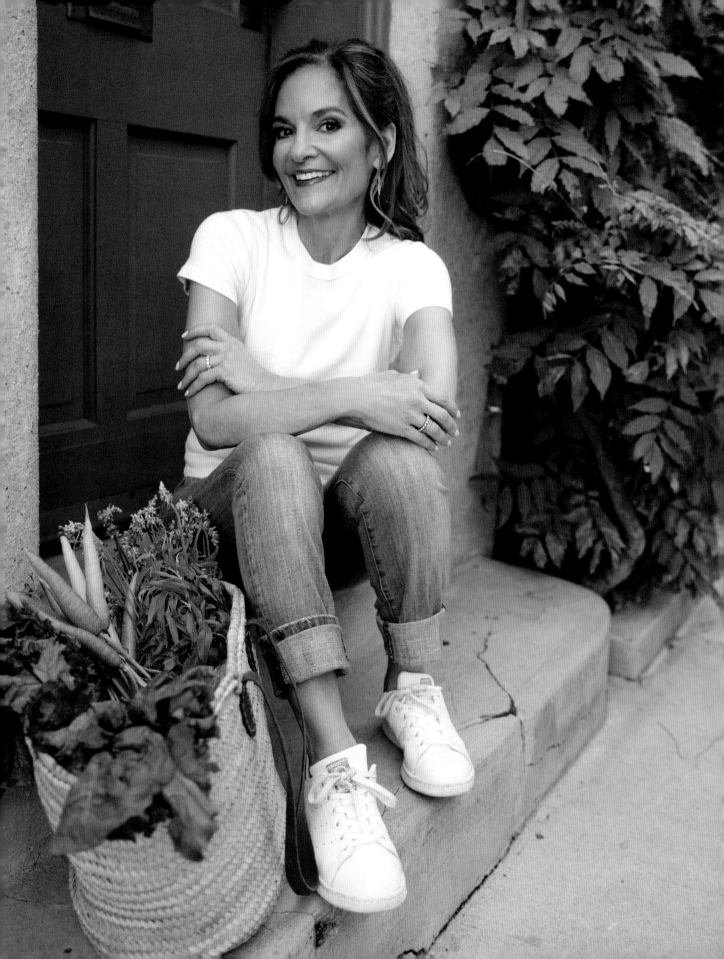

Introduction

Superfood: a wholesome food containing one or more nutrients to help elevate health.

In other words, it's a food you want on your plate.

Welcome to my Superfood fiesta! This book shines light on the most stellar superfoods—those that have been highlighted and singled out for being the most powerful, potent, and nutrient-packed. These picks have scores of quality studies behind them, supporting their prowess. They are served and devoured in Blue Zones, areas where people live the longest, healthiest lives (the five original regions in the world researchers have keyed in on are Sardinia in Italy, Okinawa in Japan, Icaria in Greece, Nicoya in Costa Rica, and Loma Linda, California; experts have studied these folks to determine the habits that help promote longevity). The people in these spots are celebrating their hundredth birthdays (and beyond)—and a large reason for this is diet. The foods they eat contain nutrients that have been identified as helping reduce the risk of the most-life threatening diseases, including heart disease and certain cancers. They've been shown to tame inflammation and ease aches and pains. They help boost your energy and mood, strengthen your immunity, and improve memory. They aid in weight control and help promote a glowing complexion and prevent wrinkles. They are *super*, indeed.

The star lineup features eight thoughtful categories: vegetables, legumes, fruit, nuts and seeds, coffee and tea, whole grains, and scrumptious extras (like cocoa powder and extra virgin olive oil). Within each category, I've identified true standouts that you'll definitely want to toss into your grocery cart.

Then these superfoods are incorporated into 150 mouthwatering recipes, so your taste buds will be delighted and your body will be showered with one power food after the next. The recipes are organized into a variety of chapters, from "Morning Meals" to "Soups and Salads" to "Enticing Entrées" to "One-Pot Wonders" to "Sweet and Savory Treats." All the work is already done—you just have to cook, eat, and enjoy. You may notice a trend toward plant-based foods. No, this isn't a coincidence—study after study shows how beneficial these nourishing items are. But you'll also find plenty of palate-pleasing protein sources, like poultry and fish—even pork and beef tenderloin make a debut—for those who need a hearty fix. I've even included chocolate, cookies, and some boozy beverages, too, so you can feel good about indulging. There's something for everyone—and every craving.

Imagine living to be one hundred—looking and feeling amazing—all while chowing down on insanely delicious food. It's entirely possible. Get set, get cooking!

Morning Meals

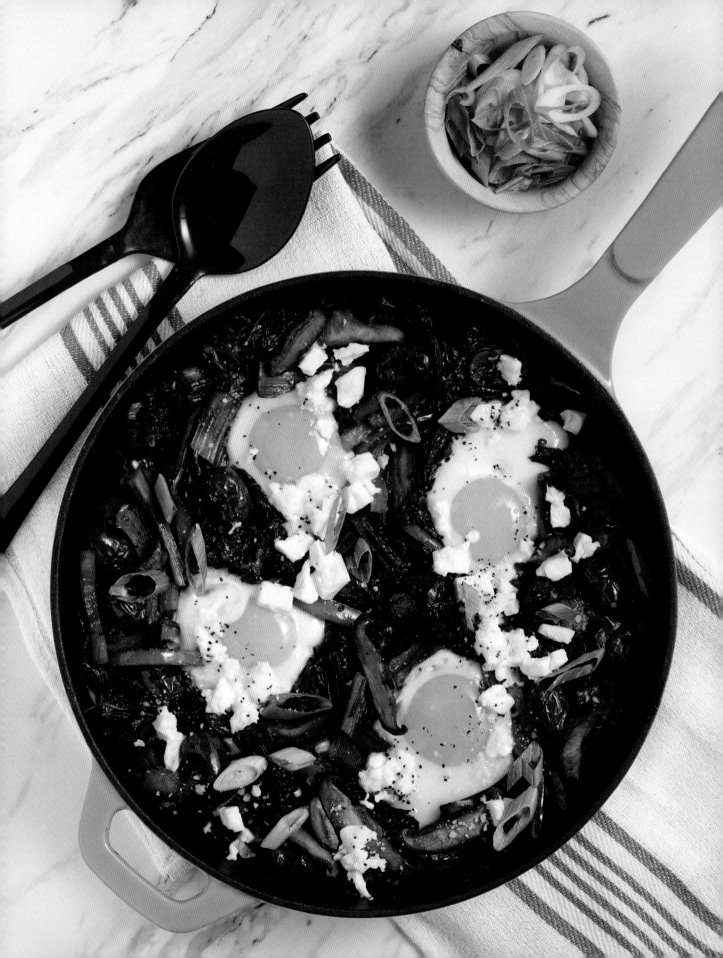

Rainbow Shakshuka

SERVES: 2 PREP TIME: 10 MINUTES COOK TIME: 20 MINUTES

I owe it to my older daughter, Jesse, for introducing me to shakshuka. I fell in love with the bold, full-flavored Middle Eastern dish while visiting her on a study-abroad program in Israel, and it became one of my go-to breakfasts. My rendition trades the standard brothy tomato sauce for a unique blend of textures and fresh veggies. I start by sautéing multicolored heirloom tomatoes with bright bell peppers, and then incorporating meaty shiitake mushrooms—ideal for their dense consistency and immunity-boosting properties—and rainbow Swiss chard, a beautiful leafy green that's bursting with fiber, antioxidants, and vitamins A and K. (If you prefer, take spinach or kale for a spin instead.) Then I nestle in the eggs, where they cook until the whites are set and the yolks remain runny. For an impressive presentation, transfer your skillet from the stovetop right to the table. Party of one? This amazingly delicious dish can easily be halved for a single serving.

1 pint multicolored cherry or grape tomatoes

1 yellow bell pepper, thinly sliced

1 bunch rainbow chard, stems chopped into 1-inch pieces (about 1 cup) and leaves torn into smaller pieces (2 to 3 cups)

3 ounces shiitake mushrooms (about 6), stems removed, and each torn into 3 or 4 pieces

2 large cloves garlic, minced

1 teaspoon chopped fresh rosemary

4 scallions, thinly sliced

¼ cup white wine or vegetable broth

4 large eggs

Kosher salt and ground black pepper

2 to 3 tablespoons crumbled feta cheese

2 to 3 tablespoons Parmesan cheese

1 Mist a skillet with olive oil spray and warm over medium-high heat. Add the tomatoes and bell pepper and allow the veggies to sit, undisturbed, for 1 to 2 minutes so they start to develop a nice charred color in certain spots. Stir and continue to cook for another 3 to 4 minutes, until the veggies are soft and the tomatoes are slightly blistered.

2 Add the chard stems and mushrooms and mist with additional olive oil spray. Continue to cook for another 3 minutes, or until the veggies are softened. Add the garlic, rosemary, chard leaves, scallions, and wine. Toss everything together to wilt the chard leaves and continue to cook for another 5 minutes, deglazing the pan and scraping up all the flavorful browned bits from the bottom of the skillet.

3 Create 4 wells within the vegetables, making room for the eggs. Mist the wells with oil spray, then carefully crack the eggs into them. Sprinkle some salt and pepper over each egg and around the vegetables. Lower the heat to medium and continue to cook until the whites are firm and set but the yolks are still runny, 4 to 5 minutes. Scatter the feta and Parmesan cheeses over the eggs. Cover and cook for about 1 minute to warm the cheese, then serve.

PER SERVING **300** CALORIES **22 g** PROTEIN **13 g** FAT (**8 g** UNSATURATED FAT, **5 g** SATURATED FAT) **380 mg** CHOLESTEROL **28 g** CARBS **8 g** FIBER **11 g** SUGAR (**11 g** NATURAL SUGAR, **0 g** ADDED SUGAR) **530 mg** SODIUM

Breakfast Coffee Cookies

MAKES: 30 COOKIES   PREP TIME: 5 MINUTES   COOK TIME: 12 MINUTES

Who doesn't love the idea of eating cookies for breakfast? It's like a dream come true. I first debuted these grab-and-go gems on the *TODAY* show and they instantly became an enormous hit—even going viral on social media. As an added bonus, they contain three brain-and-memory-boosting ingredients: cocoa powder, coffee, and blueberries. Go ahead and enjoy two or three in the A.M. with a cup of coffee . . . or channel your inner kid and go with a milk-and-cookies theme. P.S.: They're just as good as an afternoon snack.

1 cup whole wheat flour

¾ cup all-purpose flour

½ cup cocoa powder

1½ tablespoons instant coffee or finely ground coffee

1½ teaspoons ground cinnamon

1 teaspoon baking soda

½ teaspoon kosher salt

3 large eggs, lightly beaten

1 ripe banana, peeled, microwaved for 30 seconds, and mashed

½ cup plain nonfat or low-fat plain Greek yogurt

½ cup honey

1 tablespoon grapeseed or canola oil

2 teaspoons vanilla extract

1¼ cups fresh blueberries

½ to ¾ cup dark or semisweet chocolate chips

1 Preheat the oven to 350°F. Mist a large cookie sheet (or 2 standard size sheets) with nonstick oil spray. Set aside.

2 In a large bowl, combine the whole wheat flour, all-purpose flour, cocoa powder, coffee, cinnamon, baking soda, and salt. Set aside.

3 In a separate bowl, combine the eggs, mashed banana, yogurt, honey, oil, and vanilla. Stir until everything is well combined and the banana is thoroughly blended within (if small pieces remain, that's okay).

4 Pour the wet ingredients into the dry ingredients, gently stirring until fully incorporated. Fold in the blueberries and chocolate chips (or save some of the chocolate chips to sprinkle on top before baking). Do not overmix.

5 Place 1 heaping tablespoon of batter, one at a time, onto the prepared baking sheet, leaving space between each small pile. The batter will be very sticky, so mist the spoon and your fingers with nonstick oil spray as needed. Flatten each cookie by gently pressing the top with your fingers or the back of a fork (mist the fork with oil spray, too, to prevent sticking). Top each cookie with a sprinkling of reserved chocolate chips. Bake for 12 to 15 minutes. Let cool on the baking sheet and enjoy.

PRO TIP: To freeze the cookies, cool for at least 1 hour, then wrap each one individually or put 2 or 3 together in small storage bags and stash in the freezer. When you're ready to eat, thaw at room temperature or defrost in the microwave for about 30 seconds.

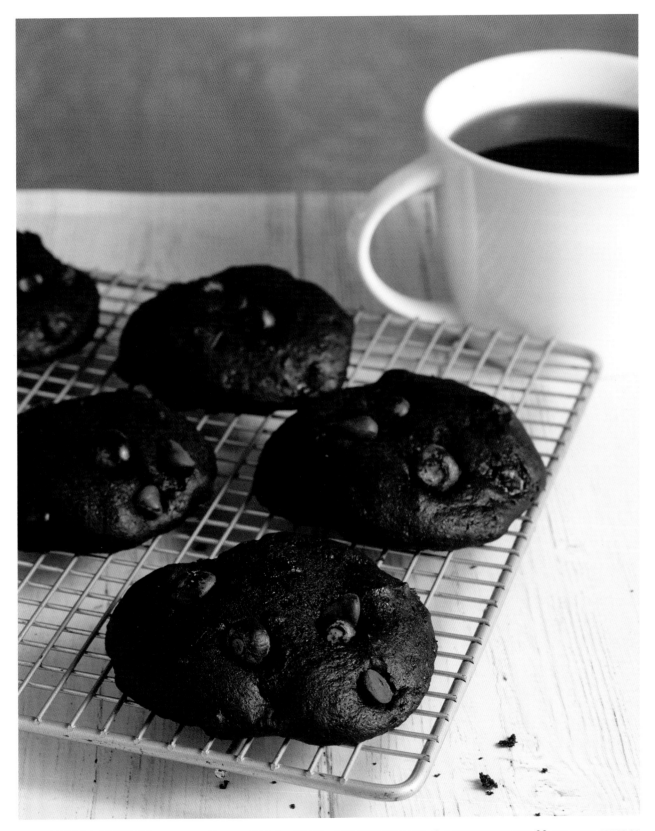

PER SERVING 1 COOKIE **80** CALORIES **3 g** PROTEIN **2 g** FAT (**2 g** UNSATURATED FAT, **0 g** SATURATED FAT) **20 mg** CHOLESTEROL **14 g** CARBS **2 g** FIBER **7 g** SUGAR (**2 g** NATURAL SUGAR, **5 g** ADDED SUGAR) **90 mg** SODIUM

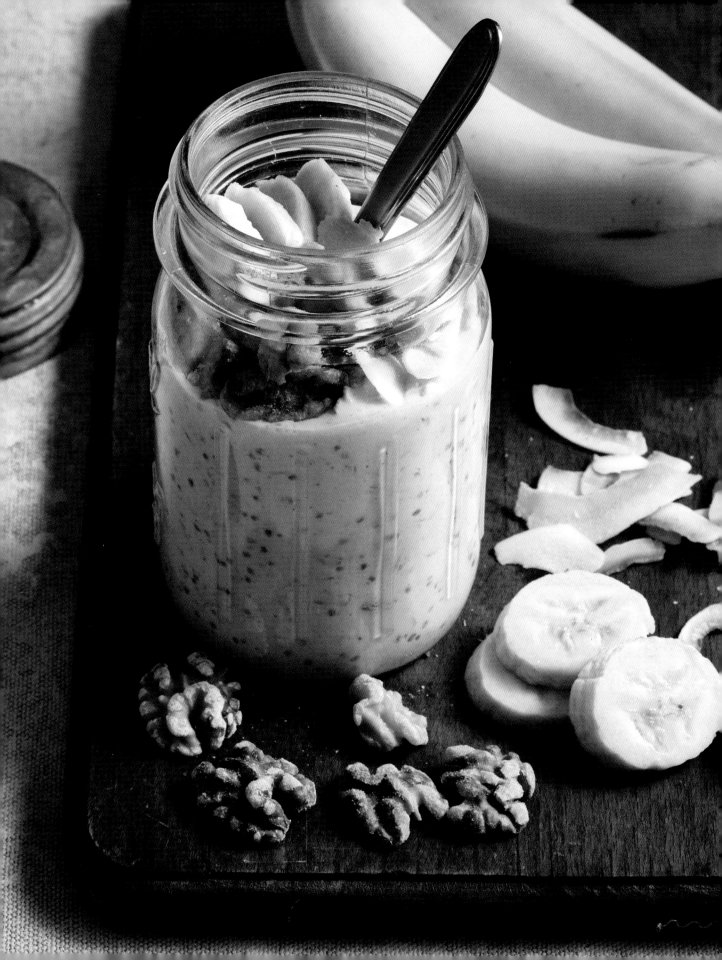

Banana Cream Pie Overnight Oats

SERVES: 1   PREP TIME: 5 MINUTES, PLUS AT LEAST 6 HOURS SOAKING

My husband and son are both huge fans of bananas . . . and of pie. Why not marry the two in one delicious and winning recipe? That's how this dish was born! Of course, it stars potassium-packed banana, which, in my opinion, is one of the most versatile ingredients out there. It's more than just a convenient snack; it lends sweetness to smoothies, creaminess to ice cream, and the perfect flavor to this nutrient-rich morning meal. This recipe also features oats, which are filled with fiber; the cottage cheese delivers satiating protein and bone-strengthening calcium; and chia seeds help it all gel together. Admittedly, my guys would probably prefer the real McCoy (a la mode), but they happily spoon this up in the morning before rushing out the door. The girls and I go bananas over it, too.

1 ripe banana, peeled

½ cup low-fat cottage cheese (preferably whipped, but any type with curds will work)

¼ cup unsweetened almond milk (or milk of choice)

¼ cup uncooked old-fashioned oats

1 teaspoon vanilla extract

1 tablespoon chia seeds

OPTIONAL TOPPERS

Sliced bananas, toasted walnuts, shredded coconut, dash of ground cinnamon

1 Microwave the banana in a bowl for about 30 seconds to soften it up. Remove from the microwave, add the cottage cheese, and mash the two ingredients until they're well combined. (Whipped cottage cheese will provide a completely smooth texture, while traditional small curd cottage cheese will provide a lumpier consistency; both taste delicious.)

2 Add the milk, oats, vanilla, and chia seeds. Stir everything together, cover, and refrigerate for at least 6 hours or overnight. Garnish with your choice of sliced banana, toasted walnuts, shredded coconut, cinnamon, or any other topping you like.

PER SERVING ~1½ CUPS **340** CALORIES **21 g** PROTEIN **9 g** FAT (**7.5 g** UNSATURATED FAT, **1.5 g** SATURATED FAT) **5 mg** CHOLES-TEROL **46 g** CARBS **10 g** FIBER **16 g** SUGAR (**16 g** NATURAL SUGAR, **0 g** ADDED SUGAR) **550 mg** SODIUM

Dirty Chai Overnight Oats

SERVES: 2   PREP TIME: 5 MINUTES, PLUS AT LEAST 6 HOURS SOAKING

Chai isn't just for tea. I love working its Indian-inspired flavors—cardamom, cinnamon, ginger, allspice, and cloves—into foods because of their complexity and warmth. The standard dirty chai recipe gets its "dirty" moniker because it features a shot of espresso. My version actually calls for brewed coffee—but you can use whichever you prefer. When I'm rushing to an early morning TV shoot or meeting and I don't have time to prepare breakfast, I've come to rely on *overnight* oats. There's nothing easier: I prep them the night before in a sealable jar, refrigerate, and then simply give a quick shake or stir when I wake up. Don't expect a sugary sweet experience; this delivers a creamy bowl of goodness filled with several distinct layers of flavorful spice—pretty darn fabulous, IMO! Of course, you can easily sweeten it up with additional honey, if you prefer.

Pro tip: This overnight creation is delicious straight from the fridge, but you can warm it up, too. Just stir in ½ cup extra milk and microwave for a minute or so.

1 cup unsweetened almond milk (or milk of choice)

¼ cup brewed coffee, cooled

2 teaspoons honey

1 teaspoon vanilla extract

¼ teaspoon kosher salt

1 teaspoon ground cinnamon

½ teaspoon ground cardamom

¼ teaspoon ground ginger

¼ teaspoon ground allspice

⅛ teaspoon ground cloves

1 cup uncooked old-fashioned oats

2 tablespoons chia seeds

1   In a small bowl, combine the milk, coffee, honey, vanilla, salt, cinnamon, cardamom, ginger, allspice, and cloves. Whisk to dissolve the honey. Stir in the oats and chia seeds until everything is evenly incorporated and the oats are submerged. Cover and refrigerate for at least 6 hours or overnight for the mixture to soften and firm.

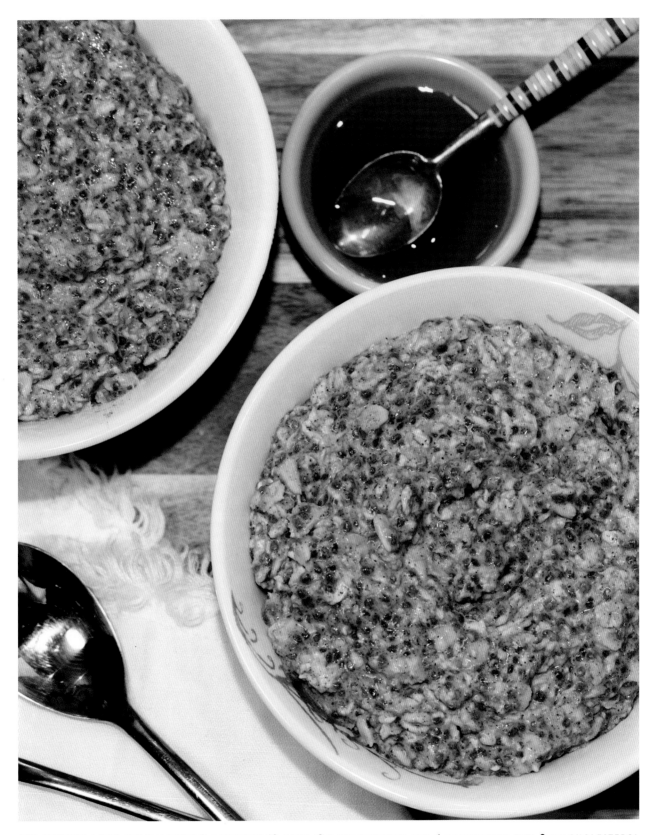

PER SERVING 1 CUP **270** CALORIES **9 g** PROTEIN **10 g** FAT (**9 g** UNSATURATED FAT, **1 g** SATURATED FAT) **0 mg** CHOLESTEROL **42 g** CARBS **11 g** FIBER **7 g** SUGAR (**1 g** NATURAL SUGAR, **6 g** ADDED SUGAR) **380 mg** SODIUM

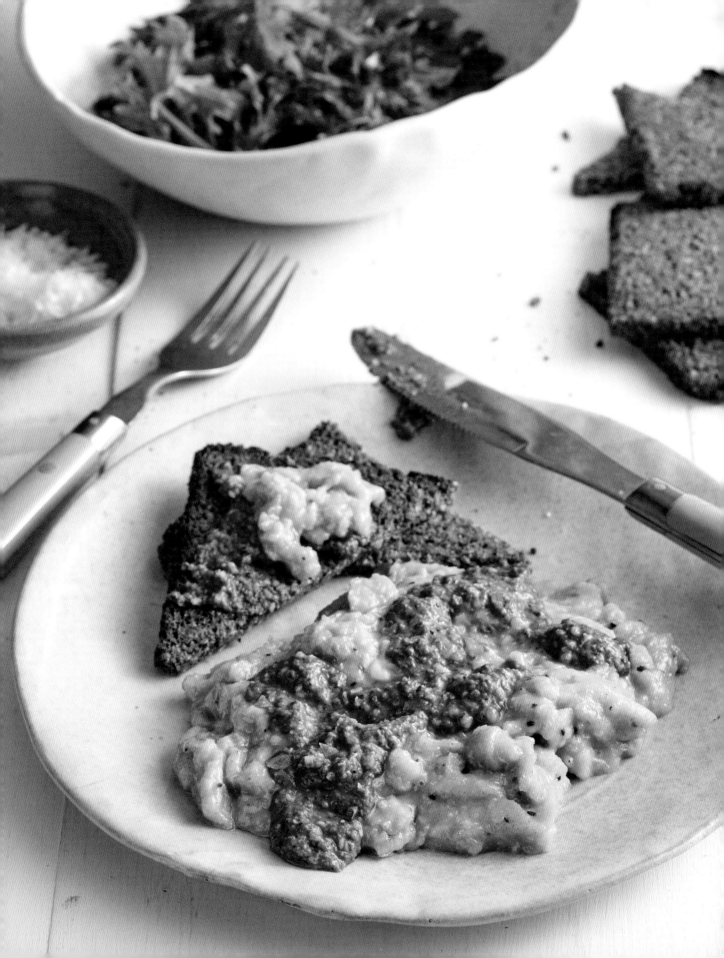

Creamy Scrambled Eggs with Kale Spinach Pesto

SERVES: 4   PREP TIME: 10 MINUTES   COOK TIME: 5 MINUTES

How do I love pesto . . . let me count the ways. Pesto is typically made with flavorful and aromatic basil, but I also added some kale and spinach to up the nutritional ante (if you like arugula, you can try swapping that in). A couple other pesto pointers: I toss in a single small ice cube while blending to maintain the bright green color. And you can easily make this nut-free by using pumpkin seeds in place of the almonds, walnuts, or pine nuts. P.S.: You'll have plenty of yummy pesto leftover for future meals.

If you're looking to manage your cholesterol, I suggest using olive oil instead of butter when scrambling the eggs and mixing four whole eggs with six egg whites instead of using eight whole eggs. It's still amazing!

PESTO
makes 1½ cups

2 cloves garlic, peeled

¼ cup blanched, toasted almonds (or toasted walnuts or pine nuts)

¾ to 1 teaspoon kosher salt

¼ teaspoon ground black pepper, or more to taste

½ cup grated Parmesan or pecorino cheese

1 tablespoon lemon juice

2 cups loosely packed baby kale leaves

2 cups loosely packed baby spinach leaves

1 cup loosely packed fresh basil leaves

5 tablespoons extra virgin olive oil

CREAMY SCRAMBLED EGGS

1 tablespoon butter or olive oil

8 large eggs, beaten

Kosher salt and ground black pepper

1 **FOR THE PESTO:** Combine the garlic, nuts, salt, pepper, cheese, lemon juice, kale, spinach, and basil in a food processor or blender and pulse until the greens are finely chopped. Add 3 to 4 tablespoons water and scrape down the sides as needed to ensure everything is well combined. Then drizzle in the oil while you continue to pulse until everything is evenly blended. Toss in a small ice cube while blending to maintain the bright green color. Taste and season with additional salt and pepper if needed.

2 **FOR THE EGGS:** In a large skillet, melt the butter or warm the oil over medium heat. Once the butter is foaming (or the oil is heated), add the eggs and reduce the heat to medium-low. As the eggs begin to set, use a spatula to gently drag the eggs to the center. Continue to gently pull the eggs away from the sides to create curds of egg, and cook until just about set, about 3 minutes.

3 Transfer the eggs to a serving dish and season with salt and pepper to taste. Drizzle the pesto over the top.

PER SERVING 2 EGGS WITH 2 TABLESPOONS PESTO **210** CALORIES **14 g** PROTEIN **17 g** FAT (**11 g** UNSATURATED FAT, **6 g** SATURATED FAT) **380 mg** CHOLESTEROL **2 g** CARBS **0 g** FIBER **1 g** SUGAR (**1 g** NATURAL SUGAR, **0 g** ADDED SUGAR) **230 mg** SODIUM

Chicken and Zucchini-Carrot Waffles with Spicy Maple Syrup

SERVES: 5   PREP TIME: 10 MINUTES, PLUS 30 MINUTES MARINATING
COOK TIME: 30 MINUTES

There are two traditional versions of this dish, both equally tempting. You can go the Southern, pure soul food route: waffles topped with melted butter, sweet syrup, and, of course, finger-licking-good fried chicken. Or enjoy a rendition like the one served in Pennsylvania Dutch Country, with pulled stewed chicken, smothered in gravy on top of your waffles. My spin, inspired by the former, incorporates—you guessed it!—veggies like zucchini and carrots mixed right into the waffle batter, and oven "fried" chicken marinated in creamy buttermilk and coated in crispy and flavorful whole grain breading. And I don't skip the syrup, but I do mix it with sriracha because anyone who knows me knows I'm all about the heat. It's gooey-good; sweet and spicy, drippy and delicious.

ZUCCHINI-CARROT WAFFLES

- 3 cups roughly chopped carrots
- 3 cups roughly chopped unpeeled zucchini
- 1 large egg, lightly beaten
- 1 large egg white
- ¼ cup chopped fresh dill
- 2 to 3 teaspoons onion powder
- ¾ cup chickpea flour (or flour of choice)
- ¾ teaspoon kosher salt
- ¼ teaspoon black pepper

OVEN "FRIED" CHICKEN TENDERS

- ½ cup low-fat buttermilk
- 1 tablespoon hot sauce
- 1 pound chicken tenders (5 pieces)
- 1½ cups crispy brown rice cereal
- 1 tablespoon ground flaxseeds
- 2 teaspoons paprika
- 1 teaspoon dried thyme
- ½ teaspoon kosher salt
- ¼ teaspoon black pepper

SPICY MAPLE SYRUP

- ½ cup maple syrup
- 2 teaspoons sriracha

1 FOR THE WAFFLES: Preheat a waffle iron and mist nonstick oil spray on the top and bottom.

2 Add the carrots and zucchini to the bowl of a food processor and gently pulse until finely chopped (being extra careful to not puree them). Transfer to a large mixing bowl and add the egg and egg white, dill, onion powder, chickpea flour, salt, and pepper and stir until everything is well blended into a batter.

3 Add ½ cup batter to each heated waffle iron compartment, close the lid, and cook for about 15 minutes. Because this is a *veggie* batter, they will take much longer to cook than traditional flour waffles. When the waffles are ready, use a fork or bamboo stick to carefully loosen the edges and lift them out of each compartment. Serve immediately, or place on a baking sheet in a low oven to keep warm until your batches are complete and you're ready to eat.

RECIPE CONTINUES

PER SERVING 250 CALORIES 27 g PROTEIN 3 g FAT (3 g UNSATURATED FAT, 0 g SATURATED FAT) 50 mg CHOLESTEROL 29 g CARBS 5 g FIBER 12 g SUGAR (8 g NATURAL SUGAR, 4 g ADDED SUGAR) 800 mg SODIUM

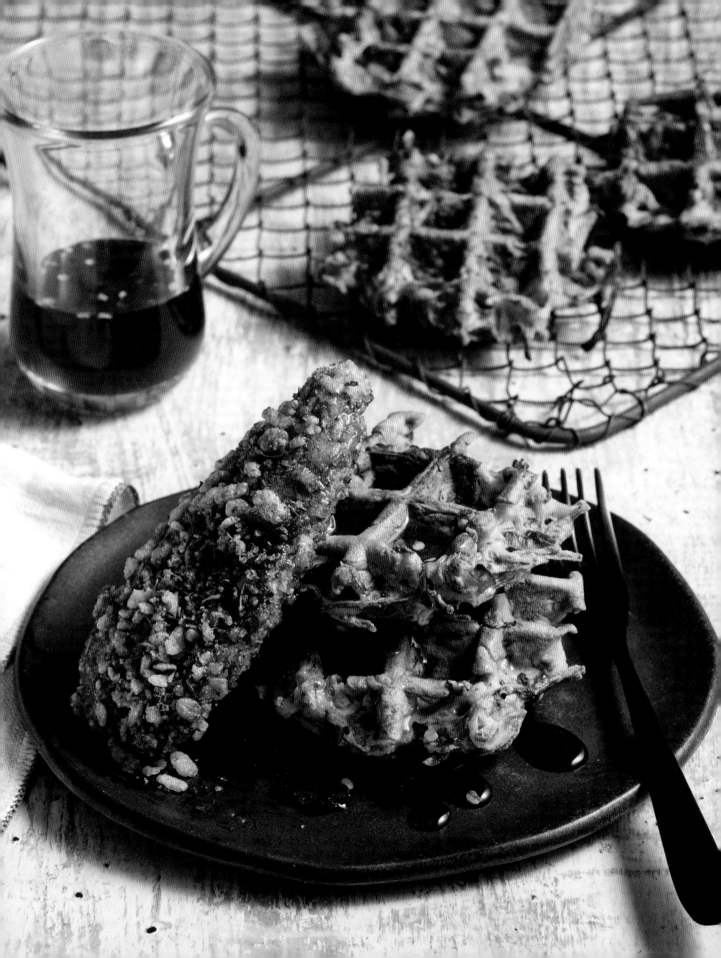

4 **FOR THE CHICKEN:** Combine the buttermilk and hot sauce in a zip-top bag. Place the chicken in the bag, move it around to coat, and marinate in the fridge for at least 30 minutes or overnight.

5 Preheat the oven to 375°F. Mist a small baking sheet with nonstick oil spray and set aside.

6 Place the cereal in a zip-top bag and lightly crush with a soup can, rolling pin, or meat mallet. Don't pulverize it; you want it to look like coarse breadcrumbs, so be sure to leave pieces and texture to it. Open the bag and add the flaxseeds, paprika, thyme, salt, and pepper.

7 Working in batches, lift one piece of chicken from the buttermilk marinade at a time and place in the cereal bag. Shake it around to coat in cereal crumbs and place on the baking sheet, being careful to keep them from touching. Mist the tops with oil spray and bake for 10 to 15 minutes, or until the chicken is cooked through and they're golden brown.

8 **FOR THE SYRUP:** In a small bowl, stir together the maple syrup and sriracha. **TO SERVE:** Stack 2 waffles with 1 piece of chicken on each plate and drizzle on 1 teaspoon spicy maple syrup.

Toast and Chia Jam

This homemade jam has replaced the traditional jarred stuff in my house. We use it on just about everything, including toast, pancakes, my Protein Bagels (page 44), scones, PB&J sandwiches, and even stirred into yogurt and oatmeal to boost the flavor and nutrition. It's super easy to make (the addition of chia seeds forms a jelly-like consistency as it sits in the fridge overnight), and everyone has a favorite variety. Plus, it's insanely jammy and delicious without any added sugar.

You can use fresh or frozen fruit to whip these up. The option for frozen gives you a lot of freedom, since you're not locked in and limited to a specific season and its offerings. The only caveat is the Peach Mango & Ginger flavor—I prefer to use fresh ripe mango and canned peaches in natural juice, because they work much better than frozen in this recipe. Once you start making these scrumptious jams and stashing them in the fridge, you can experiment with all sorts of amazing creations and combos: Try mixing the Wild Blueberry with the PB Coconut Cookie Dough Dip (page 260) spread for an epic PB&J sandwich. Or pair Strawberry Orange with fresh sliced mango for a delicious spin to top your waffle. Or prep a yogurt parfait with one thin layer of Peach Mango Jam and a second layer of Cherry Jam for a gorgeous and good-for-you presentation. The options are endless!

Note: A fresh batch of jam will keep in the fridge in a sealed container for up to two weeks, or you can freeze in a sealed container for 2 months; simply defrost overnight in the fridge before using.

STRAWBERRY ORANGE CHIA JAM
makes about 1¾ cups

3 cups fresh or frozen strawberries

3 tablespoons orange juice

2 tablespoons chia seeds

1 In a medium saucepan, combine the strawberries and orange juice and cook over medium heat for about 10 minutes for frozen strawberries and 8 minutes for fresh strawberries, continuously stirring, chopping, and mashing the fruit with a potato masher or the back of a wooden spoon to break up the skin and release the natural juices.

2 Remove the pan from the heat. Add chia seeds to the fruit and mix well. Transfer the mixture to a mason jar or other container, seal, and refrigerate overnight.

PER SERVING 1 TABLESPOON **10** CALORIES **0 g** PROTEIN **0 g** FAT **0 mg** CHOLESTEROL **2 g** CARBS **1 g** FIBER **1 g** SUGAR (**1 g** NATURAL SUGAR, **0 g** ADDED SUGAR) **0 mg** SODIUM

RECIPES CONTINUE

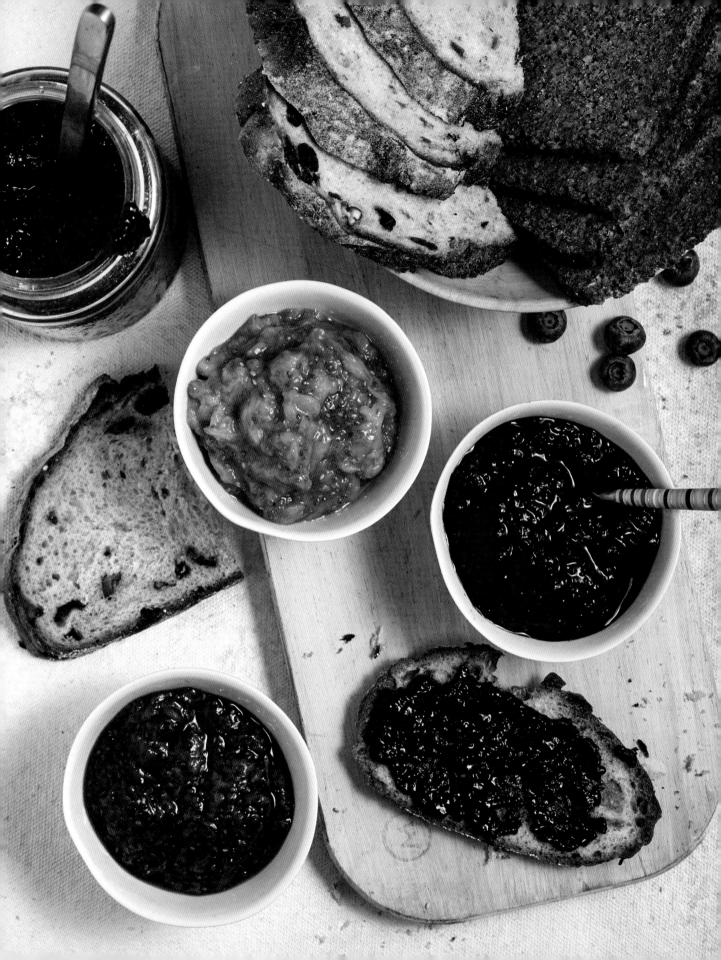

CHERRY CHIA JAM
makes about 1¾ cups

2 cups pitted fresh or frozen sweet cherries

1 cup fresh or frozen pineapple cubes

2 tablespoons chia seeds

1 In a small saucepan, combine the cherries and pineapple. (If you're using frozen fruit, thaw it slightly first.) Cook over medium heat for about 7 minutes, continuously stirring, chopping, and mashing it with a potato masher or the back of a wooden spoon to break up the skin of the cherries and release the natural juices of the fruit.

2 Remove the pan from the heat and pick out any remaining large pineapple chunks. (Don't discard them—they're delicious mixed into oatmeal, yogurt, or cottage cheese.)

3 Add the chia seeds to the fruit and mix well. Transfer the mixture to a mason jar or other container, seal, and refrigerate overnight.

PER SERVING 1 TABLESPOON **15** CALORIES **0 g** PROTEIN **0 g** FAT **0 mg** CHOLESTEROL **3 g** CARBS **1 g** FIBER **1 g** SUGAR (**1 g** NATURAL SUGAR, **0 g** ADDED SUGAR) **0 mg** SODIUM

PEACH, MANGO, AND GINGER CHIA JAM
makes about 1¾ cups

2 cups sliced mango (from 1 to 2 fresh mangoes)

1 cup canned peaches in natural juice, drained, with juice reserved

1 tablespoon grated fresh ginger root

2 tablespoons chia seeds

1 In a medium saucepan, combine the mango, peaches, 3 tablespoons of reserved peach juice, and the ginger. Cook over medium heat for about 6 minutes, continuously stirring, chopping, and mashing the fruit with a potato masher or the back of a wooden spoon to break up the skin and release the natural juices.

2 Remove the pan from the heat. Add chia seeds to the fruit and mix well. Transfer the mixture to a mason jar or other container, seal, and refrigerate overnight.

PER SERVING 1 TABLESPOON **10** CALORIES **0 g** PROTEIN **0 g** FAT **0 mg** CHOLESTEROL **2 g** CARBS **0 g** FIBER **1 g** SUGAR (**1 g** NATURAL SUGAR **0 g** ADDED SUGAR) **0 mg** SODIUM

WILD BLUEBERRY AND RASPBERRY CHIA JAM
makes about 1¾ cups

1¾ cups fresh or frozen wild blueberries

2 cups fresh or frozen raspberries

1 tablespoon lemon juice

½ to 1 teaspoon lemon zest

2 tablespoons chia seeds

1 In a small saucepan, combine the blueberries, raspberries, lemon juice, and lemon zest and cook over medium heat for 5 to 6 minutes, continuously stirring, chopping, and mashing the fruit with a potato masher or the back of a wooden spoon to break up the skin and release the natural juices.

2 Remove the pan from the heat. Add chia seeds to the fruit and mix well. Transfer the mixture to a mason jar or other container, seal, and refrigerate overnight.

PER SERVING 1 TABLESPOON **15** CALORIES **0 g** PROTEIN **0 g** FAT **0 mg** CHOLESTEROL **2 g** CARBS **1 g** FIBER **1 g** SUGAR (**1 g** NATURAL SUGAR, **0 g** ADDED SUGAR) **0 mg** SODIUM

Apple and Sage Breakfast Sausage

MAKES: ABOUT 28   PREP TIME: 10 MINUTES   COOK TIME: 16 MINUTES

Apples are one food you'll always find in my kitchen. (During apple-picking season, my house resembles an applesauce factory . . . one of my family's most beloved uses!) With so many different types, it's hard to choose my favorite. In this dish, I've used Granny Smith—tart, yet subtly sweet—but you can certainly substitute what you like best. Mixing grated Granny Smith with a number of flavorful seasonings and protein-rich ground poultry—turkey or chicken— creates the ultimate flavor combo. I prefer cooking with 90 to 93% lean ground poultry for juicier patties (99% lean typically yields a dryer end result). And while I normally leave the peel on when I cook with apples, it works better without it in this recipe.

Pro tip: Typically, chefs avoid overmixing ground meat (for burgers or meatloaf), but in this case, doing so ensures that the mixture holds together without any starchy binder and results in the distinct texture of moist, meaty sausage. These flavorful patties can be served for breakfast (alongside eggs or pancakes, or on their own with a side of fruit as they're so protein-packed), or any other time of day. Sweet and savory sausage satisfaction!

1 pound ground turkey or chicken (90 to 93% lean)

1 medium Granny Smith apple, peeled, cored, and grated (about 1 cup)

2 teaspoons ground sage

½ teaspoon fennel seeds, roughly chopped

½ teaspoon red pepper flakes, or more to taste

½ teaspoon garlic powder

½ teaspoon smoked paprika

½ teaspoon onion powder

1¼ teaspoons kosher salt

1 tablespoon maple syrup

1 In a large bowl, combine all the ingredients. Be sure to evenly distribute the seasonings and create a smooth consistency.

2 One at a time, create small (golf ball–size) balls using the palms of your hands, then flatten each into ⅛- to ¼-inch-thick patties, or form them into 2-inch-long sausage links. You will have about 28.

3 Mist a large skillet with nonstick oil spray and warm over medium heat. Add the first batch of patties and cook for about 2 minutes per side, searing the outsides so they become nicely browned and have a slight caramelized appearance. As they cook, do not press down on the tops with a spatula or they'll become too dry. If making sausage links, move them around on the hot pan to brown all sides as they cook and extend the cooking time by an extra minute or so. Repeat, misting the pan with oil spray between batches, until all the sausage is cooked.

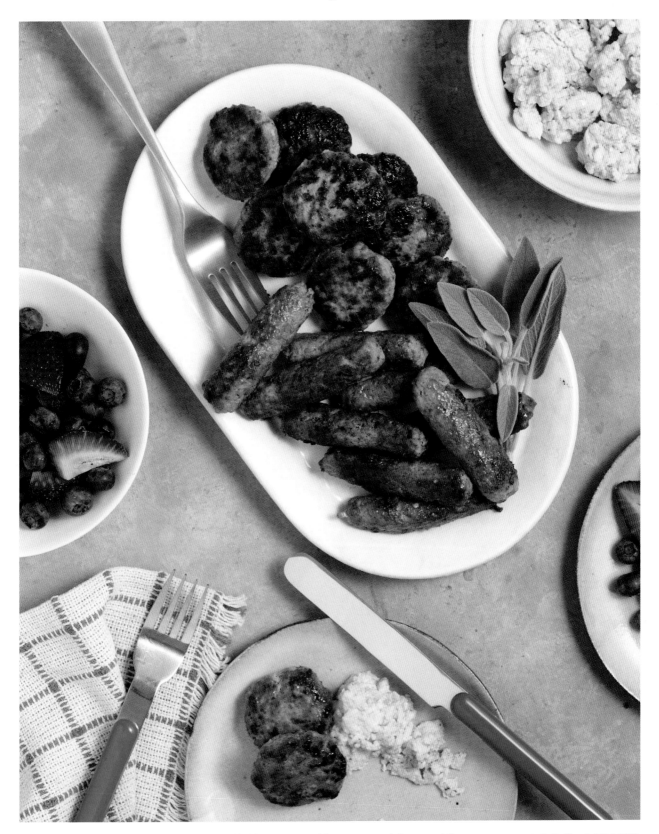

PER SERVING 4 PATTIES OR SAUSAGE LINKS **90** CALORIES **14 g** PROTEIN **1.5 g** FAT (**1.5 g** UNSATURATED FAT, **0 g** SATURATED FAT) **50 mg** CHOLESTEROL **5 g** CARBS **1 g** FIBER **3 g** SUGAR (**1 g** NATURAL SUGAR, **2 g** ADDED SUGAR) **420 mg** SODIUM

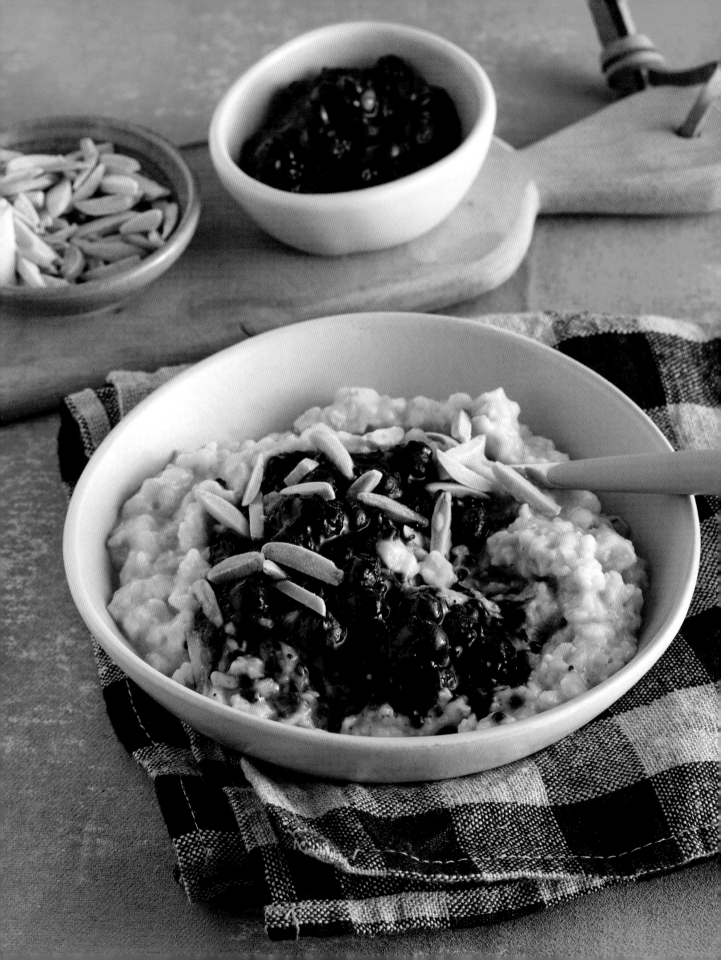

Blueberry Pie Oatmeal

SERVES: 2   PREP TIME: 3 MINUTES   COOK TIME: 5 MINUTES

The people who know me may tell you that I'm obsessed with oatmeal. They wouldn't be lying. Oatmeal is the ultimate whole grain. It's filling, delicious, nutritious, and versatile. I'm constantly experimenting with the breakfast staple, trying to come up with new and out-of-the-box ways to serve it up. When I was creating this blueberry breakfast bowl, I was aiming for a dessert-like feel, sort of like a blueberry pie filling experience, but of course, one that's good for you. Featuring two top-notch ingredients certainly gave me a solid head start. Blueberries are always atop the list of foods richest in antioxidants. And oats are high in beta-glucans, a fiber that may lower cholesterol and boost immunity. Then there's the tasty and toasty almond slivers scattered over the top, which can easily be swapped for pecans, walnuts, peanuts or any other nut you have on hand. It's an ideal recipe to whip up for a special breakfast date or a hang-in weekend with the gang. And of course, if you're dining alone, you can easily stash the leftover blueberry sauce in the fridge and make one bowl at a time.

BLUEBERRY SAUCE
makes about ¾ cup

1 cup fresh or frozen blueberries

2 tablespoons cranberry juice (or juice of choice)

1 tablespoon chia seeds

OATMEAL
makes about 2 cups

1 cup unsweetened almond milk (or milk of choice)

1 cup uncooked old-fashioned oats

¼ cup toasted almond slivers*

Fresh blueberries for garnish (optional)

* *If starting with raw almond slivers, spread them out on a baking sheet and toast in a 350°F oven for 3 to 4 minutes.*

1 FOR THE BLUEBERRY SAUCE: In a small microwave-safe bowl, combine the blueberries, cranberry juice, and chia seeds. Cover and microwave for 2 minutes. Give the mixture a good stir and let it sit and thicken while you prepare the oats.

2 FOR THE OATMEAL: In a medium saucepan, combine the milk, 1 cup water, and the oats. Bring to a boil over medium-high heat, reduce heat to medium-low, and cook for about 5 minutes, stirring occasionally, until you reach your desired thickness and creaminess. TO SERVE: Divide the oatmeal between 2 bowls and top each with half of the blueberry sauce. Scatter the toasted almonds over the top and garnish with fresh blueberries, if desired.

PER SERVING **320** CALORIES **10 g** PROTEIN **13 g** FAT (**12 g** UNSATURATED FAT, **1 g** SATURATED FAT) **0 mg** CHOLESTEROL **45 g** CARBS **10 g** FIBER **10 g** TOTAL SUGAR (**10 g** NATURAL SUGAR, **0 g** ADDED SUGAR) **90 mg** SODIUM

Blender Carrot Cake Pancakes with Cream Cheese Frosting

SERVES: 4   PREP TIME: 5 MINUTES   COOK TIME: 10 MINUTES

On those days when it's hard to get out of bed, let this be your motivation: the flavors of carrot cake with cream cheese frosting for breakfast. Oh yeah, things just got interesting!

While the flavor is fantastic, the health perks are even more impressive, thanks to a few power ingredients. The banana delivers potassium to help manage blood pressure and bloating. The eggs contain protein to help steady blood sugar, which in turn can balance appetite and mood. Whole grain oats introduce cholesterol-lowering capability. And the carrots chip in some beta-carotene, which boosts immunity among other benefits. These gems are also flourless and gluten-free.

Note that while you can use precut matchstick carrots from the grocery store, I prefer to grate my own carrots for a moister result.

PANCAKES

- ½ cup unsweetened almond milk (or milk of choice)
- 1 ripe banana
- 1 large egg
- 4 large egg whites
- ¾ cup uncooked old-fashioned oats
- 1 tablespoon ground cinnamon
- 1 teaspoon ground ginger
- ½ teaspoon ground nutmeg
- 1 teaspoon baking powder
- ½ teaspoon kosher salt
- 2 tablespoons maple syrup
- 2 teaspoons vanilla extract
- ½ teaspoon maple extract or maple flavor
- 1¼ cups grated carrots (from 2 medium carrots, grated on the largest holes)

CREAM CHEESE FROSTING

- ¼ cup reduced-fat cream cheese, at room temperature
- 1½ tablespoons maple syrup
- ¼ teaspoon vanilla extract
- ⅛ teaspoon kosher salt

1 FOR THE PANCAKES: Combine the almond milk, banana, whole egg and egg whites, oats, cinnamon, ginger, nutmeg, baking powder, salt, maple syrup, and vanilla and maple extracts to the blender and puree, about 20 seconds. Stop and scrape down the sides of the blender if necessary. Then, with the motor turned off, use a spoon to carefully mix in the grated carrots.

2 Liberally coat a large skillet with nonstick oil spray and warm over medium-low heat. Working in batches, add the batter, a scant ¼ cup at a time, and cook for about 2 minutes per side, until browned on the outside and completely cooked through on the inside. If the pancakes become too browned before they're cooked through, reduce the heat to low.

3 FOR THE FROSTING: In a small bowl, mix the cream cheese, maple syrup, vanilla, salt and 2 tablespoons warm water until well blended. Drizzle over stacks of pancakes or enjoy on the side.

PER SERVING 3 PANCAKES WITH 1 TO 2 TABLESPOONS FROSTING **200** CALORIES **8 g** PROTEIN **4.5 g** FAT (**3 g** UNSATURATED FAT, **1.5 g** SATURATED FAT) **50 mg** CHOLESTEROL **32 g** CARBS **4 g** FIBER **14 g** SUGAR (**5 g** NATURAL SUGAR, **9 g** ADDED SUGAR) **410 mg** SODIUM

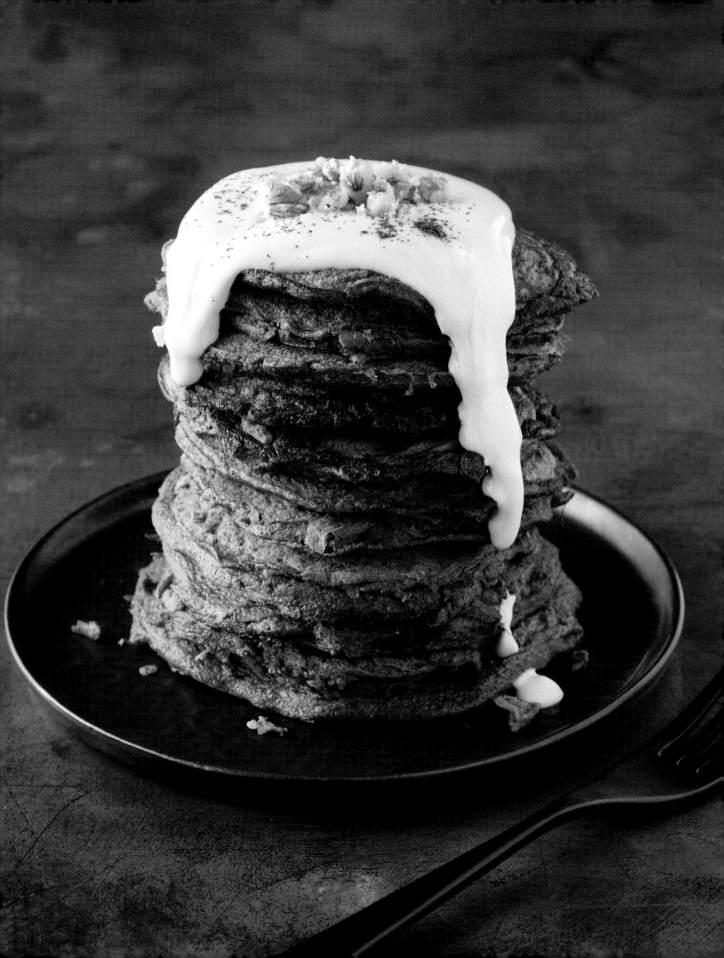

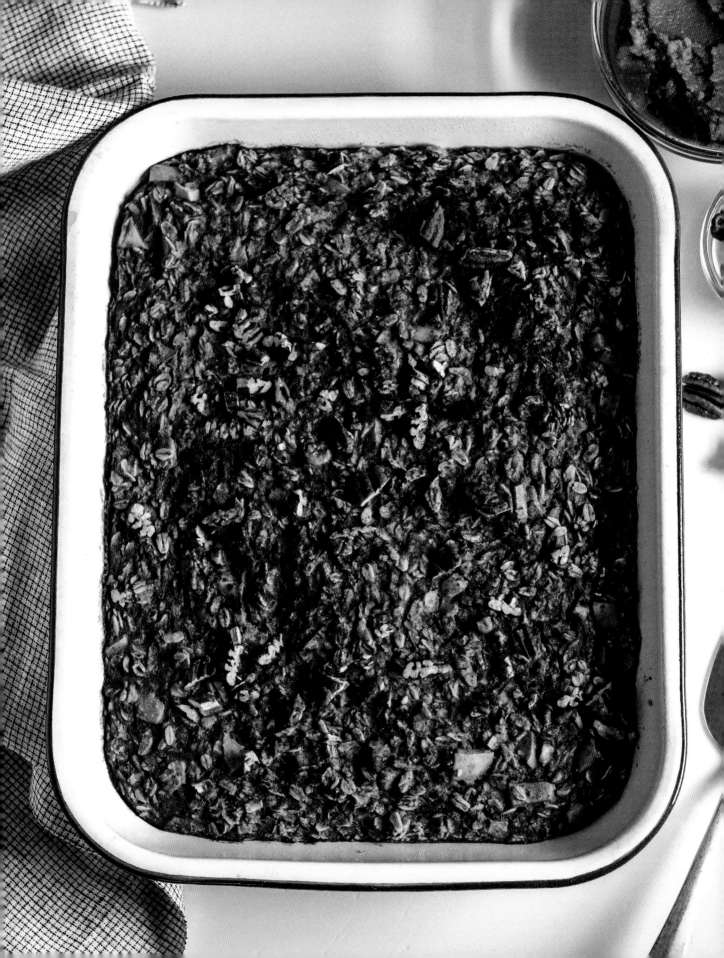

Pumpkin Pie Maple Oatmeal Bake

SERVES: 12   PREP TIME: 5 MINUTES   COOK TIME: 35 MINUTES

Imagine what you'd get if you combined creamy pumpkin pie with a comforting bowl of maple oatmeal. I'd always wondered myself, and that's exactly how this recipe came about. I originally created this dish in the fall, when I couldn't get enough of the classic flavor combinations of pumpkin, cinnamon, apple, maple, pecans and walnuts. Fall in New York is one of my favorite times of year. The weather finally turns cooler after the hot, humid, sticky summer. The leaves start to change color, more beautiful than I can ever even try to describe. And fall produce—apples, pumpkins, pears, grapes, to name just a few—begin to grace grocery store and supermarket shelves, inspiring tons of new and flavorful recipes, like this one. It's sweet and hearty, warm and comforting; you'll want to lick the fork clean (no judgment here).

4 large eggs

3 large egg whites

1½ cups unsweetened almond milk (or milk of choice)

2 teaspoons vanilla extract

1 teaspoon maple extract or maple flavor

1 cup canned pumpkin puree

2 teaspoons pumpkin pie spice, plus more for topping

¼ cup maple syrup

3 cups uncooked old-fashioned oats

1 teaspoon baking powder

½ cup toasted wheat germ

2 tablespoons ground flaxseeds

1 apple, such as Honeycrisp, Fuji, or Gala, skin on, finely diced (about 1½ cups)

½ cup pecans or walnuts, roughly chopped and toasted, plus more

OPTIONAL TOPPERS

Toasted pecans or walnuts, natural applesauce, maple syrup or honey

1 Preheat the oven to 350°F. Mist a 9 by 13-inch baking dish with nonstick oil spray and set aside.

2 In a large bowl, whisk together the eggs, egg whites, almond milk, vanilla, maple extract or flavor, pumpkin puree, pumpkin pie spice, and maple syrup. Add the oats, baking powder, wheat germ, flaxseeds, apple, and pecans or walnuts and mix until combined.

3 Transfer the batter to the prepared baking dish and even it out using a spatula. Sprinkle some pumpkin pie spice (or you could swap in cinnamon) and additional nuts, if using, over the top.

4 Bake for 35 to 40 minutes, until golden brown, slightly puffed, and there is no liquid remaining in the middle. Serve immediately, hot from the oven, with an optional dollop of applesauce and a drizzle of maple syrup or honey on each slice. Store leftovers covered in the refrigerator for up to 2 days. Or wrap well and freeze for up to 2 months (add a splash of milk and reheat in the oven or microwave).

PER SERVING 190 CALORIES 7 g PROTEIN 7 g FAT (6 g UNSATURATED FAT, 1 g SATURATED FAT) 45 mg CHOLESTEROL 26 g CARBS 3 g FIBER 7 g TOTAL SUGAR (3 g NATURAL SUGAR, 4 g ADDED SUGAR) 60 mg SODIUM

Butternut Ginger Porridge

SERVES: 4   PREP TIME: 5 MINUTES   COOK TIME: 10 MINUTES

This porridge includes fiber-rich oats, potassium-packed butternut squash, and fragrant ginger, cinnamon, nutmeg, and cloves. Ginger is one of my favorites because aside from lending an earthy flavor, it also possesses anti-inflammatory properties so it can help ease aches and pains. Contrary to one of the favorite stories, this porridge *isn't* too hot and *isn't* too cold—it's just right. And unlike Goldilocks, my family gobbles it up and asks for seconds— I'm hoping yours will too.

Note: If you are making this in a pressure cooker, be sure to use nondairy milk, because dairy milk tends to scorch in the pot.

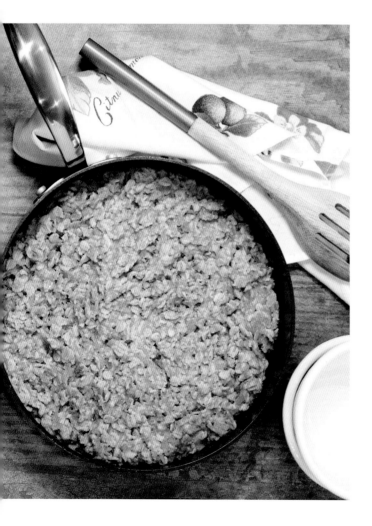

1 (13.5-ounce) can lite coconut milk (or 2 cups milk of choice)

2 cups uncooked old-fashioned oats

1½ tablespoons grated fresh ginger root (or 1 teaspoon ground ginger)

½ teaspoon kosher salt

1 teaspoon ground cinnamon

¼ teaspoon ground nutmeg

⅛ teaspoon ground cloves

2 cups grated fresh butternut squash (about ½ small squash)

½ teaspoon vanilla extract

½ teaspoon maple extract or maple flavor

3 tablespoons maple syrup

1 In a large pot, combine 2 cups water and the coconut milk and bring to a boil over medium-high heat. Add the oats, ginger, salt, cinnamon, nutmeg, cloves, and squash to the pot, stir everything to combine, reduce the heat to low, and simmer for about 8 minutes, stirring occasionally.

2 Remove from the heat and let sit for 2 minutes to thicken up. Stir in the vanilla and maple extracts along with maple syrup and serve.

PER SERVING 1¼ CUPS **210** CALORIES **7 g** PROTEIN **4.5 g** FAT (**4 g** UNSATURATED FAT, **0.5 g** SATURATED FAT) **0 mg** CHOLESTEROL **37 g** CARBS **6 g** FIBER **3 g** SUGAR (**1 g** NATURAL SUGAR, **2 g** ADDED SUGAR) **340 mg** SODIUM

Winter Waffles with Root Vegetables

MAKES: 12 WAFFLES   PREP TIME: 10 MINUTES   COOK TIME: 15 MINUTES

Here I've given the starchy favorite a latke-like spin by filling them with savory winter vegetables—think butternut squash and beets. (Feel free to change the ratio and/or swap in your favorites.) To save time, you can purchase precut or spiralized veggies at the grocery store. Bonus: These waffles are wheat-free, gluten-free, and dairy-free . . . but the total opposite of flavor-free!

1 medium Spanish or yellow onion, roughly chopped

6 generous cups roughly chopped butternut squash and beets*

2 large egg whites

¼ cup chopped fresh dill

¾ cup chickpea flour

¾ teaspoon kosher salt

¼ teaspoon black pepper

OPTIONAL TOPPERS

Natural applesauce, yogurt, poached eggs

*   *You can also use spiralized veggies and chop them up by hand.*

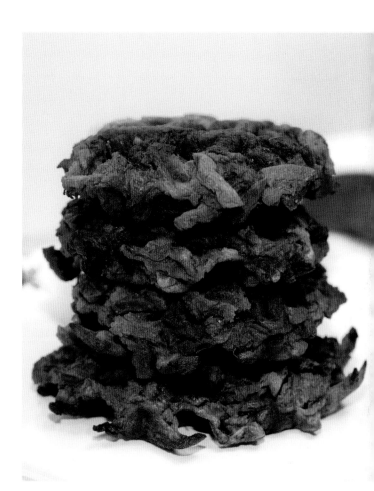

1 Preheat a waffle iron and mist with nonstick oil spray on the top and bottom.

2 Add the onion, squash, and beets to the bowl of a food processor and gently pulse until finely chopped, being extra careful not to puree them. Transfer to a mixing bowl and add the eggs, dill, chickpea flour, salt, and pepper and stir until everything is well blended into a batter.

3 Add ½ cup batter to each heated waffle iron compartment, close the lid, and cook for about 15 minutes. Because this is a *veggie* batter, they will take much longer to cook than traditional flour waffles. When the waffles are ready, use a fork or bamboo stick to carefully loosen the edges and lift them out of each compartment. Serve immediately, or place on a baking sheet in a low oven to keep warm until your batches are complete and you're ready to eat.

PER SERVING 1 WAFFLE **70** CALORIES **3 g** PROTEIN **0.5 g** FAT (**0.5 g** UNSATURATED FAT, **0 g** SATURATED FAT) **0 mg** CHOLES-TEROL **14 g** CARBS **3 g** FIBER **5 g** SUGAR (**5 g** NATURAL SUGAR, **0 g** ADDED SUGAR) **150 mg** SODIUM

Breads, Bagels, Muffins, and Biscuits

Bagel Bites with
Scallion Cream Cheese Filling 37

Mediterranean Rosemary-Olive Bread 39

Low-Carb Quiche Biscuits
with Bacon, Cheddar, and Chives 43

Protein Bagels
(Plain and Cinnamon Raisin) 44

Ginger-Spiced Pear Bread 47

Poblano Cornbread
with Spiced Honey Drizzle 48

Low-Carb Tortilla Wraps 50

Flaxseed Pita Triangles 51

Whole Grain Naan with Super Seeds 52

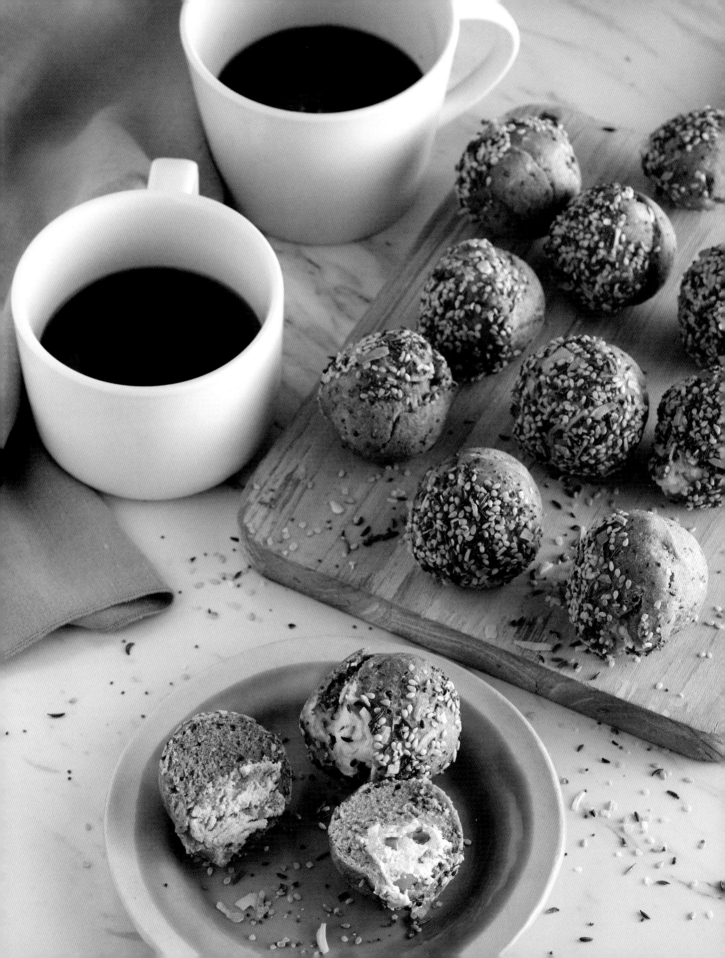

Bagel Bites with Scallion Cream Cheese Filling

MAKES: 16 BAGEL BITES   PREP TIME: 20 MINUTES
(PLUS AT LEAST 2½ HOURS RISING)   COOK TIME: 15 MINUTES

These stuffed bagel bites are a labor of love for your next brunch or a lazy weekend morning. Here's how I simplify prep: The night before, I make the dough and stash it in a covered bowl in the fridge. While it typically takes only two hours to rise, you can easily let it sit overnight. I also freeze the cream cheese filling the night before; that way, a lot of the work is front-loaded and there's minimal prep in the a.m.

The filling can be whatever you want: plain cream cheese, cream cheese with scallions (or jalapeños or lox), or no filling at all. I personally love using scallions for their oniony flavor and because they contain prebiotics, beneficial compounds that promote gut health. A dose of lox offers up omega-3s. And the topping is more than just a pretty sprinkling of seeds—it adds heart-healthy fats, flavor, and a satisfying crunch.

SCALLION CREAM CHEESE

4 ounces (½ cup) light cream cheese, at room temperature

2 scallions, sliced

2 ounces lox or smoked salmon, coarsely chopped (optional)

SUPER SEED TOPPING
makes about ⅔ cup

1 tablespoon sesame seeds

1 tablespoon poppy seeds

1 tablespoon dry minced onion

1 tablespoon chia seeds

1 tablespoon hemp seeds

1½ teaspoons caraway seeds

1 teaspoon kosher salt

BAGEL DOUGH

1 (¼ oz) packet instant or fast-rise yeast (~ 2 teaspoons)

1 teaspoon honey

2 cups white whole wheat flour*

2 tablespoons ground flaxseeds

2 tablespoons hemp seeds

⅛ teaspoon kosher salt

* *If you can't find white whole wheat flour, use standard whole wheat.*

1 FOR THE CREAM CHEESE: Line a small baking sheet with parchment paper. In a small bowl, mix the cream cheese, scallions and lox, if desired, using a rubber spatula or spoon. Drop ½-tablespoon piles onto the parchment paper, creating a total of 16. Cover and place in the freezer to harden for at least 30 minutes or overnight.

2 FOR THE SEED TOPPING: Combine all the ingredients in a bowl, cover, and set aside.

3 FOR THE BAGEL DOUGH: Pour 1 cup lukewarm water into a small bowl. Add the yeast and honey and mix until no lumps remain and everything is well combined. Let sit for about 10 minutes to foam and bubble up. This indicates that it has become active.

RECIPE CONTINUES

PER SERVING 1 BAGEL BITE **90** CALORIES **4 g** PROTEIN **3 g** FAT (**2 g** UNSATURATED FAT, **1 g** SATURATED FAT) **5 mg** CHOLESTEROL **13 g** CARBS **2 g** FIBER **1 g** SUGAR (**1 g** NATURAL SUGAR, **0 g** ADDED SUGAR) **75 mg** SODIUM

4 In a large bowl, combine the flour, flaxseeds, hemp seeds, and salt. Make a well in the center. Pour the active yeast mixture into the well and stir, incorporating all of the flour to form a dough ball. Then scrape the dough ball onto a lightly floured countertop or cutting board and knead the dough for about 2 minutes. (**NOTE**: I like to use a large enough bowl so I can knead the dough right inside without messing up the countertop.)

5 Mist the bottom and inner sides of the bowl with olive oil spray. Place the dough ball back inside and cover with a slightly dampened dish towel. Let it sit undisturbed for 2 hours (or overnight in the fridge) to rise.

6 **TO ASSEMBLE AND BAKE:** Set an oven rack to the middle position and preheat the oven to 375°F. Remove the cream cheese balls from freezer.

7 When the dough is done resting, cut it into 4 equal pieces, then cut each quarter into 4 equal pieces to make 16 pieces. Working with one at a time, flatten each piece of dough and wrap it around a frozen cream cheese ball, pinching the tops to seal each seam. Roll between your palms to create a smooth bagel "ball" and dip the top into your seed topping, then place on the baking sheet with the seed side facing up. (I use the same baking sheet from the cream cheese balls and simply swap in fresh parchment paper.) Repeat until all 16 bagel bites are on the baking sheet. Let rest for about 30 minutes to rise a bit more.

8 Place in the oven and bake for 15 to 20 minutes. Serve warm or at room temperature.

Mediterranean Rosemary-Olive Bread

SERVES: 12   PREP TIME: 25 MINUTES,
PLUS 2¼ HOURS RISING TIME   COOK TIME: 35 MINUTES

The secret to bread baking is in the kneading, which I actually find both relaxing and therapeutic (and, heck, it's also a good workout!). The first time I made traditional yeast bread, I searched online to find a video on kneading techniques, and you might be surprised by just how many good ones there are out there (browse a few for more pointers if you're unsure). You can also use a mixer—a stand mixer with a dough setting is a great option—but I really prefer to use my hands, the best and most reliable kitchen tool there is! Whenever I'm kneading, I like to imagine my great grandmother in her kitchen doing the same thing. It makes me feel connected to my ancestors.

Whole grain flour results in a denser chew than standard flour. It's a texture I've come to love and appreciate, but if you'd like a lighter loaf, feel free to use white whole wheat flour. It's a softer type of whole grain and is still 100 percent whole wheat. Or you could go with a 50-50 mix of whole wheat flour and any other everyday flour.

A quick tip: As tempting as it might be to cut corners when it comes to resting time (at least 1½ hours for the first rise and 45 minutes for the second), I strongly recommend against it. Whole grain flour is dense and takes longer than refined flours to rise (even when using instant yeast). Be patient and you'll enjoy the payoff. I like to bake my breads on a preheated pizza stone or a baking sheet on the lower rack of the oven. The crust will be deep golden brown and possess a toasty and crackly texture. You can give the bottom of the loaf a tap to see if it's done—it should sound hollow when it's baked. In terms of flavor and health perks, this bread boasts heart-healthy olives, fresh fragrant rosemary, and fiber- and mineral-rich whole grains. This combo converts an everyday loaf into a Mediterranean masterpiece!

RECIPE CONTINUES

Here's a little kneading know-how: Place the dough on a counter sprinkled with flour to prevent sticking. Take the part farthest from you and fold it in half toward you, back down into itself, using the heels of your hands to flatten it out again. Keep working and pressing the dough until it's a flat circle. Give the dough a slight turn and repeat the process, adding a sprinkling of flour (without going crazy) to prevent sticking as needed. Continue this kneading and turning cycle until your dough is smooth and elastic.

1 (¼-ounce) packet instant or fast-rise dry yeast (~ 2 teaspoons)

½ teaspoon honey

2¼ cups plus 2 tablespoons whole wheat flour, plus more as needed

3 tablespoons ground flaxseeds

¾ teaspoon kosher or coarse sea salt

1 tablespoon olive oil

1 heaping tablespoon chopped fresh rosemary

¾ cup pitted, halved kalamata olives, patted dry

OPTIONAL GARNISH

Coarse salt

Chopped fresh rosemary

1 Pour 1¼ cups lukewarm water into a small bowl. Add the yeast and honey and mix until no lumps remain and everything is well combined. Let sit for 10 to 15 minutes to foam and bubble up. This indicates that the yeast has become active.

2 In a large bowl, combine the flour, flaxseeds, and salt. Add the yeast mixture, oil, and rosemary to the flour bowl and stir, incorporating all of the flour until a sticky, flexible dough starts to form. Sprinkle in more flour if the dough sticks to the sides of the bowl.

3 Prepare a large cutting board or a flat countertop with a sprinkling of flour and place the dough on top. Knead with both hands, pressing and folding, for about 10 minutes, adding the olives at the midway mark. Sprinkle more flour as needed if the dough sticks to your hands or the surface.

4 Mist the bottom and inner sides of the bowl you've been using with olive oil spray. Place the dough back in the bowl, cover with a dampened towel, and set in a warm area to rise for 1½ to 2 hours. It will nearly double in size.

5 Mist a baking sheet with olive oil spray and place the dough on top. Gently press down on the dough to release any air pockets. Reshape into a ball with the seam side down, cover again with the dampened towel, and let rest for another 45 to 60 minutes, until it rises by about one third.

6 Set an oven rack to the lowest position and preheat the oven to 425°F.

7 Using a sharp knife, gently score the top of the bread in a crisscross pattern. Mist with olive oil spray and garnish with a sprinkling of coarse salt and chopped rosemary, if desired. Bake for 35 minutes, or until golden brown. Allow to cool for at least 10 minutes before slicing so the inside has time to settle in and dry.

Serve fresh or freeze (to freeze, completely cool, then tightly wrap the loaf and store in the freezer for up to 2 months).

PER SERVING 1 SLICE **130** CALORIES **4 g** PROTEIN **6 g** FAT (**6 g** UNSATURATED FAT, **0 g** SATURATED FAT) **0 mg** CHOLESTEROL **18 g** CARBS **3 g** FIBER **0 g** SUGAR **220 mg** SODIUM

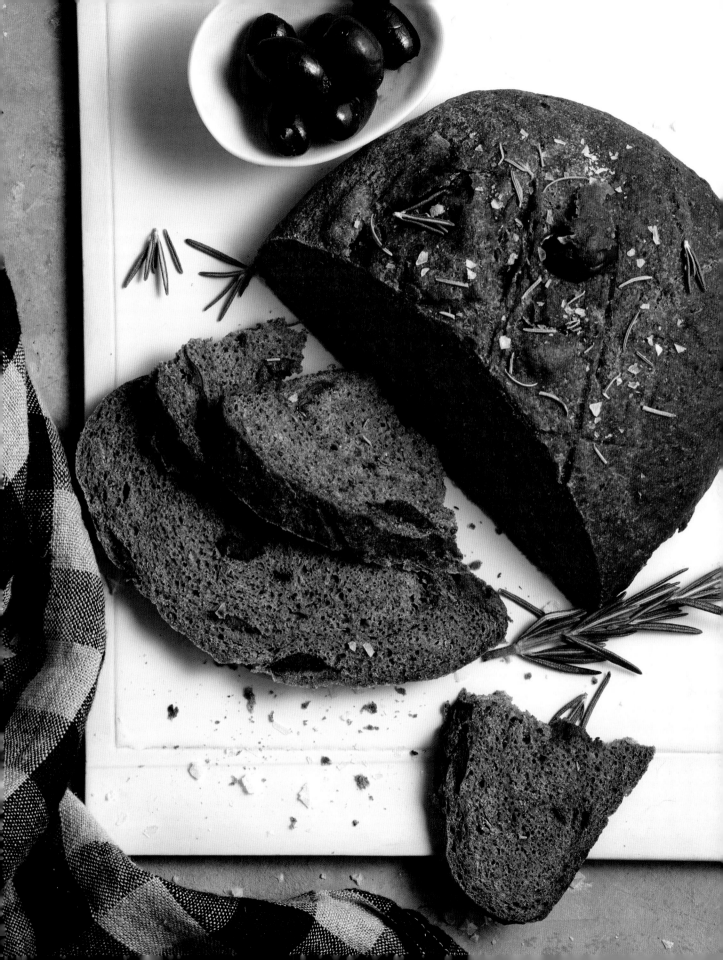

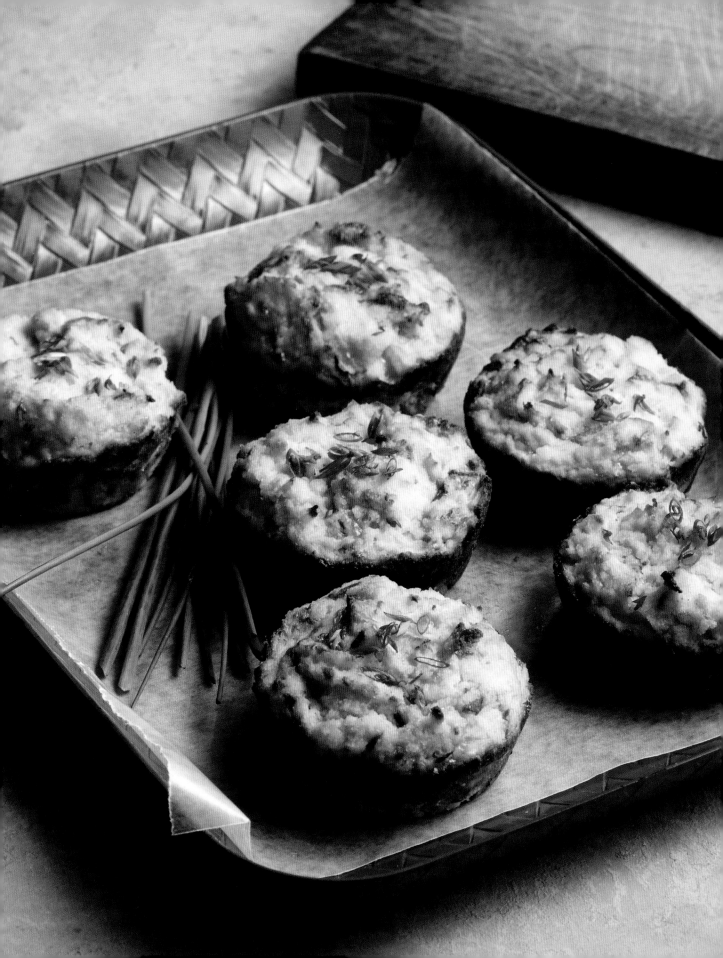

Low-Carb Quiche Biscuits with Bacon, Cheddar, and Chives

MAKES: 6 BISCUITS   PREP TIME: 10 MINUTES   COOK TIME: 25 MINUTES

These easy-to-make biscuits deliver on taste *and* nutrition: They're flourless, gluten-free, and hey, I even snuck in some cauliflower (what can I say, I'm a dietitian). I like to whip up a double batch and freeze each biscuit individually. Then, on hectic mornings, I pop one or two in the microwave for about a minute and I have a satisfying breakfast to take on the road.

4 cups cauliflower florets (or 3 cups packaged cauliflower rice)

½ cup blanched almond flour

1 teaspoon baking powder

½ teaspoon kosher salt

½ cup 2% reduced-fat shredded sharp cheddar cheese

2 large egg whites, lightly beaten

2 tablespoons butter, melted*

3 to 4 strips turkey bacon, cooked and crumbled

2 tablespoons chopped fresh chives

*   *If you're watching cholesterol, swap in soft tub (trans fat–free) spread.*

1 Preheat the oven to 400°F. Mist 6 compartments of a muffin tin with nonstick oil spray and set aside.

2 Place the cauliflower florets or rice in a microwave-safe bowl, add a splash of water, cover, and microwave for about 6 minutes, until the cauliflower is soft and mushy. Mash with a fork until smooth. Drain out as much water as possible by placing the cauliflower in a kitchen towel or between a bunch of layered paper towels and squeezing. Once the cauliflower is drained, add the almond flour, baking powder, and salt and stir well. Mix in the cheese, egg whites, and butter. Add the bacon and chives and mix to create a batter.

3 Using your hands, form 6 balls and place them into the prepared muffin tin. The muffin compartments will be almost full. Bake for 23 to 25 minutes, until the tops are slightly browned.

To freeze, wrap each biscuit individually and place in the freezer for up to two months. When you're ready to enjoy, microwave for 60 to 90 seconds to warm.

PER BISCUIT **150** CALORIES **8 g** PROTEIN **11 g** FAT (**7 g** UNSATURATED FAT, **4 g** SATURATED FAT) **20 mg** CHOLESTEROL **6 g** CARBS **2 g** FIBER **2 g** SUGAR (**2 g** NATURAL SUGAR, **0 g** ADDED SUGAR) **320 mg** SODIUM

Protein Bagels (Plain and Cinnamon Raisin)

MAKES: 8 BAGELS   PREP TIME: 10 MINUTES   COOK TIME: 25 MINUTES

In New York (where I'm from), bagels are a way of life—and they're totally delicious. But let's face it, these doughy delights are typically made with refined, junky white flour, are void of nutrition, and can set you back more calories and carbs than you care to count—and that's before you spread on your topping of choice. These better-for-you bagels pack 10 grams of protein, 4 grams of fiber, and a whole host of vitamins and minerals. That's because they're made with whole grain flour, which contains more fiber and minerals than standard flour; chia seeds, which are filled with fiber and omega-3 fats; and protein-rich Greek yogurt. Now that's a good morning!

Note: These freeze wonderfully. When ready to enjoy, simply thaw in the microwave, slice, and toast in the toaster oven. Alternatively, you can slice them before freezing and place them directly in the toaster oven from the freezer.

PLAIN

2 cups white whole wheat flour*

1 tablespoon baking powder

1 tablespoon chia seeds

1½ teaspoons kosher salt

2 cups nonfat plain Greek yogurt (thicker brands work best)

* *You can also use standard whole wheat flour.*

1 FOR PLAIN BAGELS: Preheat the oven to 350°F. Line a baking sheet with parchment paper.

2 Combine the flour, baking powder, chia seeds, and salt in a large bowl. Add the yogurt and mix until all the ingredients are incorporated into a batter. Knead the dough with clean hands until it's dry and elastic (this will take about 1 minute). Divide into 8 balls.

3 One at a time, roll each ball between your palms and form into a long rope (if it breaks apart, just squish it back together). Lay the rope on the parchment paper and form it into a circular shape, cinching the ends to complete a closed bagel. Leave space between each bagel on the baking sheet so they're not touching. Dip the tops into any preferred

seasonings, if desired. (I love to use my Super Seed Topping [page 37], as shown in the photo, right.)

4 Place in the oven and bake for 25 minutes. Let cool before slicing.

CINNAMON RAISIN

2 cups white whole wheat flour*

1 tablespoon baking powder

1 tablespoon chia seeds

1 teaspoon kosher salt

2 cups nonfat plain Greek yogurt (thicker brands work best)

3 tablespoons packed brown sugar

1 tablespoon ground cinnamon

¼ to ½ cup raisins

* *You can also use standard whole wheat flour.*

1 FOR CINNAMON RAISIN BAGELS: Preheat the oven to 350°F. Line a baking sheet with parchment paper.

2 Combine the flour, baking powder, chia seeds, and salt in a large bowl. Add the yogurt and mix until all the ingredients are incorporated into a

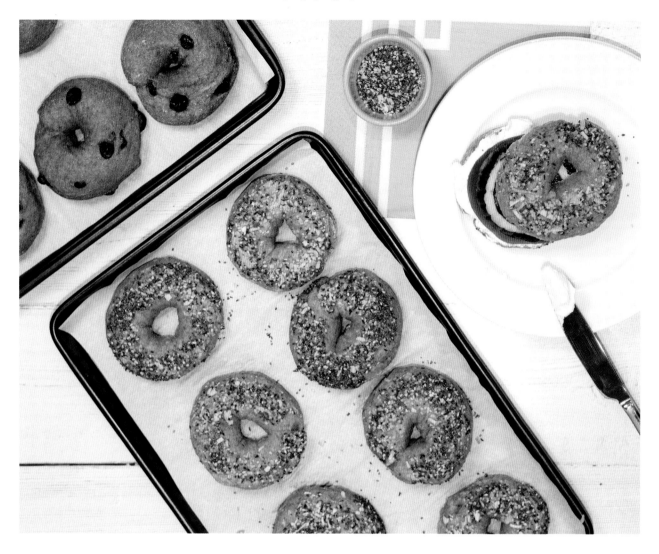

batter. Knead the dough with clean hands until it's dry and elastic (this will take about 1 minute). In a small bowl, combine the brown sugar and cinnamon until well incorporated and knead into the dough. Then knead in the raisins until evenly distributed and divide the dough into 8 balls.

3 One at a time, roll each ball between your palms and form into a long rope (if it breaks apart, just squish it back together). Lay the rope on the parchment paper and form it into a circular shape, cinching the ends to complete a closed bagel. Leave space between each bagel on the baking sheet so they're not touching. Place in the oven and bake for about 25 minutes. Let cool before slicing.

NOTE: These freeze wonderfully. When ready to enjoy, simply thaw in the microwave, slice, and toast in the toaster oven. Alternatively, you can slice before freezing and place in the toaster oven directly from the freezer.

PER PLAIN BAGEL **140** CALORIES **10 g** PROTEIN **1.5 g** FAT (**1.5 g** UNSATURATED FAT, **0 g** SATURATED FAT) **5 mg** CHOLES-TEROL **24 g** CARBS **4 g** FIBER **2 g** SUGAR (**2 g** NATURAL SUGAR, **0 g** ADDED SUGAR) **390 mg** SODIUM

PER CINNAMON RAISIN BAGEL **180** CALORIES **10 g** PROTEIN **1.5 g** FAT (**1.5 g** UNSATURATED FAT, **0 g** SATURATED FAT) **5 mg** CHOLESTEROL **35 mg** CARBS **5 g** FIBER **10 g** SUGAR (**5.5 g** NATURAL SUGAR, **4.5 g** ADDED SUGAR) **280 mg** SODIUM

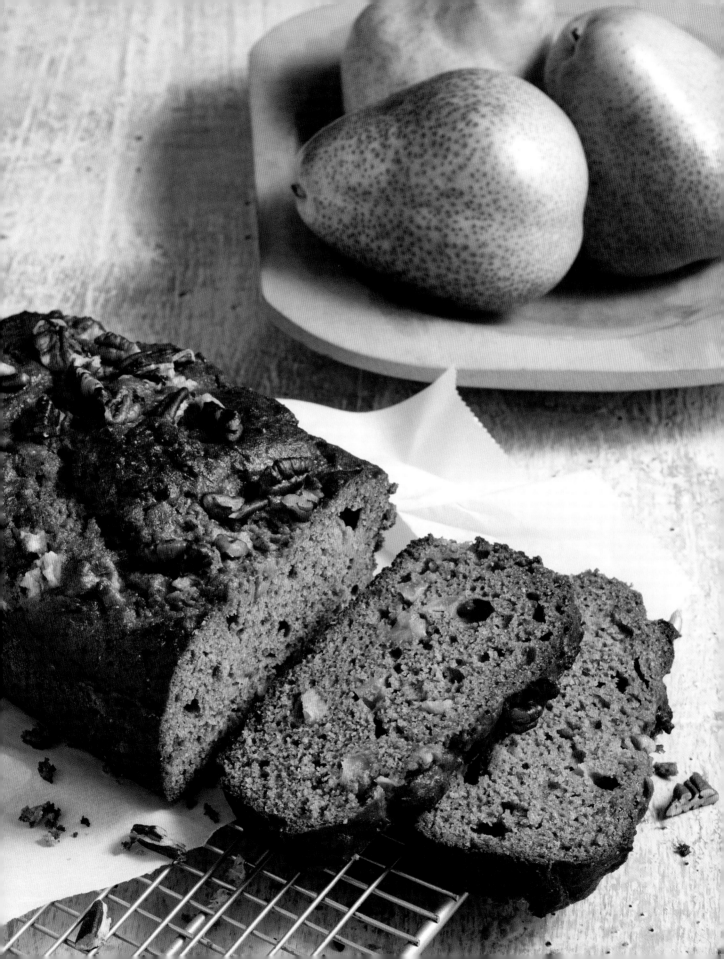

Ginger-Spiced Pear Bread

MAKES: 12 SLICES   PREP TIME: 15 MINUTES   COOK TIME: 45 MINUTES

This bread is un-*pear*-alleled. Pears are so great because they're rich in vitamin C, potassium, and fiber. This cozy recipe is reminiscent of gingerbread, with its luscious and flavorful pear, thick molasses, and warm spices. It is sweet, yet wholesome, featuring a handful of good-for-you ingredients, including pecans, yogurt, wheat germ, and whole grain flour. (I usually use white–whole wheat flour or whole wheat pastry flour for this recipe, but you can easily swap in another favorite—or create a blend of two different flours.) I dare you to resist a fresh-out-of-the-oven slice. In fact, even though it's in the "bread" category, it's more like a moist, indulgent cake.

1¼ cups white whole wheat flour*

⅓ cup toasted wheat germ

2 teaspoons baking powder

½ teaspoon kosher salt

1½ teaspoons ground cinnamon

1 teaspoon ground ginger

⅛ teaspoon ground nutmeg

⅛ teaspoon ground cloves

2 large eggs

1 teaspoon vanilla extract

3 tablespoons molasses

2 tablespoons honey

¼ cup grapeseed or canola oil

½ cup plain or vanilla nonfat yogurt, Greek or traditional

1 large ripe pear, peeled and finely diced into uniform pieces (1½ cups)

⅓ cup chopped pecans or walnuts

*   *You can swap for whole wheat pastry flour, but standard whole wheat flour works well, too.*

1   Preheat the oven to 350°F. Mist the bottom and sides of a 9- by 5-inch loaf pan with nonstick oil spray. Alternatively, you can line it with parchment paper for easy removal. Set aside.

2   In a medium bowl, combine the flour, wheat germ, baking powder, salt, cinnamon, ginger, nutmeg, and cloves. Set aside.

3   In a separate medium bowl, whisk together the eggs, vanilla, molasses, honey, oil, and yogurt. Then pour the wet ingredients into the bowl with the flour and spices and mix to create a fluffy batter. Fold in the chopped pears, taking care not to overmix; stir no more than 10 to 15 times.

4   Add the batter to the prepared loaf pan and smooth out the top so that it's evenly distributed. Sprinkle the chopped pecans or walnuts over the loaf. Bake for 45 to 55 minutes, until a toothpick inserted into the middle comes out clean.

PER SERVING 1 SLICE **170** CALORIES **4 g** PROTEIN **8 g** FAT (**7 g** UNSATURATED FAT, **1 g** SATURATED FAT) **30 mg** CHOLESTEROL **22 g** CARBS **3 g** FIBER **11 g** SUGAR (**5 g** NATURAL SUGAR, **6 g** ADDED SUGAR) **100 mg** SODIUM

Poblano Cornbread with Spiced Honey Drizzle

SERVES: 12   PREP TIME: 10 MINUTES   COOK TIME: 30 MINUTES

When I first took a shot at creating cornbread for our Thanksgiving feast, I stayed true to the original and whipped up a plain version. You'd be surprised by how delicious it is . . . even without all the sugar and butter that traditional recipes call for. I added whole corn kernels along with the cornmeal for extra texture. Corn is rich in filling fiber as well as two antioxidants, lutein and zeaxanthin, that help protect your eyes.

On the second go-around, I decided to spice things up a bit with chile peppers. OMG . . . so good! Whether you make this as a plain-traditional cornbread or a spicy rendition, it's a win-win, but the charred poblanos do add great flavor and gentle heat to the savory home-style bread. Bonus: The active ingredient, capsaicin, offers impressive benefits, including a slight elevation to your metabolism and a boost to heart health.

1 poblano chile, seeded and finely chopped

1 cup whole wheat flour

1 cup yellow cornmeal

1 tablespoon baking powder

1½ to 2 teaspoons kosher salt

1 (15-ounce) can sweet corn, rinsed and drained

3 tablespoons butter, melted

2 large eggs

1 cup low-fat plain yogurt

¼ cup honey

1 Preheat the oven to 375°F. Mist an 8-inch square baking pan or glass dish with nonstick oil spray. Set aside. (Alternatively, you can bake the cornbread in a preheated cast-iron skillet.)

2 Mist a small skillet with nonstick oil spray and warm over medium-high heat. Add the poblano and cook, stirring frequently, until browned or charred on the edges, 5 to 6 minutes. Remove from the heat and set aside to cool.

3 In a large bowl, combine the flour, cornmeal, baking powder, and salt. Stir in the corn kernels and cooked poblano.

4 In a medium bowl, add the melted butter and eggs and lightly beat. Add the yogurt and honey and mix until everything is well combined.

5 Add the wet ingredients to the dry ingredients and stir together; do not overmix. Pour the batter into the prepared pan and, using a spatula or the back of a spoon, smooth the top so it's evenly distributed. The batter will be thick and fluffy. Bake for 30 to 35 minutes, until the center of the bread springs back when gently pressed. Serve warm with an optional spread of whipped butter or spiced honey. To make spiced honey, warm ¼ cup honey with ½ teaspoon crushed red pepper flakes in a saucepan over medium-low heat until gently bubbling.

PER SERVING 1 SLICE 170 CALORIES 5 g PROTEIN 4.5 g FAT (2 g UNSATURATED FAT, 2.5 g SATURATED FAT) 35 mg CHOLES-TEROL 30 g CARBS 2 g FIBER 9 g SUGAR (3 g NATURAL SUGAR, 6 g ADDED SUGAR) 270 mg SODIUM (ADD 40 CALORIES PER TEASPOON OF SPICED HONEY DRIZZLE OR WHIPPED BUTTER)

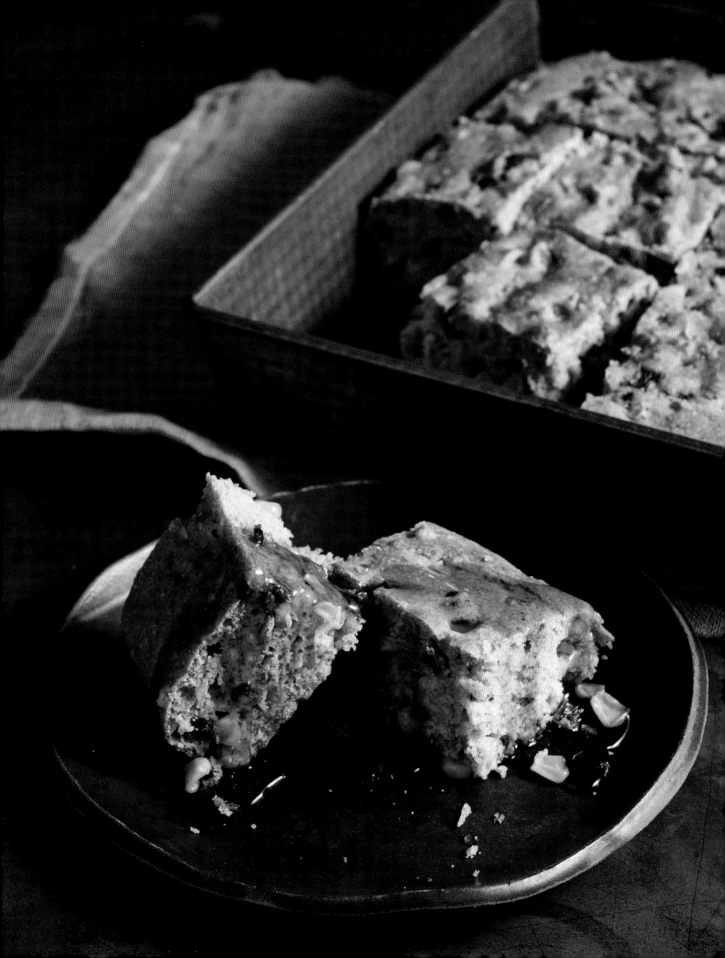

Low-Carb Tortilla Wraps

MAKES: 4 (5-INCH) TORTILLAS   PREP TIME: 6 MINUTES   COOK TIME: 5 MINUTES

DIY tortillas! They're surprisingly simple to assemble (just five ingredients including salt!) and they're healthier, lower in carbs and calories, and higher in satiating protein than most store-bought brands. They're also gluten-free.

I used two different types of flour in the recipe, because I prefer the mixture of the two—in my opinion, the combo offers the best texture and flavor. But if you only have one of the flours on hand, double up and it will still turn out great.

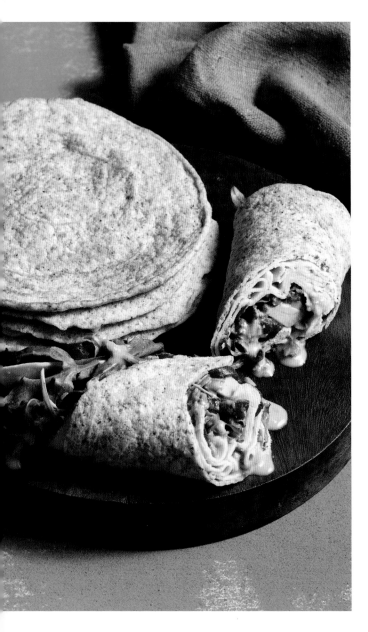

4 large egg whites

2 tablespoons ground flaxseeds

2 tablespoons tapioca flour or arrowroot

2 tablespoons blanched almond flour

¼ teaspoon kosher salt

1 In a small bowl, combine the egg whites and ground flaxseeds and whisk with a fork. Set aside for 5 minutes to allow the mixture to gel.

2 In a separate small bowl, combine the tapioca flour, almond flour, and salt. Once the egg-flax mixture has gelled, whisk the flour mixture into it. It will be lumpy at first, but keep whisking until it's smooth, about 1 minute total.

3 Mist an 8-inch skillet with nonstick oil spray and warm over medium heat. Add about ¼ cup of the tortilla batter to the pan, and with a spatula or the back of a spoon, smooth out the top until it is about 5 inches in diameter. Cook for 1 to 2 minutes per side. Repeat until all of the batter is used up and you have 4 round tortillas.

PER SERVING 1 TORTILLA **70** CALORIES **5 g** PROTEIN **3.5 g** FAT (**3.5 g** UNSATURATED FAT, **0 g** SATURATED FAT) **0 mg** CHOLESTEROL **5 g** CARBS **1 g** FIBER **0 g** SUGAR **180 mg** SODIUM

Flaxseed Pita Triangles

SERVES: 4   PREP TIME: 5 MINUTES   COOK TIME: 12 MINUTES

These low-carb pita triangles are high in protein and fiber thanks to the flaxseeds and egg. Bonus: You'll also score some omega-3 fatty acids from the flaxseeds. And they're so easy to pull together; they take just fifteen minutes from start to finish. A quick heads up that the mixture will thicken if you let it sit too long, so be sure to use the batter shortly after making. If you find the batter is too thick, you can add 1 to 2 teaspoons of water to help thin it out.

Pro tip: Trace 4 circles (5 inches each) or 2 circles (8 inches each) on the underside of the parchment paper to use as a guide to spread your mixture into the perfect circle. (You'll cut these circles into wedges after they're cooked.)

1 large egg

1 large egg white

2 tablespoons olive oil

½ teaspoon garlic powder

½ teaspoon Italian seasoning

¼ teaspoon kosher salt, plus more to sprinkle on top (optional)

¾ teaspoon baking powder

⅔ cup ground flaxseeds

1 Set an oven rack to the lowest position and preheat the oven to 400°F. Line 2 baking sheets with parchment paper. Set aside.

2 In a medium bowl, whisk together the egg, egg white, oil, garlic powder, Italian seasoning, salt, baking powder, and 2 tablespoons water. Be sure to mash any small clumps of seasoning or baking soda. Add the flaxseeds and whisk until smooth.

3 Place 4 even piles (or 2 piles if you're making larger pitas) of batter on the prepared baking sheets and, using a spatula, butter knife, or the back of a spoon, spread each pile into an even 5-inch circle (or 8-inch circle if you're making 2 larger pitas). Leave a little space in between each one so they're not touching. Sprinkle some extra salt over the top, if desired.

4 Bake for 8 minutes. Then carefully flip the pitas and bake for another 4 minutes, or until desired crispness (4 minutes will result in softer pitas and 5-plus minutes will be toastier). Allow the pitas to cool slightly, then slice each round into wedges. Serve with hummus, guacamole, or any preferred dip. These will keep, refrigerated, in an airtight container for up to 4 days or in the freezer for up to 2 months.

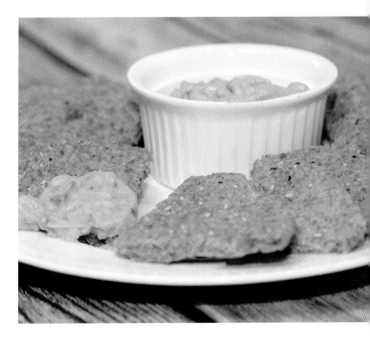

PER SERVING **180** CALORIES **6 g** PROTEIN **16 g** FAT (**14 g** UNSATURATED FAT, **2 g** SATURATED FAT) **45 mg** CHOLESTEROL **6 g** CARBS **5 g** FIBER **0 g** SUGAR **160 mg** SODIUM

Whole Grain Naan with Super Seeds

SERVES: 6   PREP TIME: 15 MINUTES, PLUS 2 HOURS FOR RISING

COOK TIME: 10 MINUTES

Naan is an oven-baked flatbread. Its pull-apart-doughy deliciousness makes it one of my favorite offerings at Indian restaurants, especially when it's served warm from a clay oven. While I've taken a few liberties and shortcuts, this whole grain, seedy spin tastes delectable fresh off the griddle (no oven required). I usually serve it alongside my Turmeric Hummus (page 124), which is a match made in heaven. But truth be told, it's a rock-star bread that doesn't need any backup.

SEED MIX*

2 tablespoons chia seeds

2 tablespoons sesame seeds

2 tablespoons pumpkin seeds, sunflower seeds, or hemp seeds

* *You may use any combination of the above seeds.*

NAAN

1 teaspoon honey

1 (¼-ounce) packet active dry yeast (~ 2 teaspoons)

½ cup nonfat or low-fat plain Greek yogurt

1 tablespoon extra virgin olive oil

2¼ cups whole wheat flour, plus more for rolling†

1 teaspoon kosher salt

† *You may use a combo of whole wheat and all-purpose flour for a less dense chew.*

1 **FOR THE SEED MIX:** In a small bowl, combine all the seeds and set aside.

2 **FOR THE NAAN:** Pour ¾ cup lukewarm water into a small bowl. Add the honey and yeast and mix until no lumps remain and everything is well combined. Let it sit for 10 to 15 minutes to foam and bubble up. This indicates that the yeast has become active. Now add the yogurt and oil to the mixture and combine.

3 In a large bowl, combine the flour and salt and make a well in the center. Then add the yeast-

yogurt mixture to the well in the flour bowl and stir to incorporate the flour into the dough and create a shaggy dough ball. Scrape the dough ball onto a lightly floured countertop or cutting board and knead the dough for about 2 minutes. (NOTE: If your mixing bowl is large enough, you can knead the dough right inside without messing up the countertop.)

4 Mist the bottom and inner sides of the mixing bowl with olive oil spray. Place the dough ball back inside and cover with a slightly dampened dish towel. Let sit undisturbed for 2 hours to rise (it will roughly double in size).

5 When the dough is finished rising, cut the ball into 6 even pieces. One by one, gently roll each of the pieces to the shape of your choice. I like to make oblong shapes, about 4 by 7 inches. If the dough is sticky, sprinkle a small amount of flour on the counter or your hands. After you achieve your desired shape, sprinkle 1 tablespoon of the seed mixture over the top of each piece, pressing down with your hands to incorporate the seeds into the dough. This will help them adhere when the naan is on the skillet.

6 Mist a large skillet or griddle with oil spray and warm over medium heat. Add 2 breads at a time to the hot pan (seeds facing up) and cook for 2 minutes, or until golden brown underneath. Carefully flip with a wide spatula and cook for another 1 minute. Transfer to a serving dish and repeat with the remaining dough. Serve warm or at room temperature.

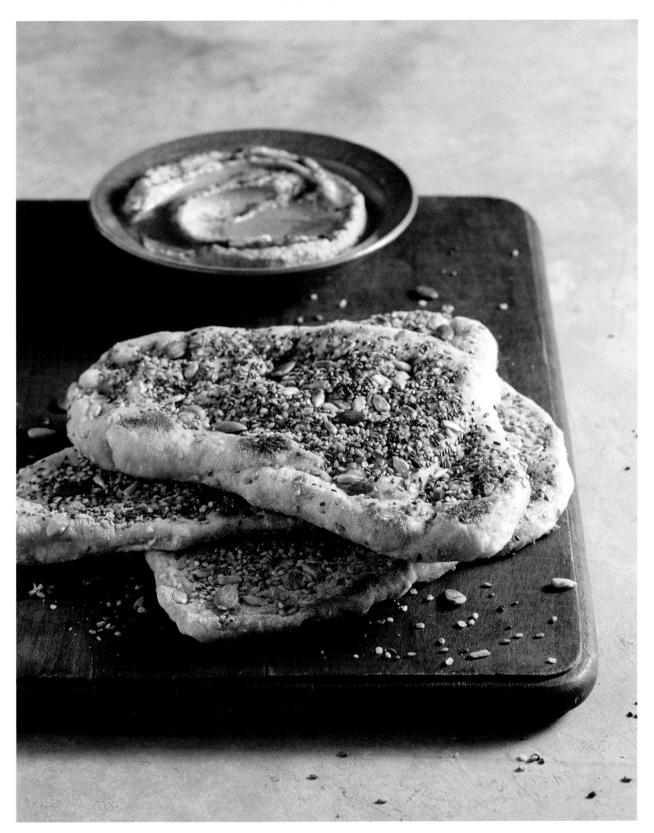

PER SERVING 1 NAAN **250** CALORIES **11 g** PROTEIN **8 g** FAT (**7 g** UNSATURATED FAT, **1 g** SATURATED FAT) **0 mg** CHOLESTEROL **37 g** CARBS **7 g** FIBER **2 g** SUGAR (**1 g** NATURAL SUGAR, **<1 g** ADDED SUGAR) **330 mg** SODIUM

Soups and Salads

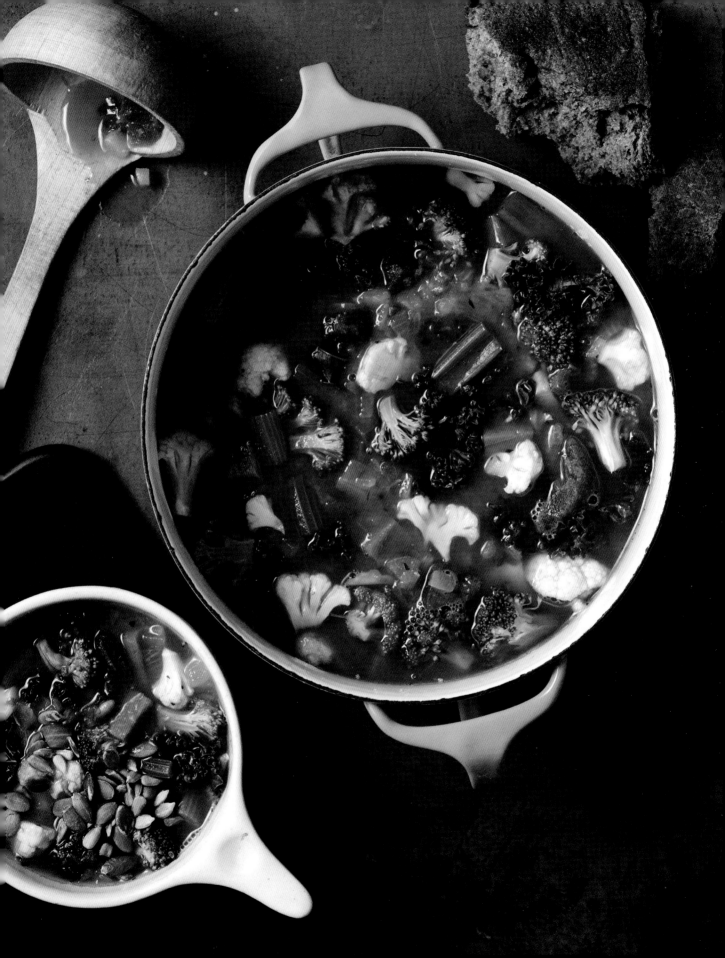

Longevity Soup

MAKES: 7 CUPS PREP TIME: 15 MINUTES COOK TIME: 40 MINUTES

Each spoonful of this soothing soup is loaded with foods that can help promote longevity. Bite after bite boasts hearty beans, cruciferous vegetables (hello, broccoli and cauliflower!), lycopene-rich tomato broth, leafy greens, and nuts and/or seeds. Research from the Blue Zones, areas of the world where people tend to live the longest, suggests that a nutritious diet featuring these star foods can help you feel and look amazing well into your golden years.

The pot is almost overflowing with fresh veggies—carrots, celery, onions, tomatoes, and leafy greens in addition to the broccoli and cauliflower. I thicken the soup by pureeing some of the beans with a bit of broth and the tomato paste adds a wonderfully rich touch. Each cup provides 7 grams of protein and 7 grams of fiber, but trust me, you'll want to slurp up much more than a cup. Topped with nuts or seeds, this soup is sure to satisfy—I'm betting it makes a regular appearance in your weekly menu rotation.

2 (15-ounce) cans small white beans, rinsed and drained, divided

4 cups reduced-sodium vegetable or chicken broth, divided

1 onion, finely chopped

3 cloves garlic, minced

2 stalks celery, chopped

3 medium carrots, chopped

1 to 2 cups broccoli florets, chopped

1 to 2 cups cauliflower florets, chopped

2 cups canned crushed tomatoes

1 (14.5-ounce) can stewed tomatoes

1 teaspoon dried oregano

1 teaspoon dried basil

2 fresh rosemary sprigs

1 teaspoon kosher salt, plus more to taste

2 to 3 handfuls fresh kale or spinach leaves, roughly chopped

Ground black pepper

Chopped toasted nuts or seeds for garnish (optional)

1 In a blender, combine 1 can of the white beans with 1 cup of the broth and blend until smooth. Set aside.

2 Liberally coat a pot with nonstick oil spray and warm over medium heat. Add the onion and garlic and cook until softened, about 5 minutes. Add the celery, carrots, the remaining 3 cups broth, the broccoli, cauliflower, crushed tomatoes, stewed tomatoes, oregano, basil, the second can of beans, the rosemary, and salt. Bring to boil, then reduce heat and simmer, uncovered, for about 25 minutes.

3 Remove the rosemary sprigs from the pot. Add the pureed white beans from the blender and kale or spinach and simmer for another 10 minutes, or until the greens wilt. Season with additional salt and pepper and top each serving with a sprinkling of nuts or seeds, if desired.

PER SERVING 1 CUP **140** CALORIES **7 g** PROTEIN **1 g** FAT (**1 g** UNSATURATED FAT, **0 g** SATURATED FAT) **0 mg** CHOLESTEROL **26 g** CARBS **7 g** FIBER **8 g** SUGAR (**8 g** NATURAL SUGAR, **0 g** ADDED SUGAR) **550 mg** SODIUM

Smoky Chicken and Quinoa Soup

MAKES: 10 CUPS   PREP TIME: 15 MINUTES   COOK TIME: 45 MINUTES

This soup was a lucky accident! One chilly, rainy Sunday afternoon, I set out to use up a few leftover cooked chicken breasts that I had in the fridge, and decided on creating a hearty soup. I tossed a hodgepodge of items into the pot, including onions, bell peppers, corn, canned tomatoes, broth, and quinoa. It was nothing out of the ordinary, but then I added a spice blend similar to one I use for a favorite chili I make, and wow, did it turn out amazing. It's smoky and addictive, light in calories, and packed with nutrition. It's also high in protein and keeps me feeling full for hours. This one-pot wonder is proof that when you combine leftovers with a little imagination you can end up with mouthwatering magic.

1 medium onion, finely diced

1 medium red, yellow, or orange bell pepper, finely diced

¾ teaspoon kosher salt, or more to taste

¼ teaspoon ground black pepper

2 to 3 cloves garlic, minced

2½ tablespoons mild chili powder

2 teaspoons ancho chile powder

1 teaspoon ground cumin

½ teaspoon dried oregano

1 teaspoon smoked paprika

4 cups reduced-sodium chicken broth

1 (28-ounce) can diced fire-roasted tomatoes

3 cups cooked and shredded chicken breast*

1 cup fresh, frozen, or canned corn kernels

⅓ cup dry quinoa

3 scallions, thinly sliced (optional)

1 lime, cut into wedges (optional)

* If starting with raw chicken, use this recipe: Place 2 chicken breasts (bone-in and skin on) on a rimmed baking sheet. Mist the tops with nonstick olive oil spray and sprinkle on some kosher salt and ground black pepper. Roast in an oven set at 400°F for 40 to 45 minutes or until cooked through. The skin should appear golden brown in color and slightly crisp. Set aside and allow to cool. Remove the skin from the chicken and discard. Separate the meat from the bones and shred into bite-sized pieces.

1 Liberally coat a Dutch oven or large pot with nonstick oil spray and warm over medium-high heat. Add the onion, bell pepper, salt, and black pepper and cook for 6 to 7 minutes, stirring occasionally. Add the garlic, mild chili powder, ancho chile powder, cumin, oregano, and paprika and stir everything together. Cook until fragrant, 1 to 2 minutes. Add the broth and tomatoes and bring to a boil. Reduce the heat and simmer for 20 minutes, stirring occasionally.

2 Add the shredded chicken, corn, and quinoa to the pot. Stir to combine and simmer, uncovered, for another 20 minutes, or until the quinoa has puffed and cooked through. Serve each bowl of soup with a sprinkling of scallions and a lime wedge, if desired.

PER SERVING 1 CUP **140** CALORIES **17 g** PROTEIN **2 g** FAT (**1 g** UNSATURATED FAT, **1 g** SATURATED FAT) **25 mg** CHOLESTEROL **13 g** CARBS **3 g** FIBER **5 g** SUGAR (**5 g** NATURAL SUGAR, **0 G** ADDED SUGAR) **490 mg** SODIUM

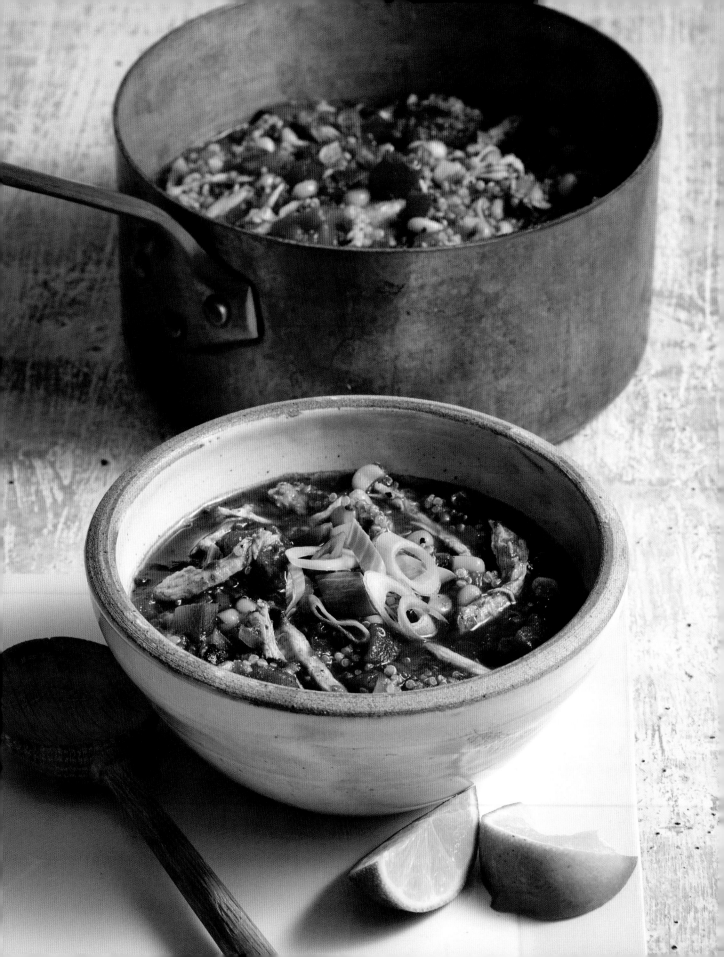

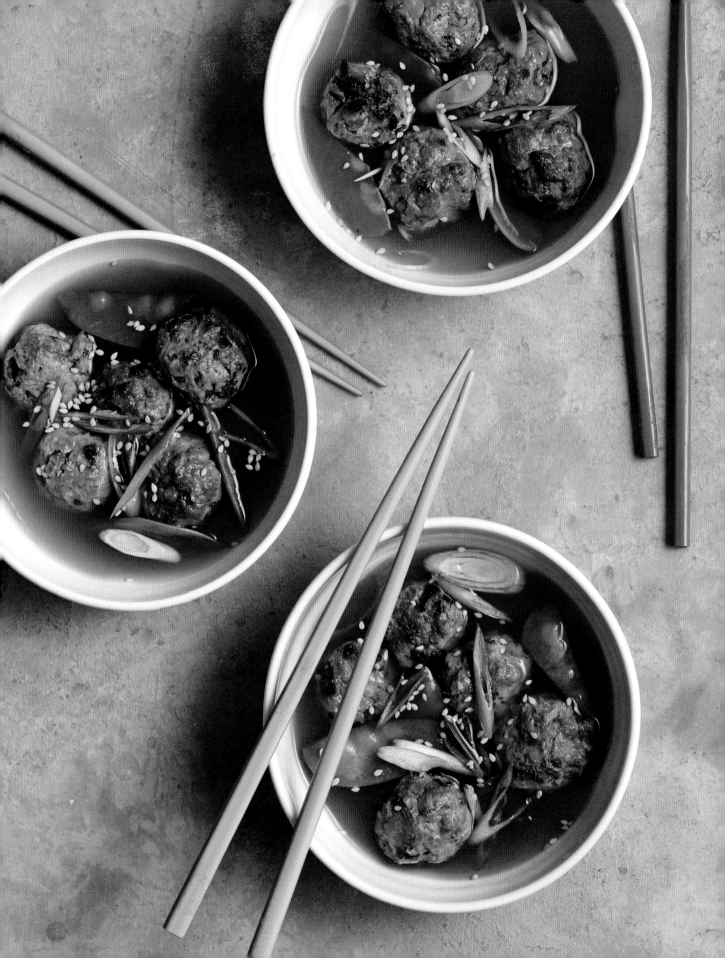

Miso Soup with Mushroom Scallion Meatballs

SERVES: 6   PREP TIME: 15 MINUTES   COOK TIME: 15 MINUTES

Chinese dumplings (aka wontons) are delicious in their own right. Add them to a steaming bowl of miso soup, and they soak in all the yummy flavors of the broth, seasonings, veggies, and all the other ingredients. I created my own healthified and dough-free "wontons" using lean turkey meat and immune-boosting mushrooms. I drop them into this miso soup, which is a traditional Japanese soup consisting of stock and miso paste, a type of seasoning made from fermented soybeans. If you don't like snap peas, you can substitute for snow peas, baby bok choy, or your favorite vegetable. Your fortune says: You are in for one tasty soup!

Note: Miso paste is super high in sodium. While my miso soup is significantly less salty than most restaurant versions, it's still relatively high, so if you have high blood pressure enjoy this only on occasion.

TURKEY MEATBALLS
makes 28

1 pound ground turkey (90 to 93% lean)

1 cup shiitake mushroom caps, finely chopped

1 scallion, minced

¼ cup minced cilantro or parsley

4 cloves garlic, minced

2 tablespoons reduced-sodium soy sauce

¼ teaspoon fish sauce (optional)

½ teaspoon toasted sesame oil

½ teaspoon rice vinegar

SOUP

8 cups reduced-sodium mushroom or vegetable broth

2 cups snap peas, strings removed and cut in half

2 teaspoons rice vinegar

½ cup plus 2 tablespoons miso paste

1 scallion, thinly sliced (optional)

1. Preheat the oven to 450°F. Line a baking sheet with parchment paper and set aside.

2. FOR THE MEATBALLS: In a large bowl, combine the ground turkey, mushrooms, scallion, cilantro, garlic, soy sauce, fish sauce (if using), oil, and vinegar with your hands. Mix until the turkey gets a little sticky. Roll the mixture into 1-tablespoon-size meatballs and line them up on the baking sheet (you should have 28 meatballs). If the mixture starts to stick to your hands, dampen your hands with cold water. Bake for 10 minutes, or until cooked through.

3. FOR THE SOUP: Bring the broth to a simmer in a large pot over medium-high heat. Add the snap peas and cook for 1 to 2 minutes, until cooked through and vibrant green. Turn off the heat and add the vinegar. In a small bowl, whisk the miso with ½ cup of the hot broth from the pot until the miso is dissolved and then add back to the pot. Add the cooked meatballs to the broth and simmer for 5 to 10 minutes. Ladle the soup into bowls and garnish with the scallion, if desired.

PER SERVING 1¼ CUPS SOUP AND 5 OR 6 WONTON MEATBALLS **220** CALORIES **19 g** PROTEIN **6 g** FAT (**5 g** UNSATURATED FAT, **1 g** SATURATED FAT) **35 mg** CHOLESTEROL **24 g** CARBS **9 g** FIBER **9 g** SUGAR (**9 g** NATURAL SUGAR, **0 g** ADDED SUGAR) **1,050 mg** SODIUM

Creamy Garlic Soup with Shrimp and Tofu

MAKES: 8 CUPS   PREP TIME: 15 MINUTES   COOK TIME: 20 MINUTES

This luxurious soup is easy to make but delivers an indulgent flavor with a sinfully rich texture because of the cashews, which are soaked, softened, and blended into a silky cream. I've added a good dose of garlic for flavor, but that's not its only perk. The kitchen staple can also help manage blood pressure thanks to its two active ingredients, allicin and glutamylcysteine. While I often give the option for swapping jarred garlic or garlic powder for the sake of convenience, in this case, I encourage you to use fresh garlic cloves and take the time to mince them, because it's really one of the star ingredients. But I'll offer you another time saver in its place: You can buy precut matchstick carrots. (I'm all about shortcuts!)

1 cup raw cashews, soaked in hot water for at least 30 minutes and drained

4 cups reduced-sodium vegetable or chicken broth, divided

6 large cloves garlic, minced

1 tablespoon Thai or Korean chili paste

½ cup (4 ounces) canned tomato sauce

1 to 2 tablespoons rice vinegar

1 pound medium shrimp, peeled and deveined, tail off

½ block (8 ounces) firm tofu, well drained and cut into ½-inch cubes*

2 medium carrots, cut into matchsticks (about 1 cup)

Fresh cilantro for garnish

* *If you prefer a firmer tofu consistency, sandwich the drained block between layered paper towels (or kitchen towels) and top with a heavy book. Let sit for at least 30 minutes to drain before cutting into cubes.*

1 In a blender, combine the cashews with 1 cup of the broth and blend for about 30 seconds, until completely smooth and creamy. Set aside.

2 Liberally mist a large pot with nonstick oil spray and warm over medium heat. Add the garlic and cook until lightly browned, about 2 minutes, stirring constantly so it doesn't burn. Add the chili paste and cook for 1 minute. Add the tomato sauce and stir to combine. Add the pureed cashews, the remaining 3 cups broth, and the vinegar and bring to a boil. Reduce the heat and simmer for 10 minutes.

3 Add the shrimp, tofu, and carrot sticks to the pot and continue to simmer for about 4 minutes, until the shrimp are fully cooked and the tofu absorbs all of the yummy flavors. Ladle the soup into bowls and garnish each with cilantro.

PER SERVING 1 CUP **170** CALORIES **14 g** PROTEIN **8 g** FAT (**6.5 g** UNSATURATED FAT, **1.5 g** SATURATED FAT) **55 mg** CHOLESTEROL **9 g** CARBS **1 g** FIBER **3 g** SUGAR (**3 g** NATURAL SUGAR, **0 g** ADDED SUGAR) **480 mg** SODIUM

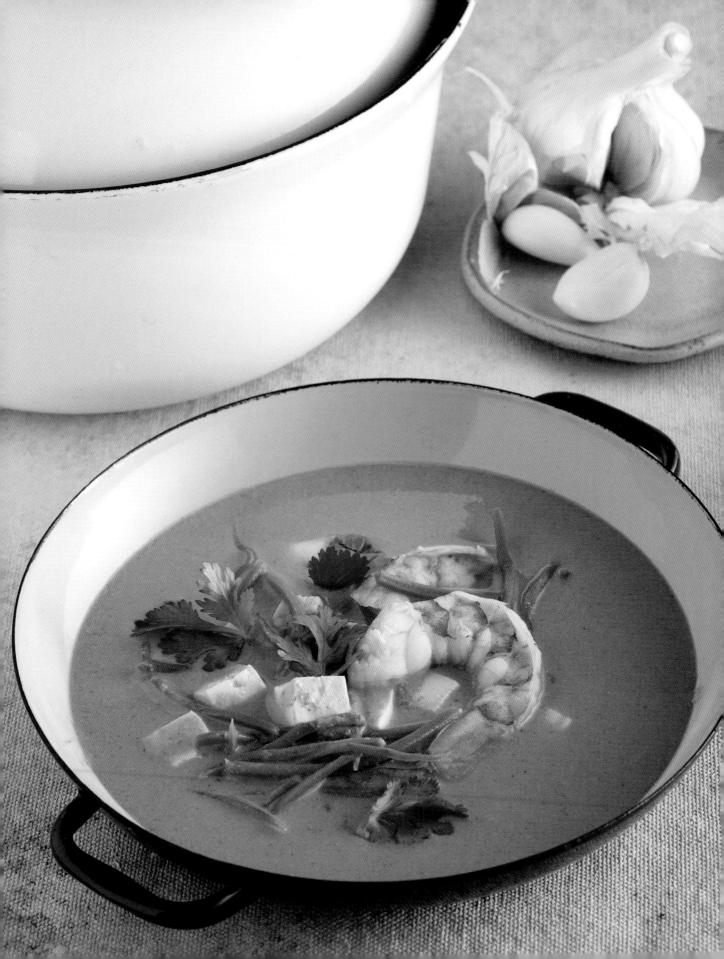

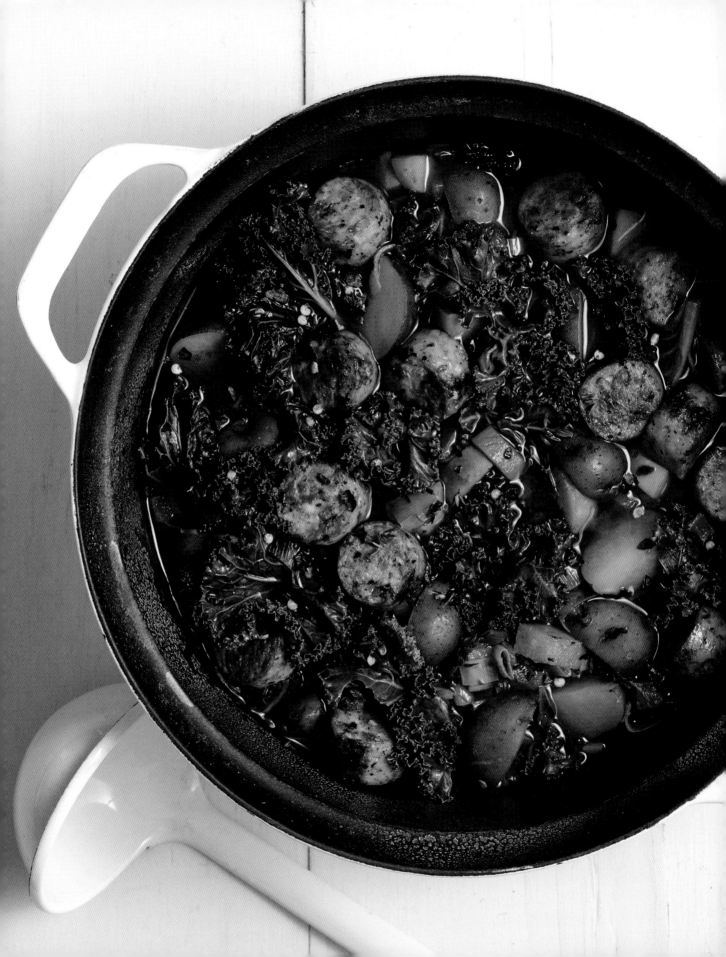

Portuguese-Style Caldo Verde with Sausage and Kale

MAKES: 9 CUPS   PREP TIME: 10 MINUTES   COOK TIME: 20 MINUTES

Stir things up with this Portuguese classic, which is sure to transport you to the streets of Lisbon with every scent and slurp. Caldo verde is a traditional Portuguese green soup that uses spicy chorizo sausage as the base. In this recipe, I've swapped the typical fatty pork sausage with a lighter chicken chorizo sausage, delivering the same great flavor in a better-for-you package. I prefer using precooked chorizo, as it saves you time in the kitchen. Whichever you choose is totally up to you—simply tweak the cooking time accordingly.

As much as I'm in love with leeks, I recognize that they require some extra cleaning, so to save time you could easily swap in extra onions or sliced scallions instead. Celery root introduces interesting character to the soup. While not nearly as well known as its similarly flavored cousin the celery stalk, its nutritional punch is nonetheless profound. The mild veggie is a solid source of fiber, as well as nutrients like potassium and manganese.

3 precooked chorizo-spiced chicken sausage links (about 9 ounces)

1 medium leek, white and green parts, cut in half lengthwise and sliced ¼ inch thick (2 to 3 cups)*

3 cloves garlic, minced

½ cup chopped onion

1½ cups peeled and diced celery root

¼ teaspoon salt, plus more to taste

½ teaspoon dried thyme

⅛ teaspoon red pepper flakes

1 large bunch kale, stems removed, coarsely chopped (about 6 cups)

4 cups reduced-sodium chicken broth

8 ounces small red potatoes, cut into ½-inch pieces

Ground black pepper

Lemon wedges (optional)

*   *If you want to skip the leek, add an extra cup of chopped onion or scallions.*

1 Mist a pot with nonstick oil spray and warm over medium-high heat. Add the sausage and cook for about 5 minutes to warm through and brown on all sides. Transfer the links to a cutting board and slice into ¼-inch rounds. Return the pieces to the pot and cook for an additional 2 minutes to sear the insides, stirring to ensure they brown evenly on all sides. Transfer the seared sausage to a plate, cover, and set aside.

2 Lower the heat to medium and reapply oil spray to the pot. Add the leeks, garlic, onion, celery root, and salt and cook for about 5 minutes, stirring occasionally, until the veggies are nice and soft. Stir in the thyme and red pepper flakes and cook for about 30 seconds. Add the kale and cook until it wilts and starts to turn bright green, about 2 minutes. Add ½ cup of the broth and stir to deglaze the pan, scraping the bottom to incorporate all of the browned bits and pieces. Add the remaining 3½ cups broth and bring to a boil. Add the potatoes and reserved sausages and reduce heat to lowest setting. Simmer uncovered for about 10 minutes, until the potatoes are fork tender. Season with salt and black pepper. Serve with lemon wedges, if desired.

PER SERVING 1 CUP **90** CALORIES **7 g** PROTEIN **2.5 g** FAT **(1.5 g** UNSATURATED FAT, **1 g** SATURATED FAT) **20 mg** CHOLESTEROL **11 g** CARBS **2 g** FIBER **2 g** SUGAR **(2 g** NATURAL SUGAR, **0 g** ADDED SUGAR) **270 mg** SODIUM

Cumin-Spiked Black Bean Soup with Spicy Okra Topping

MAKES: 8 HEAPING CUPS PREP TIME: 10 MINUTES COOK TIME: 20 MINUTES

This flavorful soup is in regular rotation in the Bauer house. I love that it takes fiber-rich black beans, a standard, cost-effective staple, and combines it with okra, a lesser known veggie that boasts a super interesting texture. Not only is okra delicious and high in soluble fiber to benefit your heart and clear your arteries; it also possesses antioxidant and anti-fatigue properties. If you haven't cooked with it yet, this is a great way to give it a go.

To make this soup thick and creamy while still keeping it light, remove a cup or two from the pot and carefully puree in a blender, then mix it back into the simmering soup pot. You can also use an immersion blender right in the pot to achieve the same result.

Pro Tip for Soaking Dried Beans

Overnight Method: Place 1½ to 2 cups dry beans in a bowl and cover with about 4 cups water. Refrigerate overnight.

Quick Method: Place 1½ to 2 cups dry beans in a pot and cover with cold water by 1 inch. Bring to a rolling boil over high heat, then put a lid on the pot and turn the heat off. Let sit for 1 hour, then drain.

SOUP

1 yellow onion, chopped (about 1½ cups)

3 cloves garlic, minced

1 teaspoon cumin seeds

¾ teaspoon kosher salt, divided

2 medium carrots, chopped (about 1 cup)

2 large stalks celery, chopped (about 1 cup)

1 red or yellow bell pepper, chopped (about 1 cup)

1 tablespoon ground cumin

1 tablespoon chili powder

1 teaspoon dried oregano

1 teaspoon dried thyme

1 medium chipotle pepper in adobo sauce (optional)

1 (15-ounce) can crushed tomatoes

3 (15-ounce) cans black beans, rinsed and drained

OKRA TOPPING
makes 1½ cups

8 ounces okra pods, thinly sliced

½ teaspoon cumin seeds

½ teaspoon red pepper flakes

¼ teaspoon kosher salt

OPTIONAL TOPPERS

Crumbled queso fresco, avocado slices, pepitas, and chopped cilantro

1 **FOR THE SOUP:** Liberally mist a medium saucepan with nonstick oil spray and warm over medium heat. Add the onion, garlic, cumin seeds, and ¼ teaspoon of the salt and cook for 3 to 4 minutes, stirring often. Add the carrots, celery, and bell pepper and cook for another minute or so (mist with additional oil spray if the pan becomes dry). Add the ground cumin, chili powder, oregano, and thyme and give it a good stir. Add the chipotle pepper, if using, crushed tomatoes, black beans, and 3 cups water. Bring to a boil, then reduce the heat to low and simmer for 15 minutes.

2 Remove 2 or 3 ladlefuls of soup (1 to 1½ cups' worth) and carefully puree in a blender. **NOTE:** The soup will be very hot, so cover the lid with a kitchen towel and slowly blend, starting with the lowest setting and gradually increasing the speed until the soup is smooth. Then pour the puree back into the soup pot and stir to combine. Alternatively, you can use an immersion blender to gently puree the soup in the pot, making sure to leave the majority chunky and whole. Cover and keep warm over the lowest heat until ready to serve.

3 **FOR THE OKRA GARNISH:** Liberally mist a large skillet with nonstick oil spray and warm over medium-high heat. Add the okra, cumin seeds, red pepper flakes, and salt and cook for about 5 minutes, stirring occasionally, until lightly browned and softened. **TO SERVE,** ladle the soup into bowls and top with the okra and your choice of garnishes.

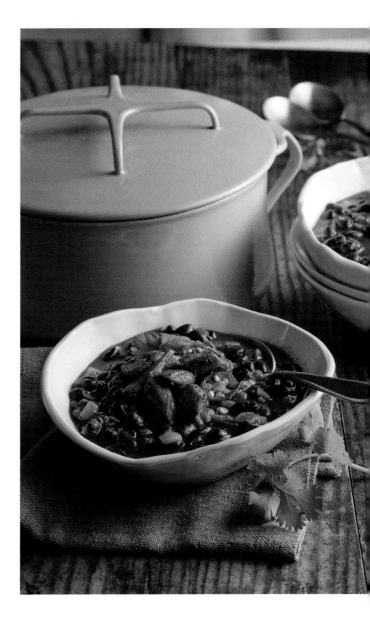

PER SERVING 1 HEAPING CUP, WITHOUT OKRA TOPPING **170** CALORIES **10 g** PROTEIN **1.5 g** FAT (**1.5 g** UNSATURATED FAT, **0 g** SATURATED FAT) **0 mg** CHOLESTEROL **30 g** CARBS **10 g** FIBER **5 g** SUGAR (**5 g** NATURAL SUGAR, **0 g** ADDED SUGAR) **320 mg** SODIUM *ADD **20** CALORIES AND **1 g** FIBER FOR OKRA TOPPING.

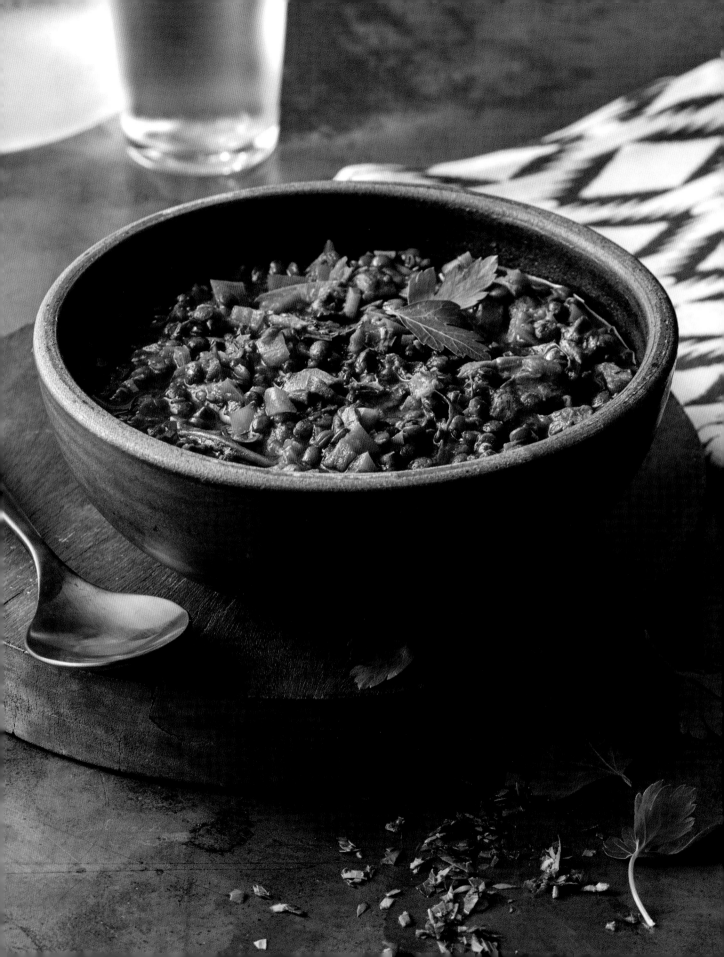

Luscious Lentil and Veggie Soup

MAKES: 10 CUPS   PREP TIME: 15 MINUTES   COOK TIME: 40 MINUTES

You'll find twelve—that's right, a dozen—superfoods in one bowl. It's like a gala of goodness! If you're trying to get your kids or spouse to eat better, this is the soup to serve. It's thick, hearty, soothing, and nutrient-packed. Don't be surprised if they ask for seconds . . . it's *that* delicious. A few notes on prep: I'm personally a hand chopper—I actually find it relaxing to manually chop each veggie—but if you're pressed for time or not as cuckoo as I am, you can give each a rough chop and then add to the bowl of a food processor and gently pulse (just be sure not to puree them). Also, if you're into your pressure cooker, it's simple to convert this recipe to your machine, and it will be ready in no time. And if you have a pot that's large enough, I recommend doubling the recipe and freezing in 2-cup containers for lots of tasty future bowls. Each serving will deliver 14 grams of protein and 10 grams of fiber (the math below is provided for one cup, but I can easily eat two). It's the ultimate comfort food that delivers serious health perks. Soup's on!

1 medium onion, finely chopped

3 stalks celery, finely chopped

2 medium carrots, finely chopped

1 medium red, yellow, or orange bell pepper, finely chopped

2 cloves garlic, minced

1¼ teaspoons kosher salt, plus more to taste

¼ teaspoon ground pepper, or more to taste

1 (8-ounce) container white button or baby bella mushrooms, roughly chopped

1 tablespoon tomato paste

1 cup canned crushed tomatoes

6 cups reduced-sodium vegetable broth

1½ cups dried green lentils, rinsed and drained

4 to 5 sprigs fresh thyme

1 bay leaf

1 to 2 cups baby spinach leaves, chopped

1 to 2 tablespoons finely chopped fresh parsley

1 to 2 tablespoons lemon juice

1 Liberally mist a large pot or Dutch oven with nonstick oil spray and warm over medium heat. Add the onion, celery, carrots, bell pepper, garlic, salt, and pepper and cook, stirring frequently, until the vegetables are softened and most of the moisture has evaporated, about 10 minutes. You will be left with a thick, rich, and slightly caramelized vegetable base. Add the mushrooms and cook for 4 minutes, stirring frequently to prevent scorching on the bottom. Reapply oil spray if the pan becomes dry. Add the tomato paste and crushed tomatoes, scraping up any bits from the bottom. Add the broth, lentils, thyme, and bay leaf.

2 Bring to a boil, then reduce the heat to low and cover the pot. Simmer for 25 to 30 minutes, until the lentils are tender. Remove the thyme sprigs and bay leaf. Add the spinach and parsley and stir until everything is well combined. Add the lemon juice and season with salt and pepper.

You can freeze this soup in an airtight container for up to 3 months.

PER SERVING 1 CUP **110** CALORIES **7 g** PROTEIN **0 g** FAT **0 mg** CHOLESTEROL **18 g** CARBS **5 g** FIBER **4 g** SUGAR (**4 g** NATURAL SUGAR, **0 g** ADDED SUGAR) **370 mg** SODIUM

Creamy Cauliflower Leek Soup with Crispy Seaweed

SERVES: 13   PREP TIME: 10 MINUTES   COOK TIME: 25 MINUTES

Cauliflower brings a bit of cruciferous magic to any recipe, helping to reduce the risk for a variety of diseases. Leeks, another star of this dish, are part of the onion family and have prebiotic power, which helps boost gut health. And celery, a standard in many soups, features luteolin, an antioxidant that can help tame inflammation. Topping it all off is a crispy seaweed garnish, aka "nori magic dust," which takes this in a whole new flavor direction. I created this topper in the spirit of the Japanese seasoning togarashi. It's a scrumptious combo of seeds, which add fiber, protein, and magnesium; and seaweed, which is also rich in fiber and protein and an alphabet soup (pun intended) of vitamins, including A, B_6, and C.

SOUP

2 tablespoons olive oil

2 large leeks, white and green parts, chopped

1 yellow onion, chopped

2 stalks celery, chopped

2 to 4 cloves garlic, minced

2 teaspoons kosher salt, plus more to taste

Ground black pepper

6 to 7 cups reduced-sodium vegetable broth

4 to 5 sprigs fresh thyme

12 heaping cups cauliflower florets (about 2 medium heads)

1 teaspoon ground nutmeg

Fresh chives or parsley (optional garnish)

CRISPY SEAWEED GARNISH (OPTIONAL)
makes about ½ cup

¼ cup pepitas (shell-off pumpkin seeds)

1 tablespoon black sesame seeds

1 (8 by 8-inch) sheet nori seaweed (or 8 snack-size sheets)

¼ teaspoon kosher salt

1 FOR THE SOUP: Warm the oil in a large pot over medium heat. Add the leeks, onion, celery, and garlic and stir to coat in the oil. Season with the salt and pepper. Cook for 8 to 10 minutes, until soft-ened, stirring frequently to prevent scorching on the bottom of the pot. Mist with oil spray as needed.

2 Add the broth and stir, scraping up any bits from the bottom. Add the thyme, cauliflower, and nutmeg. Bring to a boil, then reduce the heat to low, cover, and simmer for 15 to 20 minutes, until the vegetables are fork-tender. Remove the thyme stems and turn off the heat.

3 Using an immersion blender, puree the soup in the pot until smooth. Alternatively, carefully transfer the soup in batches to a standing blender and puree. If the soup needs thinning, add additional broth. Season with salt and pepper.

4 FOR THE CRISPY SEAWEED GARNISH: Toast the pepitas in a small dry skillet over medium heat, tossing, for 2 minutes. Add the sesame seeds and continue tossing until they start to pop, 1 minute or so. Remove the pan from the heat and allow the seeds to cool, about 10 minutes. Place into a food processor, add the nori seaweed and salt, and pulse to a coarse dust. TO SERVE: Ladle the soup into bowls and top with a sprinkling of the crispy seaweed garnish and optional chives or parsley.

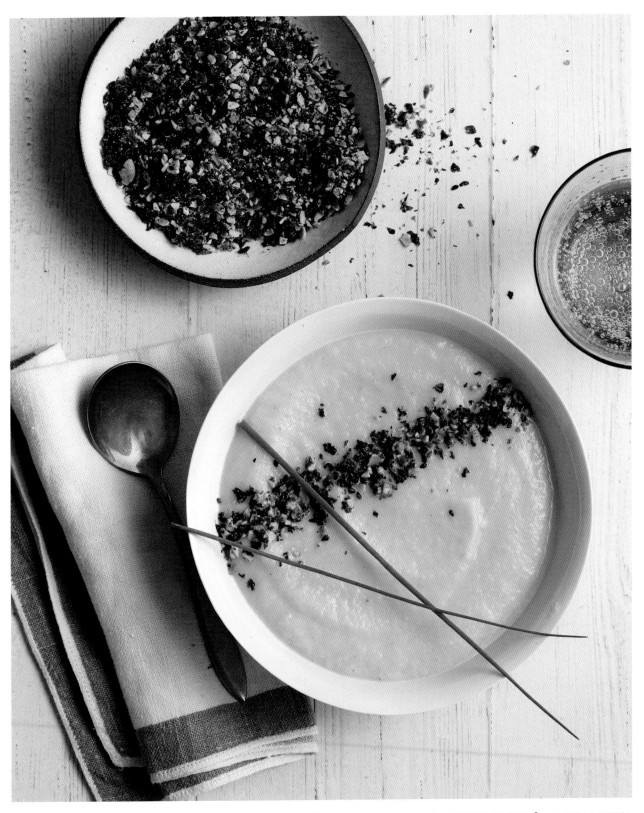

PER SERVING 1 CUP **60** CALORIES **2 g** PROTEIN **2.5 g** FAT (**2.5 g** UNSATURATED FAT, **0 g** SATURATED FAT) **0 mg** CHOLESTEROL **9 g** CARBS **3 g** FIBER **3 g** SUGAR (**3 g** NATURAL SUGAR, **0 g** ADDED SUGAR) **390 mg** SODIUM *ADD 30 CALORIES FOR EACH TABLESPOON OF CRISPY SEAWEED GARNISH.

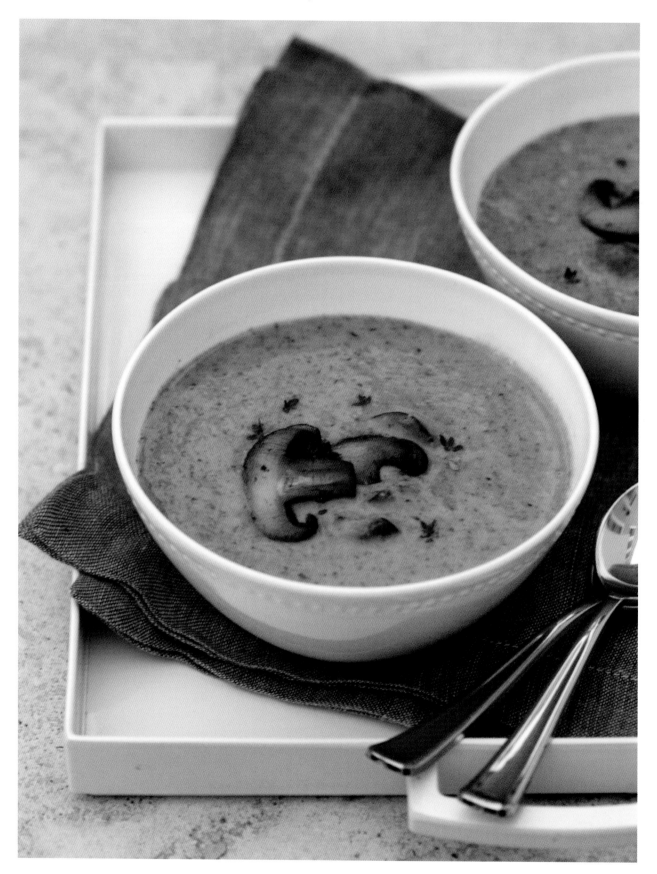

Nondairy Cream of Mushroom Soup

MAKES: 8 CUPS   PREP TIME: 5 MINUTES   COOK TIME: 30 MINUTES

Chicken noodle may be the go-to soup when you're feeling under the weather, but there's another surprising remedy: this delicious cream of mushroom soup. It's both thick and comforting, and it features a bold umami flavor that will help soothe that hacky cough and never-ending sniffles. Its immune-boosting powers come from the mushrooms. While many dismiss them as a lowly fungus, mushrooms feature antiviral properties thanks to their beta-glucans and chitosans, which can help protect against colds, flu, and other infections. Mushrooms are an inexpensive way to shower your body with a hefty dose of delicious cold-fighters.

If you prefer a thinner consistency, simply add more broth a few tablespoons at a time. You can double up the recipe and freeze extra portions for future use.

2 pounds sliced mushrooms (any type, such as button or baby bella)

2 yellow onions, finely diced (about 3 cups)

1 to 2 tablespoons olive oil

1 to 2 tablespoons fresh thyme leaves (or 1 to 2 teaspoons dried thyme)

3 cloves garlic, minced (or ¼ teaspoon garlic powder)

1 teaspoon kosher salt, or more to taste

1 (14-ounce) can cannellini beans, rinsed and drained

4 cups reduced-sodium vegetable broth

1 to 2 tablespoons balsamic vinegar

Ground black pepper

Chopped fresh parsley for garnish

1 Liberally mist a large pot with nonstick oil spray and warm over medium-high heat. Add the mushrooms and leave them undisturbed for 4 minutes. Cook for another 15 to 20 minutes, stirring occasionally. As they cook, the mushrooms will generate a lot of liquid, and then naturally absorb it as they continue to cook down. The goal is browned and caramelized mushrooms without any remaining liquid. When they're done, remove a few tablespoons and set aside to use as garnish.

2 Add the onions, oil, thyme, garlic, and salt and cook for about 5 minutes, until the onions are softened and slightly browned. Add the beans and cook, stirring, for 1 to 2 minutes. Stir in the broth and cook for another 5 minutes, reducing the heat to low when it starts to bubble.

3 Turn off the heat. Using an immersion blender, puree the soup in the pot, leaving lots of bits and pieces of mushroom for texture throughout. Alternatively, you can puree for longer to create a completely smooth soup. Stir in the vinegar and season with salt and pepper. Garnish the bowls with the reserved sautéed mushrooms and a sprinkle of parsley.

PER SERVING 1 CUP **110** CALORIES **7 g** PROTEIN **2 g** FAT (**2 g** UNSATURATED FAT, **0 g** SATURATED FAT) **0 mg** CHOLESTEROL **16 g** CARBS **5 g** FIBER **5 g** SUGAR (**5 g** NATURAL SUGAR, **0 g** ADDED SUGAR) **320 mg** SODIUM

Hearty Italian Minestrone

MAKES: 12 HEAPING CUPS   PREP TIME: 10 MINUTES   COOK TIME: 1 HOUR

Whenever a pot of minestrone is cooking up on the stove, everyone is happily waiting, spoon in hand, for their bowl to be filled. It gets slurped up in no time. The great part about classic minestrone is that the recipe has all the components of a super healthy soup. In this version, I've elevated it even more by doubling up on beans, using whole grain pasta, and packing in kale, green beans and tomatoes. You can customize it for your crew by tossing whatever veggies you have on hand and swapping in any type of bean you like, including chickpeas, edamame, black, kidney, and so on. Skip the red pepper flakes if you're sensitive to heat.

The prep is super simple—it's the cook time on the stove that takes a while. But look at it this way: That leaves you some time to take a walk, or enjoy a nice glass of Italian red wine, or plan your dream vacation to the Amalfi coast!

1 large yellow onion, cut into ½-inch pieces (about 2 cups)

2 medium carrots, cut into ½-inch pieces (about 1 cup)

2 large stalks celery, sliced ¼ inch thick (about ¾ cup)

1 teaspoon kosher salt, plus more to taste

½ teaspoon black pepper, plus more to taste

4 large cloves garlic, minced (or ½ to ¾ teaspoon garlic powder)

3 to 4 tablespoons tomato paste

1 (14-ounce) can no-salt-added diced tomatoes, with liquid

2 (15-ounce) cans cannellini beans, drained and rinsed

8 cups reduced-sodium vegetable broth

½ teaspoon dried thyme

½ teaspoon dried rosemary

¼ teaspoon dried parsley

¼ teaspoon red pepper flakes (omit if you're sensitive to heat)

2 fresh or dried bay leaves

1 cup uncooked whole grain pasta, such as elbows, shells, or penne

12 ounces green beans, ends trimmed and cut into 2-inch pieces (about 2½ cups)

4 to 5 cups chopped kale leaves

½ cup torn fresh basil (optional)

1. Liberally mist the bottom of a large pot with nonstick oil spray and warm over medium heat. Add the onion, carrots, celery, salt, and black pepper and cook for about 5 minutes, stirring occasionally, until the vegetables soften. Add the garlic and tomato paste and cook for another minute, or until the garlic is fragrant.

2. Stir in the diced tomatoes and liquid, the beans, broth, thyme, rosemary, parsley, red pepper flakes, and bay leaves and bring to a boil. Reduce the heat to low and simmer uncovered for 45 minutes.

3. While the soup is simmering, cook the pasta according to package directions for al dente minus 1 to 2 minutes (the pasta will continue to cook after it is added to the soup). Drain, rinse with cold water, and set aside.

4. When the soup is done simmering, remove the bay leaves and add the green beans and kale. Stir to combine and continue to simmer for a final 4 minutes, or until the green beans have softened slightly and the kale is wilted. Mix in the cooked pasta and season with salt and pepper. Garnish with the basil, if using, right before serving.

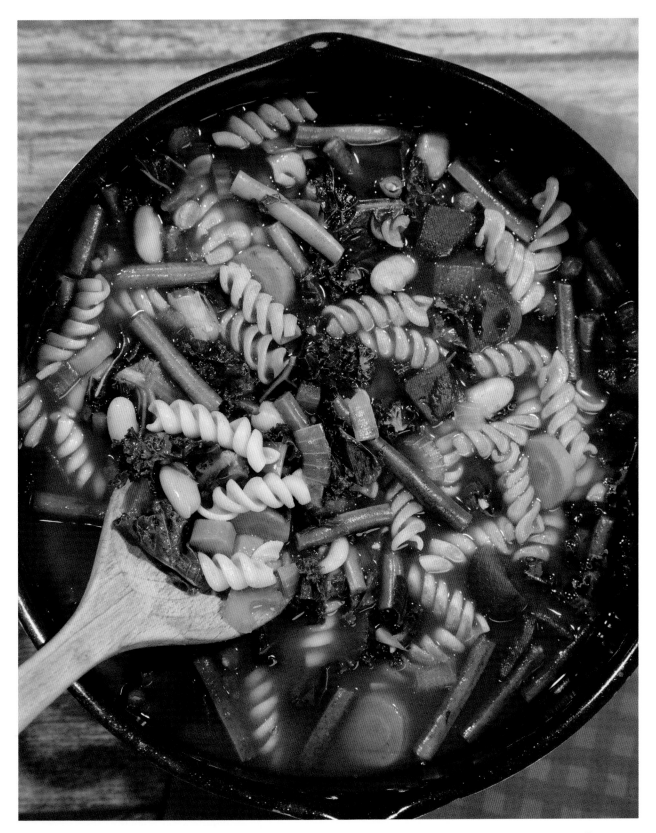

PER SERVING 1 HEAPING CUP **120** CALORIES **6 g** PROTEIN **0 g** FAT **0 mg** CHOLESTEROL **23 g** CARBS **6 g** FIBER **5 g** SUGAR (**5 g** NATURAL SUGAR, **0 g** ADDED SUGAR) **440 mg** SODIUM

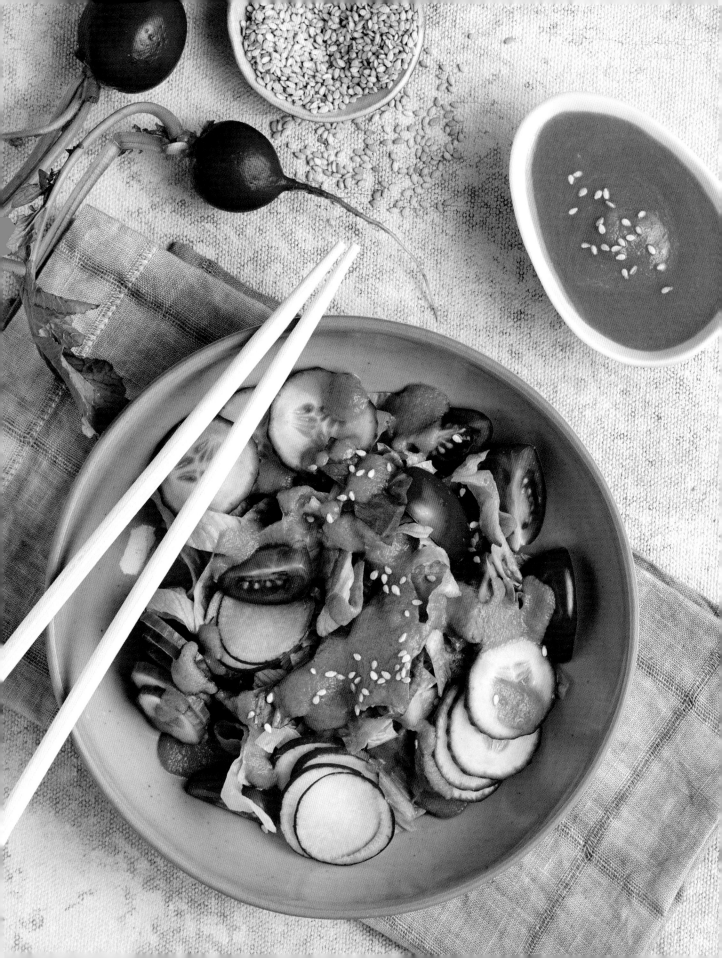

Japanese Salad with Carrot-Ginger Dressing

MAKES: 1 SALAD (AND LOTS OF EXTRA DRESSING)   PREP TIME: 10 MINUTES

As much as I love cooking, I also enjoy eating out with the fam, and Japanese food is always a crowd favorite. And boy, do we all love their signature salad. The greens are pretty basic, but the flavorful carrot-ginger dressing is WOW . . . anything but ordinary. This is my copycat version. I just toss all the ingredients into a food processor or high-speed blender and puree. My base is an easy mix of lettuce, tomato, and cucumber, but you can use whatever you have on hand. Truth be told, in this instance it's really all about the dressing anyway—the greens are just a vehicle!

This dressing is action-packed: The oil contains good-for-you fats, the ginger possesses anti-inflammatory powers, the garlic contributes to healthy arteries and blood pressure, and the carrots are rich in beta carotene to boost your immune system and promote healthy vision.

Although dressing recipes vary by restaurant, I can guarantee this one is lighter in calories, fat, sodium, and sugar—but still provides the addictive flavor we love.

SALAD
for each salad

- 2 cups chopped romaine lettuce
- 3 cherry tomatoes, halved
- 1 radish, sliced
- ¼ cucumber, thinly sliced
- Toasted sesame seeds for garnish (optional)

DRESSING
makes about 1½ cups

- ⅓ cup canola or grapeseed oil
- ¼ cup rice vinegar
- ¼ cup reduced-sodium soy sauce
- 1 teaspoon toasted sesame oil

- 3 medium carrots (or 15 baby carrots), roughly chopped
- 1 tablespoon lime juice
- 1 tablespoon honey
- 2 tablespoons peeled and roughly chopped fresh ginger root (or 1 teaspoon ground ginger)
- 2 cloves garlic, roughly chopped (or ¼ teaspoon garlic powder)
- ¼ teaspoon salt, or more to taste
- ¼ teaspoon black pepper, or more to taste

1 FOR EACH SALAD: Toss the lettuce, tomatoes, radish, and cucumber in a bowl.

2 FOR THE DRESSING: Combine all the dressing ingredients in a high-speed blender or food processor and puree. If you don't have a high-speed blender or food processor, microwave the chopped carrots for about 5 minutes to soften them before adding them to a standard blender.

TO SERVE: Toss the salad with 2 to 4 tablespoons of the dressing, and garnish with a sprinkling of sesame seeds, if desired. Store leftover dressing in a covered container in the fridge for up to 1 week. Give it a good stir before using.

PER SERVING SALAD WITH 2 TABLESPOONS DRESSING 120 CALORIES 3 g PROTEIN 7 g FAT (6.5 g UNSATURATED FAT, 0.5 g SATURATED FAT) 0 mg CHOLESTEROL 12 g CARBS 3 g FIBER 8 g SUGAR (7 g NATURAL SUGAR, 1 g ADDED SUGAR) 200 mg SODIUM *ADD 35 CALORIES FOR EACH EXTRA TABLESPOON OF DRESSING.

Bistro Wedge Salad with Mushroom Bacon and Blue Cheese Dressing

SERVES: 4   PREP TIME: 15 MINUTES   COOK TIME: 20 MINUTES

This wedge salad has so much going for it: the crisp, fresh lettuce, the creamy dressing, the addictive umami "bacon" flavor and chew—one forkful satisfies on so many different levels. My healthy hack for bacon is easy and delicious . . . just wait until you try it. The DIY blue cheese dressing cuts wayyyy back on calories and saturated fat but not flavor (and you'll have plenty left over for future meals). And while the iceberg doesn't score the highest grades for greens, it still counts as a veggie and serves up a small amount of nutrients while delivering big amounts of crunch, which makes this salad extra special.

MUSHROOM BACON

3½ ounces shiitake mushrooms, stems removed and thinly sliced (about 2½ cups)

¼ teaspoon kosher salt

BLUE CHEESE DRESSING
makes 1½ cups

1 cup low-fat buttermilk

2 tablespoons extra virgin olive oil

2 cloves garlic, roughly chopped (or ½ teaspoon garlic powder)

½ cup crumbled blue cheese, or Gorgonzola, feta, or goat cheese, divided

1 teaspoon kosher salt

¼ teaspoon black pepper

½ teaspoon onion powder

2 tablespoons minced fresh chives

SALAD

1 head iceberg lettuce, root end trimmed but left intact, cut into ¼-inch wedges

1 cup grape or cherry tomatoes, halved

Blue cheese crumbles for garnish (optional)

1 FOR THE BACON: Preheat the oven to 400°F.

2 Place the mushrooms on a baking sheet in a single layer and liberally mist with olive oil spray. Sprinkle the salt over the top and roast for about 20 minutes, tossing halfway through, until the mushrooms shrink significantly and are golden brown.

3 FOR THE DRESSING: In a high-speed blender or food processor, combine the buttermilk, oil, garlic, 6 tablespoons of the blue cheese, salt, pepper, and onion powder. Pulse until smooth, about 20 seconds. Transfer the dressing to a bowl and stir in the chives and remaining 2 tablespoons blue cheese.

TO ASSEMBLE: Arrange each lettuce wedge on a plate with the tomatoes scattered around it. Sprinkle the mushroom bacon on top and drizzle with 2 tablespoons of the dressing. Garnish with additional dressing and blue cheese crumbles, if desired.

PER SERVING SALAD WEDGE WITH 2 TABLESPOONS DRESSING 80 CALORIES 4 g PROTEIN 4.5 g FAT (3 g UNSATURATED FAT, 1.5 g SATURATED FAT) 5 mg CHOLESTEROL 10 g CARBS 2 g FIBER 4 g SUGAR (4 g NATURAL SUGAR, 0 g ADDED SUGAR) 410 mg SODIUM *ADD 25 CALORIES FOR EACH ADDITIONAL TABLESPOON OF DRESSING.

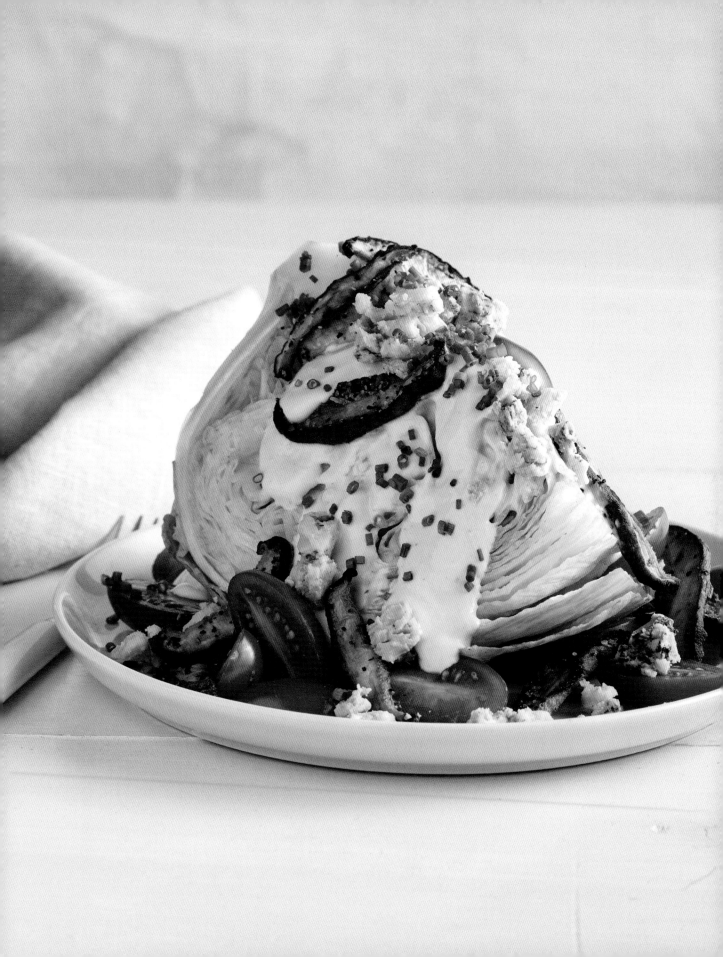

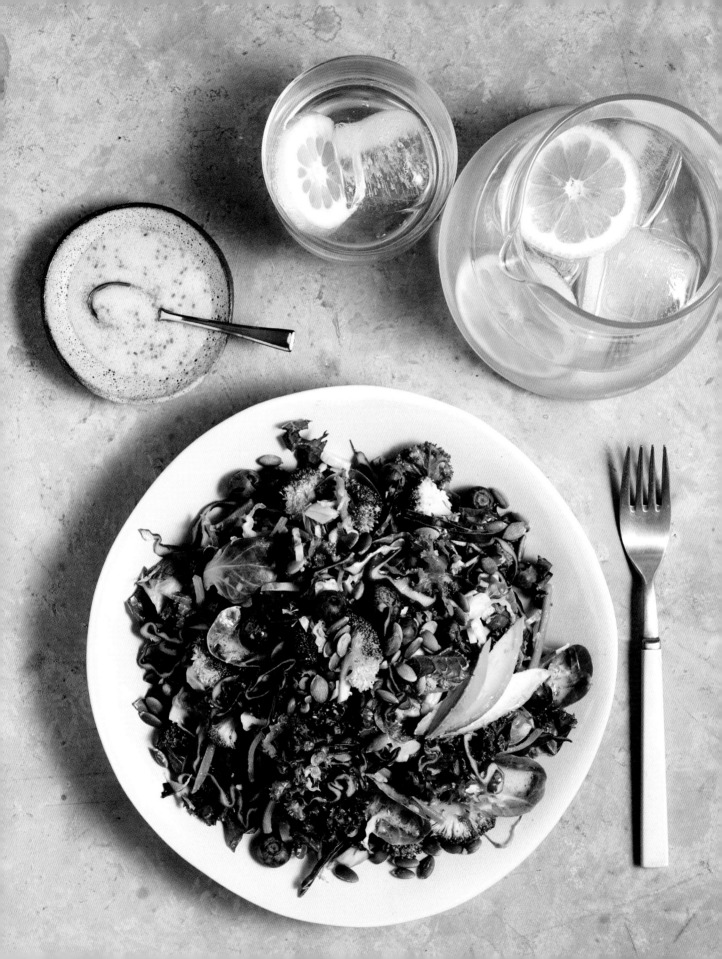

Detox Salad with Lemon-Chia Dressing

MAKES: 7 LARGE SALADS   PREP TIME: 20 MINUTES

I developed this salad as sort of a "day after" cleanse. It's intended to help you reset and refresh after a long weekend of indulgence, a vacation, or a food-filled holiday stretch. It's also a great jump-start meal if you're having trouble sticking to a healthy-eating plan. Every ingredient has been thoughtfully added to contribute something unique and effective: fiber to help promote fullness and regularity, vitamins to enhance immunity and improve overall wellness, antioxidants to tame inflammation and boost brain power, and healthy fat to increase satiety and stabilize blood sugar levels. Simply put, it's a bowl full of pure goodness. Then it's topped off with a lemon chia vinaigrette that's also designed to get you back on your A game. It has an all-star cast: vitamin-C-rich lemon juice, heart-healthy EVOO, and omega-3-rich chia seeds. And the longer it sits, the richer and thicker it gets. (If it becomes more firm than you'd like after a few days, simply add a splash of water or a dash of extra virgin olive oil and lemon juice and give it a good stir.)

While this salad requires a bit of chopping, it also yields *a lot* of volume, which means you'll have plenty of bowls to enjoy over the next couple of days. Short on time? The ingredients can easily be substituted for pre-chopped veggies, boxed or bagged salads, or pre-shredded slaw.

LEMON-CHIA VINAIGRETTE
makes 1 cup

- 2 tablespoons Dijon mustard
- 2 tablespoons chia seeds
- ½ cup fresh lemon juice
- ¼ cup extra virgin olive oil
- ¼ teaspoon kosher salt
- ⅛ teaspoon black pepper

SALAD

- 4 cups packed stemmed kale leaves, thinly sliced
- 2 medium carrots, grated
- 8 ounces Brussels sprouts, trimmed and thinly sliced (about 2½ cups)
- 2 to 3 cups finely chopped broccoli florets
- 2½ cups shredded red/purple cabbage
- 1 cup fresh blueberries
- ½ cup pumpkin seeds
- 1 avocado, sliced

1 **FOR THE DRESSING:** In a small bowl, whisk together the mustard and 2 tablespoons water until emulsified. Add the chia seeds and whisk again. Add the lemon juice, oil, salt, and pepper and whisk to combine. If the chia seeds clump together, allow the dressing to sit for 5 minutes or so and then stir. It will become smoother and thicker as it sits.

2 **FOR THE SALAD:** In a large bowl, combine the kale, carrots, Brussels sprouts, broccoli, and cabbage. Stash in a sealed container in the fridge and build each salad when you're ready to eat.

TO ASSEMBLE INDIVIDUAL SALADS: Transfer 2 cups of the veggie mixture with 2 tablespoons dressing to a plate. Top with 2 to 3 tablespoons blueberries, 1 tablespoon pumpkin seeds, and avocado. Add extra dressing if you like.

PER SERVING 2 CUPS SALAD + 2 TABLESPOONS DRESSING 250 CALORIES 9 g PROTEIN 17 g FAT (14.5 g UNSATURATED FAT, 2.5 g SATURATED FAT) 0 mg CHOLESTEROL 21 g CARBS 9 g FIBER 7 g SUGAR (7 g NATURAL SUGAR, 0 g ADDED SUGAR) 210 mg SODIUM *ADD 40 CALORIES FOR EACH ADDITIONAL TABLESPOON OF DRESSING.

Fiery Buffalo Chicken Salad in Lettuce Cups

SERVES: 4   PREP TIME: 10 MINUTES   COOK TIME: 15 MINUTES

Buffalo wings are quintessential happy hour food—greasy, comforting, and finger-licking good. I made them a little neater and whole lot healthier in this version. In fact, it's the perfect low-carb lunch or dinner wrapped in one tidy little package. You can even double up on portions because they're super light, and packed with protein. The Buffalo Ranch Dressing (which is ready in a flash) will become your new go-to recipe for everyday salads, crudité dip, or perhaps the first-of-a-kind healthy sidekick for chicken wings. Just don't skimp on the fresh herbs, because they really help tie everything together.

Shortcuts are the name of the game in this recipe: Go ahead and use leftover rotisserie or home-cooked chicken that you already have on hand. You can also follow my eaaasy instructions for roasting chicken breasts (page 58). Simply shred it with a fork, or get busy with your hands—sometimes using your fingers is easier, just saying! You can also buy pre-shredded carrots and red cabbage in the grocery store to save time.

DRESSING
makes about 1 cup

- ½ cup low-fat or nonfat plain Greek yogurt
- 2 tablespoons low-fat mayonnaise
- 1 tablespoon milk (any type)
- 1 tablespoon lemon juice
- ¼ teaspoon kosher salt
- ¼ teaspoon black pepper
- ¾ teaspoon onion powder
- ¼ teaspoon garlic powder
- 1 tablespoon finely chopped fresh chives
- 1 tablespoon finely chopped fresh parsley
- ½ teaspoon finely chopped fresh dill (or ¼ teaspoon dried dill)
- 3 to 4 tablespoons hot sauce

CHICKEN SALAD

- 4 cups shredded cooked chicken breast
- 1 head Boston or Bib lettuce (or iceberg or romaine)
- 2 stalks celery, thinly sliced
- 1 cup shredded red/purple cabbage
- 1 cup shredded carrots
- ¼ cup celery leaves (optional)

1. FOR THE DRESSING: In a small bowl, combine all the dressing ingredients and stir until well incorporated.

2. In a medium bowl, mix the chicken with two thirds of the dressing (about ⅔ cup). Set aside.

3. Break off 16 individual whole leaves from the lettuce head (making sure they are dry after rinsing and trimming away any tough stem ends). Fill each lettuce cup with 3 to 4 tablespoons of the chicken salad. Garnish with shredded vegetables and celery leaves, if using. Serve with the remaining dressing on the side for drizzling.

PER SERVING 4 LETTUCE CUPS 210 CALORIES 35 g PROTEIN 4.5 g FAT (3.5 g UNSATURATED FAT, 1 g SATURATED FAT) 100 mg CHOLESTEROL 6 g CARBS 2 g FIBER 3 g SUGAR (3 g NATURAL SUGAR, 0 g ADDED SUGAR) 490 mg SODIUM *ADD 7 CALORIES FOR EACH ADDITIONAL TABLESPOON OF DRESSING.

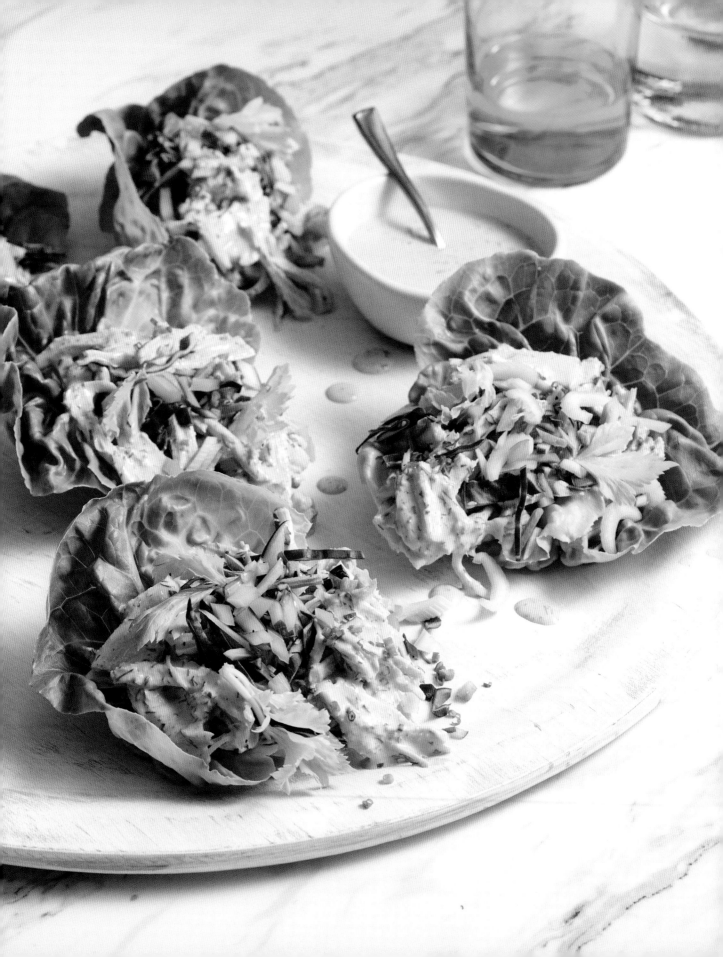

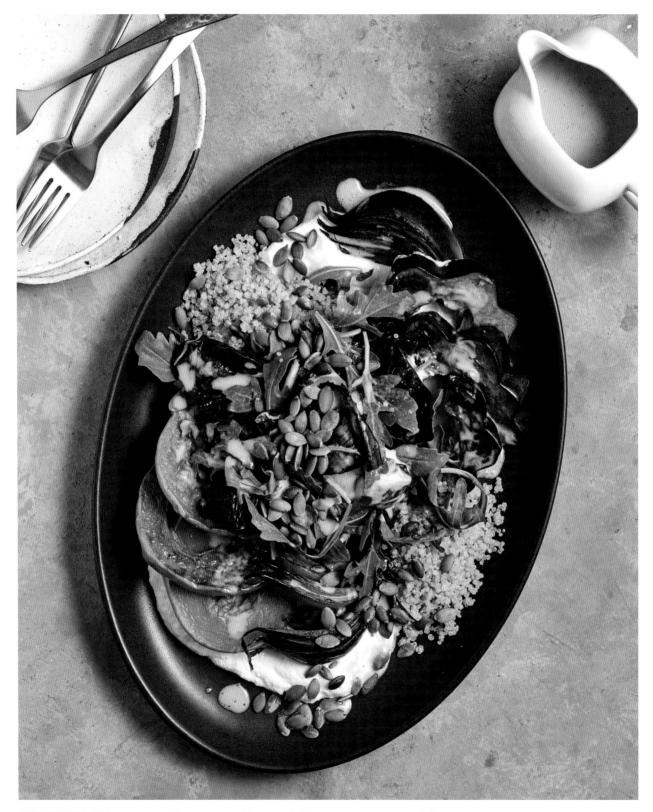

<u>PER SERVING</u> **280** CALORIES **10 g** PROTEIN **11 g** FAT (**8.5 g** UNSATURATED FAT, **2.5 g** SATURATED FAT) **5 mg** CHOLESTEROL **39 g** CARBS **6 g** FIBER **5 g** SUGAR (**5 g** NATURAL SUGAR, **0 g** ADDED SUGAR) **240 mg** SODIUM *ADD 50 CALORIES FOR EACH EXTRA TABLESPOON VINAIGRETTE.

Roasted Squash and Quinoa Salad over Ricotta Cream with Sherry Vinaigrette

SERVES: 4   PREP TIME: 10 MINUTES   COOK TIME: 25 MINUTES

When you hear "comfort food," visions of gooey mac and cheese, cheesy pizza, or crispy French fries probably come to mind. But for me, roasted acorn and butternut squash are also on the list. True, I'm a nutritionist, but give it a shot and you'll soon find out just how sweet and creamy, indulgent and insanely satisfying these produce picks are. It's a double bonus that they're also rich in nutrients that can help you feel full, promote a glowing complexion, and reduce the risk for a variety of diseases. All of the components can be made ahead of time and then tossed together whenever you're ready to eat.

SALAD

1 medium acorn squash, cut in half, seeded, and cut across the ridges into ¾- to 1-inch slices (about 8 pieces)

1 medium butternut squash, peeled, cut in half, seeded, and cut into ¾- to 1-inch half-moons (8 to 12 pieces)

1 large red onion, cut into 8 wedges through the stem end

¼ teaspoon kosher salt

½ teaspoon black pepper

3 sprigs fresh thyme (or ½ teaspoon dried thyme)

¼ cup part-skim ricotta cheese

¼ cup nonfat or low-fat plain Greek yogurt

4 cups baby arugula

2 cups radicchio leaves, torn into large pieces

1 cup cooked quinoa (⅓ cup dry, before cooking)

¼ cup toasted pepitas (shell-off pumpkin seeds)*

* *If you're starting with raw pepitas, lay them on a baking sheet and toast in the oven for 2 minutes while squash is roasting.*

VINAIGRETTE
makes about 1 cup

1 large shallot, roughly chopped (about ¼ cup)

¼ cup canned cannellini beans, rinsed and drained

¼ cup sherry vinegar

1 teaspoon Dijon mustard

¼ teaspoon kosher salt, or more to taste

¼ teaspoon black pepper, or more to taste

6 tablespoons extra virgin olive oil

1 FOR THE SALAD: Preheat the oven to 425°F. Mist a baking sheet with nonstick oil spray.

2 Spread the acorn and butternut squash slices and onions over the prepared baking sheet and mist the veggies with oil spray. Sprinkle on the salt and pepper and place the thyme sprigs on top. Roast for 15 minutes, carefully flip, and roast for another 10 to 15 minutes. Remove from the oven and set aside to cool.

3 In a small bowl, combine the ricotta cheese and yogurt. Cover and refrigerate until ready to serve.

4 FOR THE VINAIGRETTE: In a blender or food processor, combine the shallot, beans, vinegar, mustard, salt, and pepper and pulse until pureed. With the motor running, slowly drizzle in the oil through the feed tube.

5 TO ASSEMBLE: Place the arugula and radicchio in a large bowl and lightly toss with ¼ cup of the vinaigrette. Divide the ricotta-yogurt mixture evenly among the 4 plates, flattening it out with the back of a spoon. Add the quinoa, onions, acorn squash, and butternut squash around the perimeter of each plate, followed by the salad in the center. Garnish with pepitas and serve with extra vinaigrette on the side.

Shaved Fennel, Kale, Oranges, and Feta

SERVES: 4   PREP TIME: 15 MINUTES

I love thinking *out of the bowl* when it comes to salad combinations, tossing in unique produce picks and lesser known herbs. Fennel is one of those cool items that few people experiment with, and the fronds are often discarded as waste. If you're wondering, "What the heck are fronds?" you're in for a real treat. These green feathery stalk-ends that grow out of the bulb and resemble fresh dill have the same unique licorice-like flavor as fennel with a more delicate herby flair. They're terrific for garnish—just pull it right off the stalks and use it to elevate the presentation of your finished dish.

DRESSING
makes about ¾ cup

¼ cup orange juice

¼ cup white wine vinegar

1 teaspoon Dijon mustard

2 tablespoons extra virgin olive oil

¾ teaspoon kosher salt, or more to taste

¼ teaspoon black pepper, or more to taste

SALAD
makes 11 to 12 cups

1 medium fennel bulb, thinly sliced

1 bunch kale, stemmed and thinly sliced

2 medium oranges, peeled and sectioned

¼ cup shell-off toasted pistachios

⅓ cup crumbled feta

1 **FOR THE DRESSING:** In a small bowl, whisk the orange juice, vinegar, mustard, oil, salt, and pepper until well combined. Season with additional salt and pepper if needed.

2 **FOR THE SALAD:** In a large serving bowl, toss the fennel and kale with ¼ cup of the dressing to coat. Top with the oranges, pistachios, and cheese. Serve with the remaining dressing on the side to drizzle over the top.

PER SERVING **160** CALORIES **6 g** PROTEIN **9 g** FAT (**6 g** UNSATURATED FAT, **3 g** SATURATED FAT) **10 mg** CHOLESTEROL **17 g** CARBS **5 g** FIBER **9 g** SUGAR (**9 g** NATURAL SUGAR, **0 g** ADDED SUGAR) **290 mg** SODIUM *ADD 30 CALORIES IF USING THE CHEESE; ADD 25 CALORIES FOR EACH EXTRA TABLESPOON OF DRESSING.

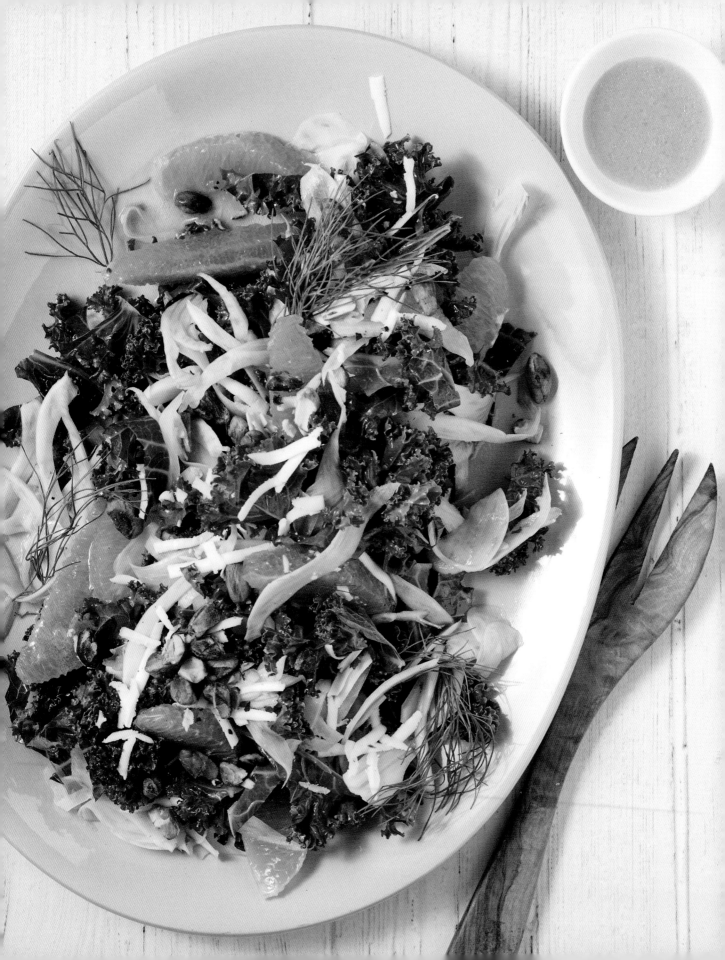

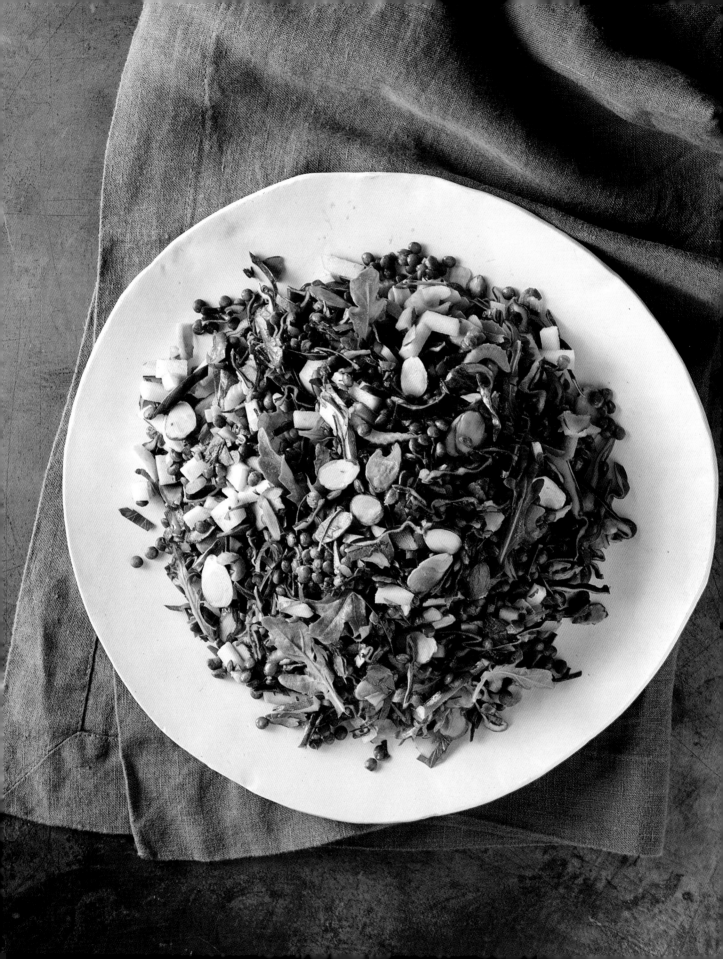

Lentil, Apple, and Purple Cabbage Salad

MAKES: 7 CUPS   PREP TIME: 5 MINUTES   COOK TIME: 20 MINUTES

Lentils are super nutritious—good for your body and the planet—yet highly underused. This scrumptious salad provides a new way to enjoy them, and I'm betting you'll be hooked. Here, I've blended the green variety with three fellow superfoods (shout out to red cabbage, apples, and almonds!) and then tossed the delicious mix in an herbaceous vinaigrette.

1 cup dry green or brown lentils, rinsed

2 to 3 sprigs fresh thyme

1¼ teaspoons kosher salt, divided, plus more to taste

2 tablespoons minced shallot

1 teaspoon honey

3 tablespoons white wine vinegar or sherry vinegar

1 teaspoon Dijon mustard

⅛ teaspoon black pepper, or more to taste

1 tablespoon minced fresh parsley

1 tablespoon minced fresh tarragon

2 tablespoons extra-virgin olive oil

2 cups shredded red/purple cabbage

2 to 3 stalks celery, diced

1 medium unpeeled Granny Smith apple, cored and diced (about 1½ cups)

¼ to ½ cup toasted sliced almonds

Arugula for garnish (optional)

1. In a large pot, bring 4 cups water to a boil. Add the lentils, thyme, and 1 teaspoon of the salt. Reduce the heat and simmer, stirring occasionally, until the lentils are tender but not mushy, 20 to 30 minutes. Drain and rinse under cold water to cool. Set aside.

2. In a small bowl, combine the shallots, honey, vinegar, mustard, the remaining ¼ teaspoon salt, the pepper, parsley, tarragon, and oil. Whisk to combine.

3. In a medium bowl, toss cooked lentils, cabbage, celery, apple, and honey-vinegar mixture. Toss in the toasted almonds and season with additional salt and pepper. You can keep the salad in a sealed container in the fridge for up to 3 days.

PER SERVING 1 CUP **170** CALORIES **7 g** PROTEIN **6 g** FAT (**6 g** UNSATURATED FAT, **0 g** SATURATED FAT) **0 mg** CHOLESTEROL **22 g** CARBS **6 g** FIBER **5 g** SUGAR (**4 g** NATURAL SUGAR, **<1 g** ADDED SUGAR) **380 mg** SODIUM

Sides, Spreads, and Dips

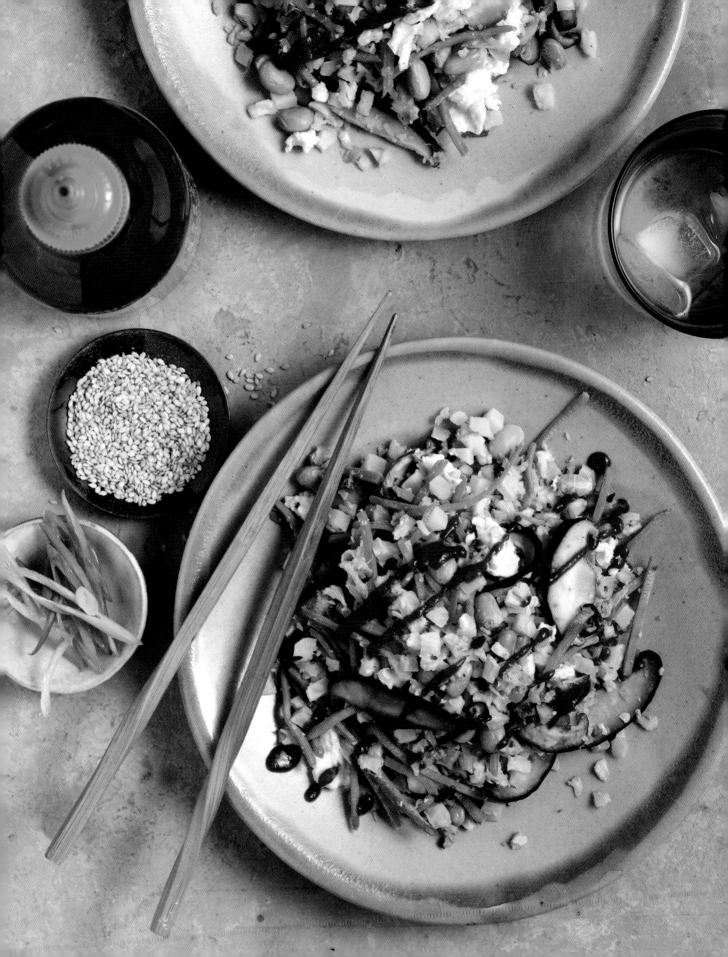

Asian Cauliflower Fried "Rice"

MAKES: 7 CUPS   PREP TIME: 15 MINUTES   COOK TIME: 15 MINUTES

I have a crush on cauliflower because of its nutrient-rich versatility. One of my favorite ways to use it is as a low-carb swap for rice. However, I found it tended to get a little mushy when I sautéed it in the skillet, so I started experimenting to see if I could find a tasty fix. The solution: roasting it in the oven. The rice maintains a firmer texture and slightly caramelizes, which enhances the flavor. Now I prep and sauté the other ingredients while the cauliflower rice is roasting, and it works beautifully. Chopsticks and sriracha are optional, but I recommend both!

5 cups raw cauliflower rice*

8 egg whites (or 1 cup liquid egg whites)

2 teaspoons toasted sesame oil

3 scallions (light and dark parts separated), thinly sliced

4 teaspoons minced fresh ginger root

3 large cloves garlic, minced (or ½ teaspoon garlic powder)

1¾ cups thinly sliced shiitake mushroom caps (from a 3½-ounce container)

1 medium carrot, grated

1 cup (8 ounces) frozen shelled edamame

½ teaspoon kosher salt, divided

½ teaspoon red pepper flakes, or more to taste

2 tablespoons reduced-sodium soy sauce

1 tablespoon rice vinegar

Sriracha for drizzling (optional)

* If you're making your own, simply add cauliflower florets to a food processor, working with small batches at a time, and gently pulse to create rice-like pieces.

1 Preheat the oven to 400°F and line 2 baking sheets with parchment paper.

2 Divide the cauliflower rice between the prepared baking sheets, mist with nonstick oil spray, and roast in the oven for 15 minutes, or until tender but not mushy. Set aside.

3 While the cauliflower cooks, mist a large skillet with nonstick oil spray and warm over medium heat. Add the egg whites and scramble them, then transfer to a plate and cover.

4 Add the oil to the hot pan and let it heat up. Add the scallions (light green and white pieces; reserving the dark green pieces) and ginger and cook for 30 to 60 seconds, until fragrant. Add the garlic and continue to cook, stirring constantly, for another 30 seconds. If the pan seems dry, add extra nonstick oil spray as needed.

5 Add the mushrooms and cook, stirring frequently, for 3 to 4 minutes, until they've softened and shrunken. Add the carrot, edamame, and ½ the salt and continue stirring for another 2 minutes, or until the carrot is tender and the edamame is heated through. Reduce the heat to the lowest setting.

6 Add the cauliflower rice to the skillet along with the dark green scallions, red pepper flakes, soy sauce, vinegar, and the remaining salt. Mix well before transferring to serving plates. Drizzle generously with sriracha, if desired.

PER SERVING 1 CUP **90** CALORIES **9 g** PROTEIN **2.5 g** FAT (**2.5 g** UNSATURATED FAT, **0 g** SATURATED FAT) **0 mg** CHOLESTEROL **10 g** CARBS **2 g** FIBER **4 g** SUGAR (**4 g** NATURAL SUGAR, **0 g** ADDED SUGAR) **350 mg** SODIUM

Twice Baked Sweet Potatoes (Savory, Sweet, Spicy)

SERVES: 4   PREP TIME: 10 MINUTES   COOK TIME: 1 HOUR AND 10 MINUTES

Most women would be less than thrilled to receive a kitchen appliance for a special occasion. Jewelry, chocolate, flowers, a romantic getaway . . . all amazing! But a juicer or blender, not so much. Me, on the other hand, I couldn't have been more elated when my husband and kids gave me a new food processor for Mother's Day. I tore the box open and started making a new recipe straightaway. I'd been mulling over a twice baked potato for a while and I christened the new gadget with these scrumptious spuds.

Sweet potatoes rock. Aside from their creamy texture and naturally sweet taste, they're loaded with goodness: potassium for blood pressure control, beta-carotene for a glowing complexion, and fiber, especially if you eat the skin. This is really a standout side, so there's no need to fuss with a complicated entrée. A simple roast chicken or fish dish, or seasoned lentils is the perfect complement. You can even pair your potato with a simple salad or steamed veggies. Truly, the spud is the star of the show. And because tastes are so varied, I've given you a base recipe for the sweet potato and three flavor options, so you can serve it up any way you want: savory, spicy, or sweet. Choose one or a combo and you're sure to satisfy all your diners.

FOR THE POTATOES

4 medium to large sweet potatoes

½ teaspoon kosher salt

⅛ teaspoon black pepper

SAVORY OPTION

1 medium shallot, finely diced

4 ounces button, baby bella, or cremini mushrooms, chopped

2 cups loosely packed baby spinach

Salt and ground black pepper

1 cup 2% reduced-fat shredded Italian five-cheese blend, divided

SWEET OPTION

4 strips cooked turkey bacon, finely chopped

½ cup pitted dried dates, chopped

½ cup toasted chopped pecans

4 teaspoons maple syrup (optional)

SPICY OPTION

½ teaspoon ground cumin

⅓ cup salsa (medium or spicy)

1 cup canned black beans, rinsed and drained

2 scallions, finely chopped, divided

1 tablespoon seeded and diced jalapeño, divided

½ cup 2% reduced-fat shredded Mexican cheese blend, divided

RECIPE CONTINUES

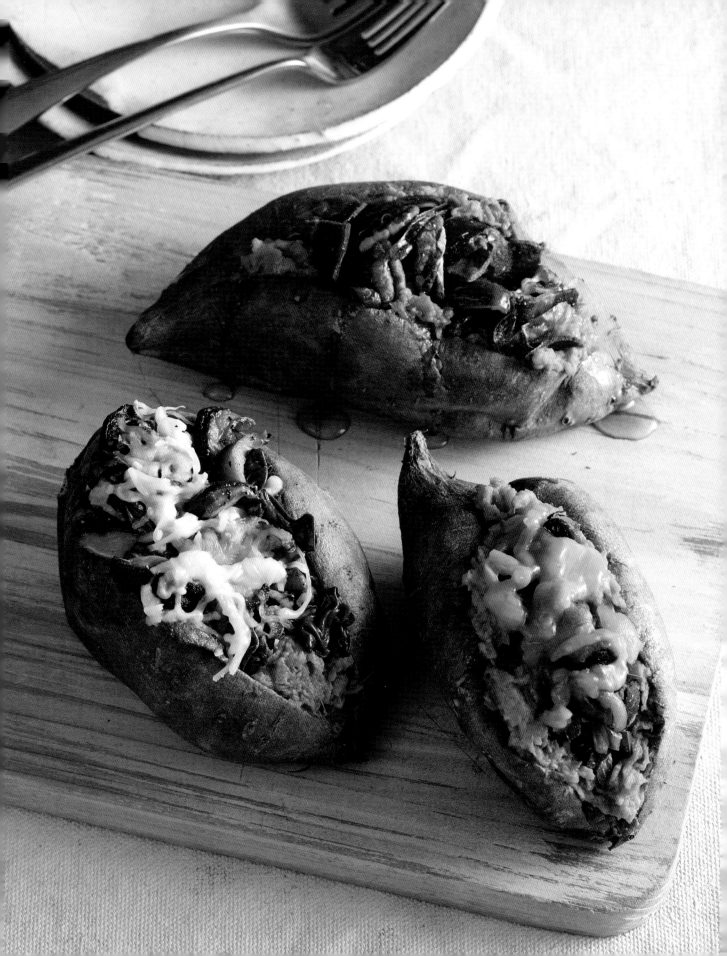

1 Preheat the oven to 400°F.

2 Pierce each sweet potato with a sharp knife a few times and place them directly on the oven rack. Place a baking sheet on the rack underneath to catch any drippings. Bake for 60 to 70 minutes, until the sweet potatoes are soft to the touch and a knife or skewer can be inserted with no resistance. Remove from the oven, along with the bottom baking sheet, and set aside to cool. Mist the baking sheet with nonstick oil spray and set aside, as you'll be using it again to warm the stuffed potatoes.

3 Once the sweet potatoes are cool enough to handle, slice off the top third and carefully scoop the flesh from the sweet potatoes (both the tops and bottoms). Be mindful to preserve the large bottom sweet potato skins, as they'll be your "bowls" for serving (you can discard—or enjoy eating—the top skin after scooping). Place all of the flesh into a food processor or blender, add the salt and pepper, and process until smooth. (If using a blender, you may need a splash of broth, milk, or water to fully whip the sweet potatoes.) Select your preferred mix-in below.

FOR *SAVORY* SWEET POTATOES: Liberally mist a medium skillet with nonstick oil spray and warm over medium-high heat. Add the shallot and cook for about 2 minutes, stirring occasionally, until it starts to become translucent. Add the mushrooms and cook for 3 to 4 minutes, until they start to soften. Add the baby spinach and stir constantly until it's wilted. Season with salt and pepper.

Fold two thirds of the cooked vegetables and ½ cup of the shredded cheese into the sweet potato puree. Divide the filling among the sweet potato skins. Top each with the reserved filling and the remaining ½ cup shredded cheese. Put on the prepared baking sheet and place back in the hot oven until the cheese is melted and the sweet potatoes are heated through, 10 to 12 minutes.

FOR *SWEET* SWEET POTATOES: In a small bowl, combine the bacon, dates, and pecans. Fold about two-thirds of the mixture into the sweet potato puree and divide among the sweet potato skins. Top with the remaining bacon-date-pecan mixture. Place on the prepared baking sheet and bake until the pecans smell fragrant and the sweet potatoes are heated through, 8 to 10 minutes. Serve drizzled with maple syrup, if desired.

FOR *SPICY* SWEET POTATOES: Add the cumin, salsa, and black beans to the sweet potato puree and stir to combine. Add two-thirds of the scallions and jalapeño. Divide the filling among the sweet potato skins and top with the remaining scallions and jalapeño. Sprinkle each sweet potato with 1 to 2 tablespoons of the cheese. Place on the prepared baking sheet and bake until the cheese is melted and the sweet potatoes are heated through, 10 to 12 minutes.

PER SERVING 1 SWEET POTATO

SAVORY 210 CALORIES 12 g PROTEIN 4.5 g FAT (1.5 g UNSATURATED FAT, 3 g SATURATED FAT) 15 mg CHOLESTEROL 31 g CARBS 5 g FIBER 7 g SUGAR (7 g NATURAL SUGAR, 0 g ADDED SUGAR) 440 mg SODIUM

SPICY 220 CALORIES 10 g PROTEIN 3.5 g FAT (1.5 g UNSATURATED FAT, 2 g SATURATED FAT) 10 mg CHOLESTEROL 39 g CARBS 8 g FIBER 7 g SUGAR (7 g NATURAL SUGAR, 0 g ADDED SUGAR) 460 mg SODIUM

SWEET 260 CALORIES 5 g PROTEIN 11 g FAT (10 g UNSATURATED FAT, 1 g SATURATED FAT) 10 mg CHOLESTEROL 39 g CARBS 6 g FIBER 15 g SUGAR (15 g NATURAL SUGAR, 0 g ADDED SUGAR) 290 mg SODIUM

Sesame-Garlic Edamame

SERVES: 3   PREP TIME: 2 MINUTES   COOK TIME: 3 MINUTES

These are *soy* good for so many different reasons. For one, the recipe takes just five minutes to make and yet it looks like a gourmet dish from a restaurant. It's a great appetizer or party plate. Second, it features nutrient-rich soybeans (aka edamame), which are a stellar source of fiber and plant-based protein. The power pair stabilizes blood sugar and helps you feel full and stay satisfied. Plus, because they're prepared in the pod, your eating pace will slow down and you'll be able to savor every tasty bite. Finally, soybeans come packaged with other good-for-you nutrients, including potassium (more than 670 mg per 1 cup shelled), calcium, and magnesium, which all enhance heart health and can also help prevent muscle cramps. And the bean benefits don't end there—they also deliver some plant-based omega-3s.

If you don't have a bag of frozen edamame in your freezer, I recommend adding it to your grocery list right now. I always keep some on hand for easy snacking. Simply steam or microwave a cup's worth, add your preferred seasonings (even just a light sprinkling of salt will do) snap them open, and pop 'em in your mouth. Or fancy it up with this four-ingredient sauce and dig in!

10 ounces edamame in the shell (frozen or fresh)

2 teaspoons toasted sesame oil

2 cloves garlic, minced

¼ to ½ teaspoon kosher salt

½ teaspoon red pepper flakes, or more to taste

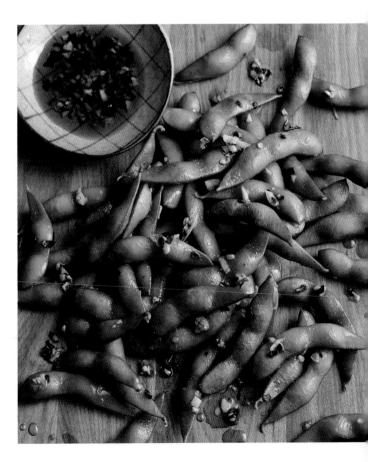

1 Steam the edamame according to the package instructions. While the edamame cooks, in a small bowl, whisk together the oil, garlic, salt, and red pepper flakes. Place the pods in a large bowl and toss with the sauce until evenly coated.

PER SERVING **155** CALORIES **10 g** PROTEIN **7 g** TOTAL FAT (**7 g** UNSATURATED FAT, **0 g** SATURATED FAT) **0 mg** CHOLESTEROL **12 g** CARBS **5 g** FIBER **1 g** SUGAR (**1 g** NATURAL SUGAR, **0 g** ADDED SUGAR) **200 mg** SODIUM

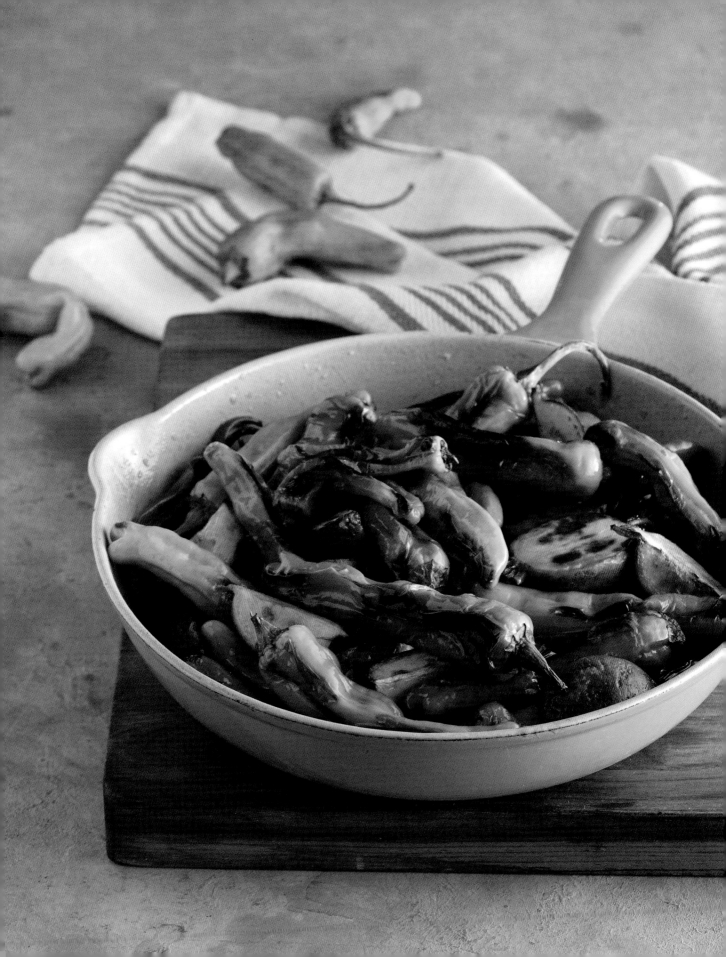

Charred Shishito Peppers and Radishes

SERVES: 4   PREP TIME: 5 MINUTES   COOK TIME: 12 MINUTES

When my husband, three kids, and I go out to eat, it's very rare that we can all agree on an appetizer to share. But when it comes to Asian food, there's always one sure thing: Blistered Shishito Peppers. When I'm able to find shishitos at the market, I prepare a version at home and let's just say they don't last very long!

If you're not familiar with shishito peppers, they're a type of pepper that's typically sweet. I say *typically* because about one in ten (or as high as one in twenty) is surprisingly hot. Part of the fun is not knowing what you're going to get. In other words, every once in a while, BOOM, you're hit with a blast of heat. The thin green skin chars up quickly, and you can eat the whole pepper, seeds and all. You can find them at most grocery stores and farmers markets.

If you don't have a large enough skillet, simply split the peppers up and make the recipe in two batches. For a fun presentation, you can leave the stems intact and use them as a handle to grab and enjoy (just don't eat the stems). I also add colorful, crunchy radishes to this dish, which contain vitamin C and compounds that may help protect against cancer.

12 ounces shishito peppers (about 30 peppers)

8 red radishes, cut in half (or quartered if they're large)

1 clove garlic, minced

¼ teaspoon kosher salt, plus more to taste

1 tablespoon lemon juice

1 Cut off the long stem from each pepper without fully removing the top. It's important to leave the stem end intact.

2 Liberally mist a large skillet with nonstick oil spray and warm over medium-high heat.

3 Add the radishes to the pan, cut-side down, and cook until they start to brown on the bottom, about 2 minutes. Push them to the outer edge of the pan and add the peppers to the middle. Mist the pan with additional oil spray if it becomes too dry. Let the peppers cook, undisturbed, in a single layer (it's okay if there's some slight overlap in the skillet), until they are browned on the bottom, about 4 minutes.

4 Reduce the heat to medium. Add the garlic and salt and toss to coat the vegetables. Continue to cook for about 5 minutes, stirring only occasionally, until they brown and blister in a few spots. Turn off the heat, squeeze on the lemon juice, and give everything a good toss. Place a cover on the skillet and let the vegetables continue to cook without the heat for 1 to 2 minutes. Remove the cover, season with salt, if desired, and serve.

PER SERVING **40** CALORIES **1 g** PROTEIN **0 g** FAT **0 mg** CHOLESTEROL **8 g** CARBS **3 g** FIBER **5 g** SUGAR (**5 g** NATURAL SUGAR, **0 g** ADDED SUGAR) **135 mg** SODIUM

Couscous Pilaf with Fresh Herbs and Feta

SERVES: 6 PREP TIME: 10 MINUTES COOK TIME: 5 MINUTES

Couscous (fun to say . . . and eat) is a small, round pasta that's made from wheat or barley. It's a staple in North African cuisines. Light and fluffy, it's prepared by steaming, boiling, or sautéing. It's tasty served with stews as well as a bazillion other recipes. Here, I use it in place of rice to create a pilaf, a Middle Eastern or Indian dish that's made with spices, veggies, or meat.

I opt for whole-wheat couscous to increase the fiber content, and I top it with a ton of yummy veggies and flavorful herbs, including fresh thyme, parsley, and dill. This sensational side comes together in a flash—it may just become one of your new weeknight favorites. Feel free to replace the couscous with cooked quinoa (to go gluten-free) or bulgur (if you're looking to try a new whole grain). If you're planning a dinner party, this pairs really well with Middle Eastern Kofta (page 194).

1¼ cups reduced-sodium vegetable or chicken broth, divided

1 tablespoon olive oil, divided

1 cup dry whole wheat couscous

¾ teaspoon kosher salt, divided

¼ teaspoon black pepper, plus more to taste

1 medium shallot, finely chopped

1 teaspoon fresh thyme leaves, finely chopped (or ¼ teaspoon dried thyme)

1 medium unpeeled zucchini, grated

½ teaspoon lemon zest

1½ cups grape or cherry tomatoes, halved

1 cup frozen peas, thawed

2 tablespoons finely chopped fresh parsley

2 tablespoons finely chopped fresh dill

1 tablespoon lemon juice

⅓ cup crumbled feta cheese

1 In a medium saucepan, bring 1 cup of the broth to a boil. Add 2 teaspoons of the oil and the couscous, stir to combine, cover immediately, and remove from heat. Allow to sit for 6 to 7 minutes, until the couscous has absorbed all the liquid. Fluff the couscous with a fork and season with ½ teaspoon of the salt and the pepper. Set aside.

2 In a large skillet, heat the remaining 1 teaspoon oil over medium-high heat. Add the shallot and thyme and cook until fragrant, about 1 minute. Add the zucchini, lemon zest, and tomatoes. Season with the remaining ¼ teaspoon salt and plenty of pepper. Cook for 2 to 3 minutes, until the vegetables start to soften but retain their color. Add the remaining ¼ cup broth and the peas and stir to heat through, 2 to 3 minutes. Remove from the heat and add the cooked couscous, parsley, dill, and lemon juice. Gently stir until well combined. Serve with the cheese on top or mixed in.

PER SERVING 1 CUP **180** CALORIES **8 g** PROTEIN **5 g** FAT (**3 g** UNSATURATED FAT, **2 g** SATURATED FAT) **10 mg** CHOLESTEROL **30 g** CARBS **6 g** FIBER **3 g** SUGAR (**3 g** NATURAL SUGAR, **0 g** ADDED SUGAR) **440 mg** SODIUM

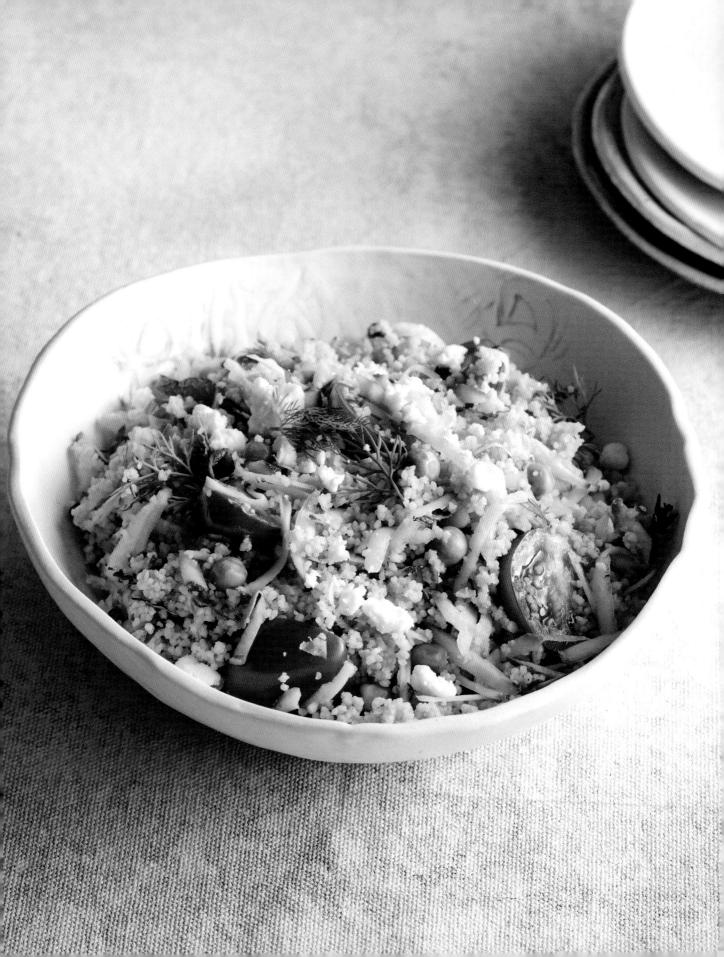

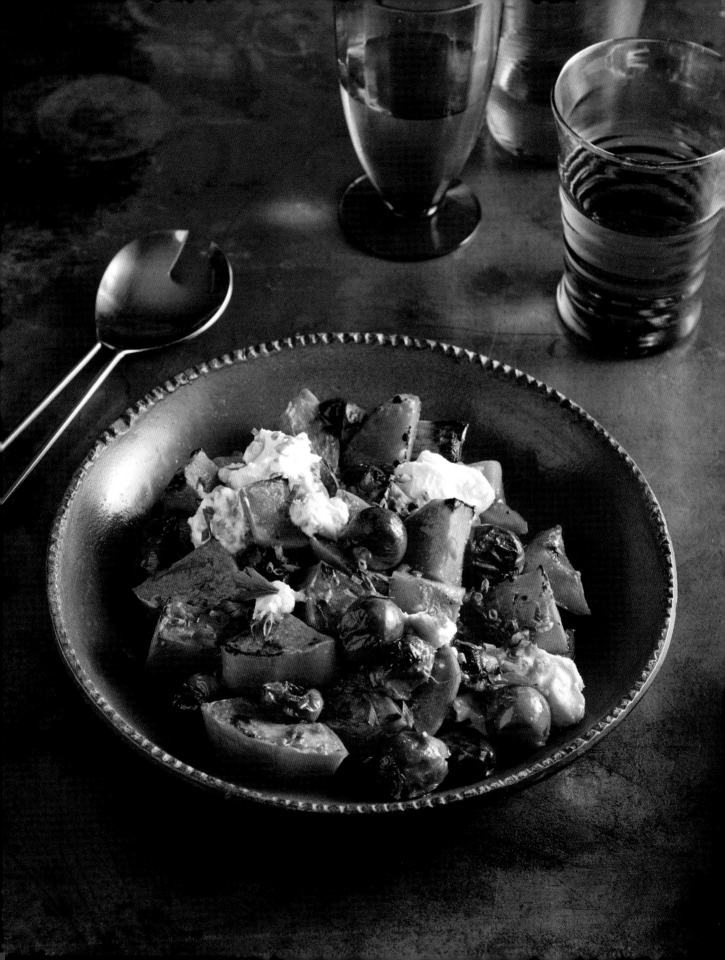

Roasted Squash with Red Grapes and Goat Cheese

SERVES: 2   PREP TIME: 10 MINUTES   COOK TIME: 45 MINUTES

This side, with five basic ingredients—including salt and pepper—is the ultimate combo of sweet and savory. It's ridiculously easy, requiring just one pan, making it ideal for busy weeknights. But it's also impressive-looking (and -tasting) enough that you can serve it for a special occasion. In other words, with minimal effort, you will look like a total pro.

You can swap in any squash variety or even sweet potatoes or yams; they're all loaded with fiber and the antioxidant beta-carotene. You can also make it your own by mixing up the cheese and herbs. For a Greek spin, use feta and mint. For a French take, use blue cheese, parsley, and tarragon. Or skip the cheese altogether and transform this into a dairy-free vegan side. It's super kid-friendly that way, too.

The squash isn't the only health-booster in this recipe. The grapes contain resveratrol, the same disease-fighting compound found in red wine. (Now that's something to toast to!) Plus, they're naturally sweet, which helps elevate the flavor of this unique combination.

You can double or triple this recipe if you're feeding a crowd or bringing this side to a party (the host will love you for it . . . just saying!).

3 cups medium to large diced seeded acorn or butternut squash*

½ teaspoon kosher salt

¼ teaspoon black pepper

1 cup red/purple seedless grapes

½ to 1 teaspoon honey

3 tablespoons goat cheese or feta cheese

1 to 2 tablespoons chopped fresh herbs, such as parsley, chives, tarragon, or mint

* *If using a whole butternut squash, remove the skin with a vegetable peeler before seeding and dicing.*

1 Preheat the oven to 450°F.

2 Mist a baking sheet with nonstick oil spray and place the squash on top in a single layer. Liberally mist the squash with additional oil spray and sprinkle the salt and pepper on top. Roast for 30 minutes, then add the grapes and honey. Stir everything together and spread it all out on the baking sheet. Return to the oven and roast for another 13 to 15 minutes, until the grapes start to pucker and burst. Remove the baking sheet from the oven and stir in the cheese, if using. Sprinkle on the fresh herbs and serve.

PER SERVING ABOUT 1¼ CUPS **90** CALORIES **2 g** PROTEIN **1.5 g** FAT (**0.5 g** UNSATURATED FAT, **1 g** SATURATED FAT) **5 mg** CHOLESTEROL **18 g** CARBS **2 g** FIBER **6 g** SUGAR (**5 g** NATURAL SUGAR, **1 g** ADDED SUGAR) **270 mg** SODIUM

Home-style Texas Baked Beans

MAKES ABOUT 5½ CUPS

PREP TIME: 15 MINUTES COOK TIME: 40 MINUTES

Sure, you can go the canned route . . . or you can whip up your own home-style baked beans—saucy, rich, and oh-so-creamy. At first glance, this recipe may look a little complicated, but it really is a simple toss and blend once you've sautéed the onions. Then pop it in the oven to get it thick, hot, and delicious.

I'm the ultimate multitasker: I often clean the kitchen and set the table while the beans are baking. Another pro-tip: I usually double the sauce recipe and store it in the fridge to use as our go-to BBQ sauce (without a drop of added sugar) for burgers, sandwiches, and roast chicken. It's nearly impossible to find store-bought BBQ sauce without added sugar, so this is a real score. My version relies on dates to lend natural sweetness and a thick, tangy flavor. And it will keep in the fridge for at least a month.

I recommend serving and enjoying this piping hot right out of the oven, but I've been known to happily gobble leftovers straight from the fridge the next day.

BARBECUE SAUCE
makes 1½ cups

- ½ cup pitted dried dates, firmly packed
- 1 (8-ounce) can no-salt-added tomato sauce
- 2 tablespoons reduced-sodium soy sauce
- 3 tablespoons balsamic vinegar
- ½ teaspoon Dijon mustard
- 2 teaspoons chili powder
- 1 tablespoon cocoa powder
- 1 teaspoon onion powder
- ½ teaspoon garlic powder
- ½ teaspoon smoked paprika

BEANS

- 1 yellow onion, finely chopped (about 1½ cups)
- ¼ teaspoon kosher salt
- 3 (15-ounce) cans pinto beans, drained and rinsed

1 FOR THE BARBECUE SAUCE: Soak the dates in boiling water for 15 minutes, then drain and add to a food processor or high-speed blender along with tomato sauce, soy sauce, vinegar, mustard, chili powder, cocoa powder, onion powder, garlic powder, and paprika. Process until smooth.

2 FOR THE BEANS: Preheat the oven to 350°F.

3 Mist a large sauté pan with nonstick oil spray and warm over medium-high heat. Add the onion and salt and cook, stirring occasionally, for 5 to 7 minutes, or until onions become soft and slightly brown. Reduce the heat to medium-low and stir in the beans, barbecue sauce, and ¼ cup water. Heat until the sauce is warm and bubbling.

4 Transfer to a baking dish, cover, and cook for 30 minutes. Serve piping hot from the oven.

PER SERVING ½ CUP **120** CALORIES **5 g** PROTEIN **0.5 g** FAT (**0.5 g** UNSATURATED FAT, **0 g** SATURATED FAT) **0 mg** CHOLESTEROL **23 g** CARBS **6 g** FIBER **7 g** SUGAR (**7 g** NATURAL SUGAR, **0 g** ADDED SUGAR) **310 mg** SODIUM

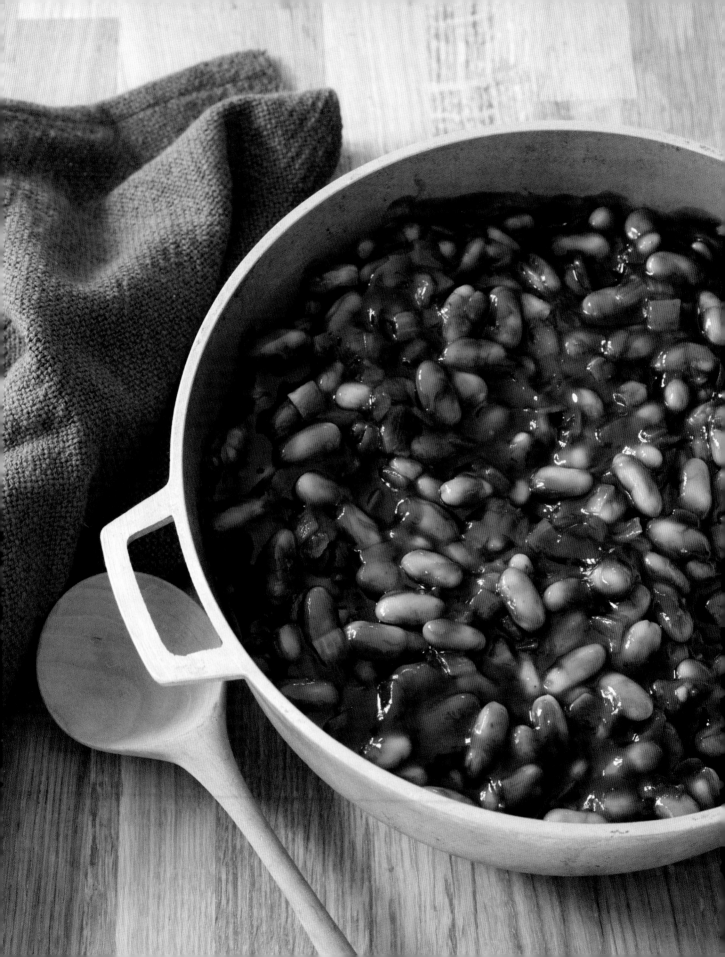

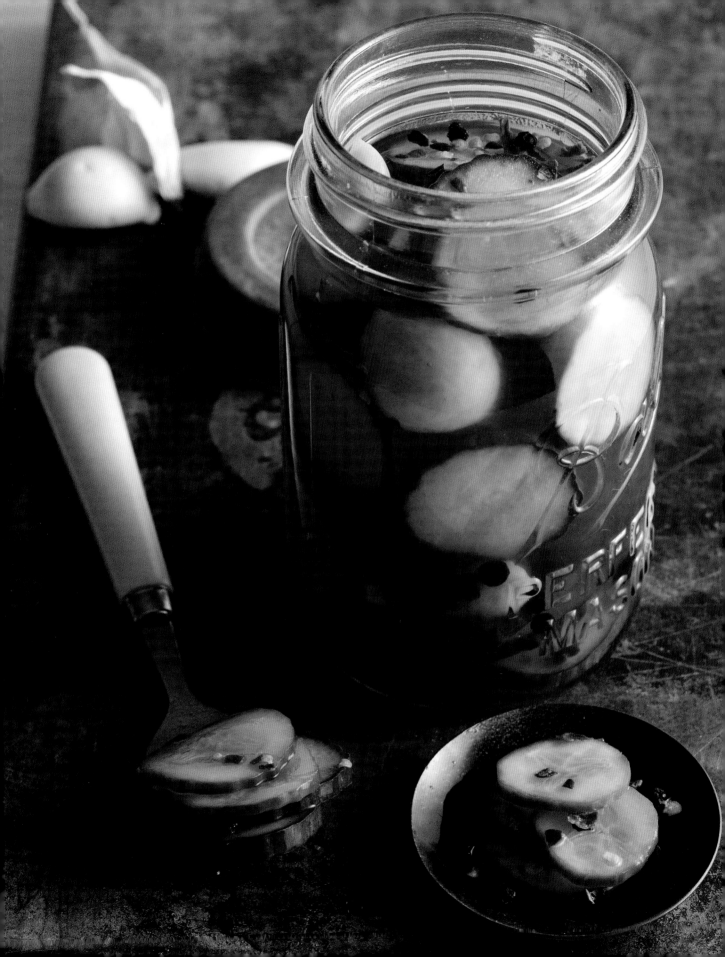

Brooklyn-style
Apple Cider Vinegar Pickles

SERVES: 4   PREP TIME: 5 MINUTES,

PLUS AT LEAST 1 HOUR IN THE REFRIGERATOR   COOK TIME: 1 MINUTE

If there were a food version of *Vogue* magazine, then apple cider vinegar would no doubt be gracing its cover. It's *that* trendy, fashionable, and popular. That's because it's super flavorful, helping lift the profile of virtually any recipe it's used in, whether it's a salad dressing, baked beans, coleslaw, or these perfect pickles. It also provides a number of health benefits, including the potential to help manage blood sugar. These pickles make a great low-carb snack or side. I personally enjoy pickles sour and extra garlicky, but feel free to experiment with different herbs or flavorings—think rosemary, dill, jalapeños . . . really, anything goes. I also include the black peppercorns and more or less red pepper flakes depending on who I'm feeding, but mix it up based on your crowd and spice rack.

1 cup apple cider vinegar

½ teaspoon kosher salt

1 teaspoon black peppercorns

1 cucumber, thinly sliced into rounds (about 2 cups)

2 to 3 cloves garlic, peeled

Dash of red pepper flakes

1 In a small pot, combine the vinegar, 1 cup water, the salt, and peppercorns. Bring to a light boil over medium heat. Place the cucumber slices into the brine mixture and stir for 1 minute.

2 Place the garlic cloves and red pepper flakes in a mason jar. Pour the cucumber slices and brine into the jar, making sure the cucumbers are fully submerged. Secure the lid and gently shake to distribute the garlic and red pepper flakes. Let cool and refrigerate for at least 1 hour (although the flavor develops over time, so I recommend letting it sit in the fridge for a few hours to overnight).

PER SERVING **10** CALORIES **1 g** PROTEIN **0 g** FAT **0 mg** CHOLESTEROL **3 g** CARBS **0 g** FIBER **1 g** SUGAR (**1 g** NATURAL SUGAR, **0 g** ADDED SUGAR) **240 mg** SODIUM

Caramelized Red Onions and Brussels Sprouts with Toasty Pecans

SERVES: 6   PREP TIME: 10 MINUTES   COOK TIME: 30 MINUTES

As much as I love to cook, I detest cleaning up. That's why I'm a huge fan of sheet pan sides. Not to mention, these types of recipes take minimal effort for huge flavor and health return.

Brussels sprouts belong to the cruciferous family, along with broccoli and cauliflower, and offer similar disease-fighting powers. Onions are considered a prebiotic, so they can help with gut health. And pecans deliver a buttery sweetness, along with phytonutrients and immune-strengthening zinc. It's truly a one-sheet wonder.

Roasting is a great way to cook vegetables, because it brings out the natural sweetness and elevates the taste of whatever you're cooking. In the case of these veggies, they become nicely browned with a delicious caramelized touch. The balsamic adds a tangy and tart sweetness. Even veggie-phobes may be won over by this dish. I always make a great big amount, because everyone wants seconds. Serve it up and watch it vanish!

2 red onions, sliced along the root into ¼-inch wedges

12 ounces Brussels sprouts, trimmed and quartered

3 tablespoons olive oil

2 tablespoons balsamic vinegar

½ teaspoon kosher salt, plus more to taste

½ teaspoon black pepper

½ cup raw pecans, roughly chopped

Chopped fresh parsley (optional)

1 Preheat the oven to 375°F.

2 In a large bowl, combine the onions and Brussels sprouts with the oil, vinegar, salt, and pepper. Gently mix with tongs to coat everything while trying to keep some of the onion wedges intact.

3 Lay everything on a large baking sheet (or 2 smaller sheets) in a single layer and roast for 20 minutes. Remove from the oven, mix the vegetables with tongs, and sprinkle the pecans over the top.

4 Increase the oven temperature to 400°F. Roast for another 10 minutes, or until the veggies are slightly charred and the pecans are toasty. Remove from the oven, season with extra salt and pepper, and garnish with parsley, if using.

PER SERVING 150 CALORIES 3 g PROTEIN 13 g FAT (11.5 g UNSATURATED FAT, 1.5 g SATURATED FAT) 0 mg CHOLESTEROL 8 g CARBS 3 g FIBER 3 g SUGAR (3 g NATURAL SUGAR, 0 g ADDED SUGAR) 170 mg SODIUM

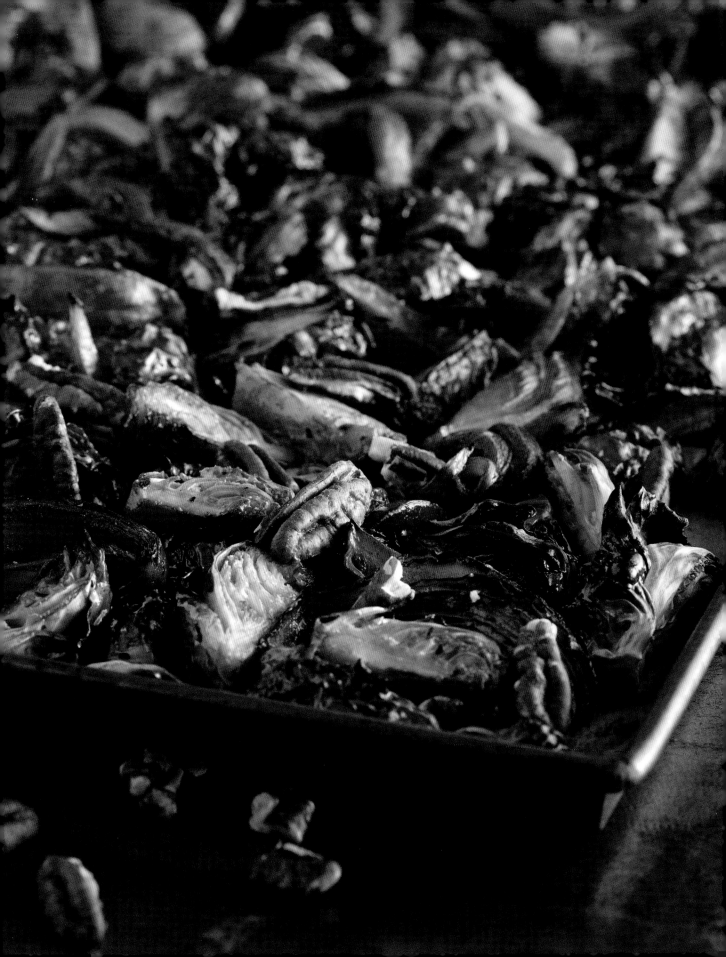

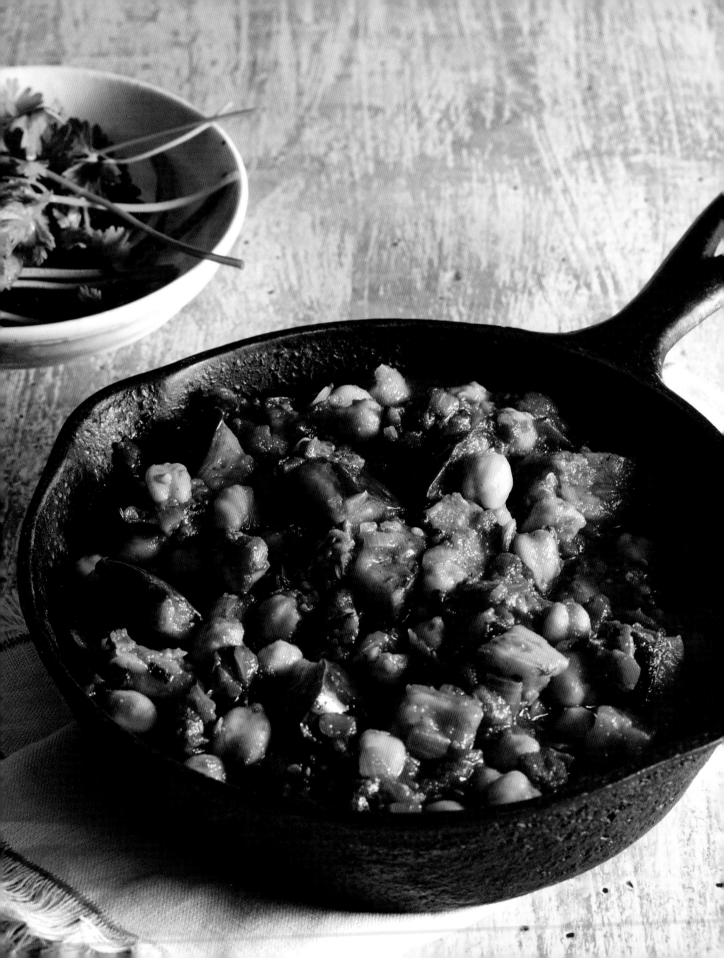

Curried Eggplant, Chickpeas, and Tomatoes

SERVES: 6   PREP TIME: 5 MINUTES   COOK TIME: 20 MINUTES

I love making Indian-inspired recipes in my kitchen because the wonderful smells linger for hours . . . long after the meal is done. Another perk: So many dishes center around plant-based foods—in this case, anthocyanin-rich eggplant, lycopene-filled tomatoes, and protein-packed chickpeas, all nutrition standouts. A note on the chickpeas: You can use dried and soak them overnight, but I typically opt for canned chickpeas in this recipe to save time. Other assets in this dish include turmeric and ginger, both of which are known for their anti-inflammatory, pain-relieving powers; onion, which research shows has prebiotic abilities and helps feed gut-benefiting probiotics; and garlic, a flavor enhancer that may also help manage blood pressure. As for the garnish, my whole house is #TeamCilantro, but I know not everyone is a fan of the polarizing herb, so if you prefer, sprinkle some parsley on top to finish it off.

If all these amazing attributes aren't enough, it's cooked in a single skillet, so the ease of prep and cleanup make this a total winner. And while it's a quick and simple side, you can easily triple (or even quadruple) up on the portion to transform it into an entrée. To me, this is true Indian-style comfort food.

1 yellow onion, finely chopped (about 2 cups)

1 large or 2 small eggplants, cut into small cubes (5 to 6 cups)

3 cloves garlic, minced (or ½ teaspoon garlic powder)

1½ teaspoons grated fresh ginger root (or ½ teaspoon ground ginger)

2 teaspoons ground cumin

1 tablespoon curry powder

1 teaspoon garam masala

2 (14-ounce) cans diced tomatoes

1 (15-ounce) can chickpeas, rinsed and drained

½ cup reduced-sodium vegetable broth

¼ teaspoon kosher salt

¼ cup minced fresh cilantro or parsley

1. Liberally mist a large skillet with nonstick oil spray and warm over medium-high heat. Add the onion and eggplant and cook for 6 minutes, or until softened and lightly browned, misting with more oil spray periodically as needed. Add the garlic and ginger and cook for about 1 minute, until aromatic. Add the cumin, curry powder, and garam masala and continue to stir for another minute, scraping the bottom of the pan to incorporate all the seasonings. Add the tomatoes, chickpeas, and broth. Bring to a gentle boil, then lower the heat and simmer for 10 to 15 minutes for the flavors to come together. Stir in the salt and garnish with the cilantro or parsley.

PER SERVING 1 HEAPING CUP **110** CALORIES **5 g** PROTEIN **1.5 g** FAT (**1.5 g** UNSATURATED FAT, **0 g** SATURATED FAT) **0 mg** CHOLESTEROL **20 g** CARBS **7 g** FIBER **7 g** SUGAR (**7 g** NATURAL SUGAR, **0 g** ADDED SUGAR) **310 mg** SODIUM

Purple Super Slaw

SERVES: 6   PREP TIME: 10 MINUTES

No cookout is complete without crunchy coleslaw. My version is a snap to make and truly allows the veggie superstars—hello, cabbage and carrots—to shine. It's sure to stand out on your spread because it's both eye-catching and mouthwatering.

I use red/purple cabbage, a cruciferous veggie that offers a trifecta of beneficial nutrients: phytochemicals, anthocyanins, and fiber. Studies show that phytochemicals found in cruciferous veggies can help protect against cancer by reducing oxidative stress. Cabbage's anthocyanins (by the way, purple grapes are rich in them, too) may help enhance memory and prevent age-related declines in cognitive function, according to research. And the veggie is high in fiber and low in calories. That means you can eat a whole lot without worrying about weight gain. A cup contains about 30 calories and 2 grams of filling fiber. While cooking purple cabbage can sometimes diminish the bright, beautiful color, raw prep, as in coleslaw, preserves its stunning hue.

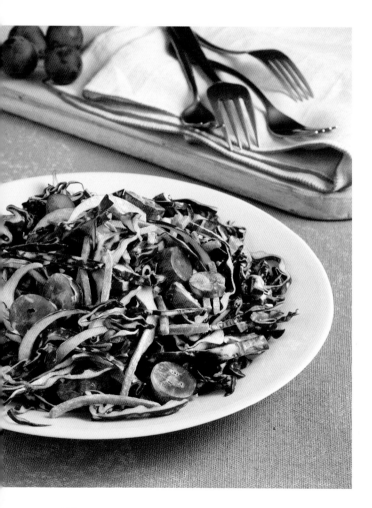

4 cups shredded purple/red cabbage

2 cups shredded carrots

¼ cup chopped red onion

1 cup sliced (into rounds) purple grapes

¼ cup low-fat mayonnaise

1 tablespoon apple cider vinegar or orange juice

1 teaspoon Dijon mustard

½ teaspoon kosher salt or coarse sea salt

Ground black pepper

1 In a large bowl, combine all the ingredients and serve.

PER SERVING 1 CUP **60** CALORIES **1 g** PROTEIN **1 g** FAT (**1 g** UNSATURATED FAT, **0 g** SATURATED FAT) **0 mg** CHOLESTEROL **13 g** CARBS **4 g** FIBER **7 g** SUGAR (**7 g** NATURAL SUGAR, **0 g** ADDED SUGAR) **300 mg** SODIUM

Kale Pesto Macaroni Salad

MAKES: 8 CUPS (WITH PLENTY OF LEFTOVER PESTO)
PREP TIME: 10 MINUTES   COOK TIME: 10 MINUTES

I decided to go green in this out-of-the-box mac salad. Here's why: kale is a leafy multivitamin, providing more than 200 percent of your daily requirement for vitamin A, and more than 100 percent for vitamin C in just one chopped cup. It also delivers two key antioxidants that promote eye health: lutein and zeaxanthin. Incorporated into a luxurious pesto tossed with whole grain macaroni, it plays double duty, by upgrading any backyard BBQ and showering your body with green goodness.

1 pound whole grain elbow macaroni

2 cloves garlic, roughly chopped

¼ cup blanched, toasted almond slivers*

¾ to 1 teaspoon kosher salt

Pinch black pepper

½ cup grated Parmesan cheese

1 tablespoon lemon juice

4 cups loosely packed baby kale leaves

1 cup loosely packed fresh basil leaves

5 tablespoons extra-virgin olive oil

*   *You may swap in pine nuts or walnuts.*

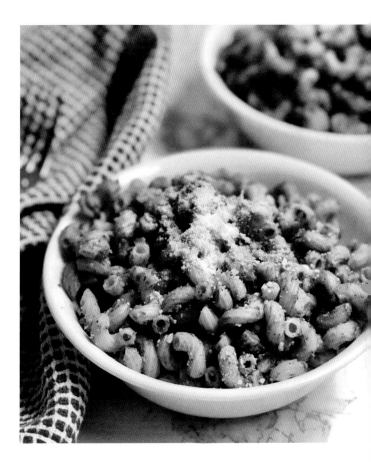

1 Cook the macaroni according to the package directions, drain, and set aside.

2 FOR THE PESTO: Place the garlic, almonds, salt, pepper, cheese, lemon juice, kale, and basil in a food processor or blender and pulse until the greens are finely chopped. Add 3 to 4 tablespoons water and scrape down the sides. Drizzle in the oil while you continue to pulse until everything is evenly blended. Toss in a small ice cube while blending to maintain a bright green color. Season with additional salt and pepper to taste.

3 Toss the pesto with cooked pasta (about 1 tablespoon pesto for 1 cup cooked macaroni). Serve chilled or at room temperature.

NOTE: You'll have plenty leftover pesto; store in a sealed jar with a thin layer of olive oil on top to prevent it from turning brown.

PER SERVING 1 CUP PESTO MACARONI 230 CALORIES 9 g PROTEIN 6.5 g FAT (5.5 g UNSATURATED FAT, 1 g SATURATED FAT) 0 mg CHOLESTEROL 40 mg CARBS 8 g FIBER 1 g SUGAR (1 g NATURAL SUGAR, 0 g ADDED SUGAR) 110 mg SODIUM

Addictive Charred Broccoli

SERVES: 3   PREP TIME: 5 MINUTES   COOK TIME: 25 MINUTES

Talk about a sure thing—this side dish is it. It's ridiculously easy to prepare and OMG delicious. Seriously, something magical happens in the oven between the combination of cook time and heat that transforms an everyday (albeit superfood) veggie into an addictive side dish worthy of seconds and thirds. My crew seriously cannot get enough. Do yourself a favor and give it a shot; you'll soon understand the drawer.

Aside from my love affair with its taste, this recipe boasts plenty of health benefits. Beloved broccoli is rich in vitamin K, which can help reduce the risk for arthritis because it protects against cartilage wear and tear. Broccoli also contains sulforaphane, to help block inflammation, and it's rich in vitamin C and fiber. Easy, tasty, and, healthy. That's a trifecta!

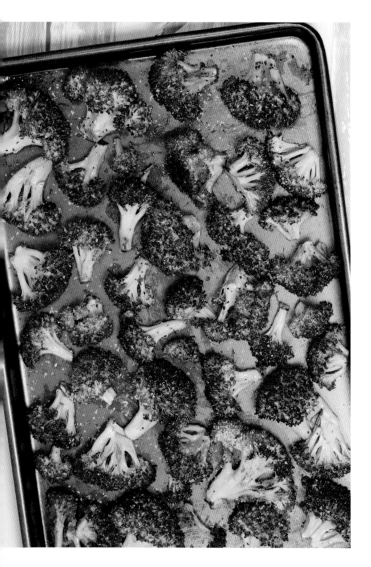

1 pound broccoli florets   **¼ teaspoon black pepper**

½ teaspoon kosher salt

1 Preheat the oven to 400°F.

2 Place the broccoli on a baking sheet in a single layer. Liberally mist the veggies with olive oil spray and sprinkle the salt and pepper evenly over the top. Feel free to add other preferred seasonings, if desired. Roast for 25 minutes, or until the tops are nicely charred and browned.

PER SERVING **40** CALORIES **5 g** PROTEIN **0.5 g** FAT (**0.5 g** UNSATURATED FAT, **0 g** SATURATED FAT) **0 mg** CHOLESTEROL **8 g** CARBS **3 g** FIBER **2 g** SUGAR (**2 g** NATURAL SUGAR, **0 g** ADDED SUGAR) **360 mg** SODIUM

Brussels Sprouts in Blankets

MAKES: 24 TO 28 PIECES   PREP TIME: 10 MINUTES   COOK TIME: 22 MINUTES

Move over, pigs in a blanket. I've given the finger food favorite a low-carb makeover using Brussels sprouts. Brussels sprouts are the bomb, boasting 4 grams each of fiber and protein per cup. Plus they deliver more than 100 percent of your daily needs for vitamin C and contain compounds that may help protect against certain types of cancers, according to some research. Let's give a well-deserved shout for sprouts!

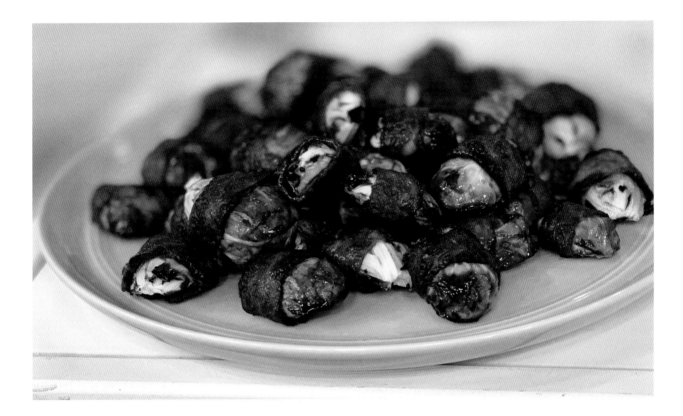

1 container (about 9 ounces) fresh Brussels sprouts, ends trimmed and cut in half lengthwise

1 tablespoon olive oil

¼ teaspoon kosher salt

⅛ teaspoon black pepper

12 to 14 strips turkey bacon, cut in half

PER SERVING 4 TO 5 PIECES **90** CALORIES **6 g** PROTEIN **7 g** TOTAL FAT (**5 g** UNSATURATED FAT, **2 g** SATURATED FAT) **20 mg** CHOLESTEROL **3 g** CARBS **1 g** FIBER **1 g** SUGAR (**1 g** NATURAL SUGAR, **0 g** ADDED SUGAR) **280 mg** SODIUM

1 Preheat the oven to 400°F.

2 In a large bowl, toss the Brussels sprouts with the oil and sprinkle on the salt and pepper. Then, one at a time, pick up each Brussels sprout and wrap it with a half slice of turkey bacon. Be sure to tuck the edges of the bacon underneath the cut side of the Brussels sprout so they stay put. Place the wrapped Brussels sprouts cut-side down on a baking sheet and bake for 22 to 25 minutes, until the bacon is crispy.

Sweet Potato Quinoa Latkes

MAKES: ABOUT 18 LATKES   PREP TIME: 5 MINUTES   COOK TIME: 10 MINUTES

During the winter holidays, I put a savory spin on potato pancakes (aka latkes) in this flourless recipe, which instead relies on cooked quinoa and one super produce pick: sweet potatoes. The orange spud is packed with beta-carotene, a plant pigment that gets converted into vitamin A, which helps boost immunity and maintain healthy vision. Plus, on the flavor front, it provides sweet creaminess to just about any recipe.

Quinoa is another welcome addition, because it's rich in protein and contains magnesium, a mineral shown to be helpful in managing migraines. Let's just say this is a pancake with perks.

Feel free to add the topping of your choice; my family likes light sour cream, Greek yogurt, or natural applesauce. Pick your fave, scoop it on, and dig in. And there's no need to enjoy these just around Hanukkah (latkes are a classic holiday food)—I make them year-round for the family. They disappear faster than I can whip them up.

1¾ cups cooked quinoa

2 cups grated sweet potato (1 to 2 sweet potatoes), grated on the largest hole and drained of excess moisture

1 small or ½ large zucchini, grated on the largest hole (about 1 cup), well drained of excess moisture

8 egg whites (or 1 cup liquid egg whites)

½ cup fresh parsley leaves, finely chopped

½ cup fresh basil leaves, finely chopped

1 teaspoon kosher salt, plus more for sprinkling on top

¼ teaspoon black pepper

OPTIONAL TOPPERS
_____

Yogurt, light sour cream, natural applesauce

1 In a large bowl, combine the cooked quinoa, sweet potato, zucchini, egg whites, parsley, basil, salt, and pepper to make a batter.

2 Liberally coat a large skillet with nonstick oil spray and warm over medium-low to medium heat. Spoon out very scant ¼-cup scoops of batter onto the skillet and cook for about 3 minutes on each side. Be sure to mist the pancake tops with oil spray between flips to prevent sticking and lightly sprinkle on additional salt over the tops of each (skip the extra salt if you're watching your sodium intake). Gently flatten the pancakes with a spatula or the back of spoon on each side as they cook. Serve with yogurt, light sour cream, natural applesauce, or any other preferred topping.

PER SERVING 1 LATKE (WITHOUT TOPPINGS) **40** CALORIES **3 g** PROTEIN **0 g** FAT **0 mg** CHOLESTEROL **7 g** CARBS **1 g** FIBER **1 g** SUGAR (**1 g** NATURAL SUGAR, **0 g** ADDED SUGAR) **135 mg** SODIUM

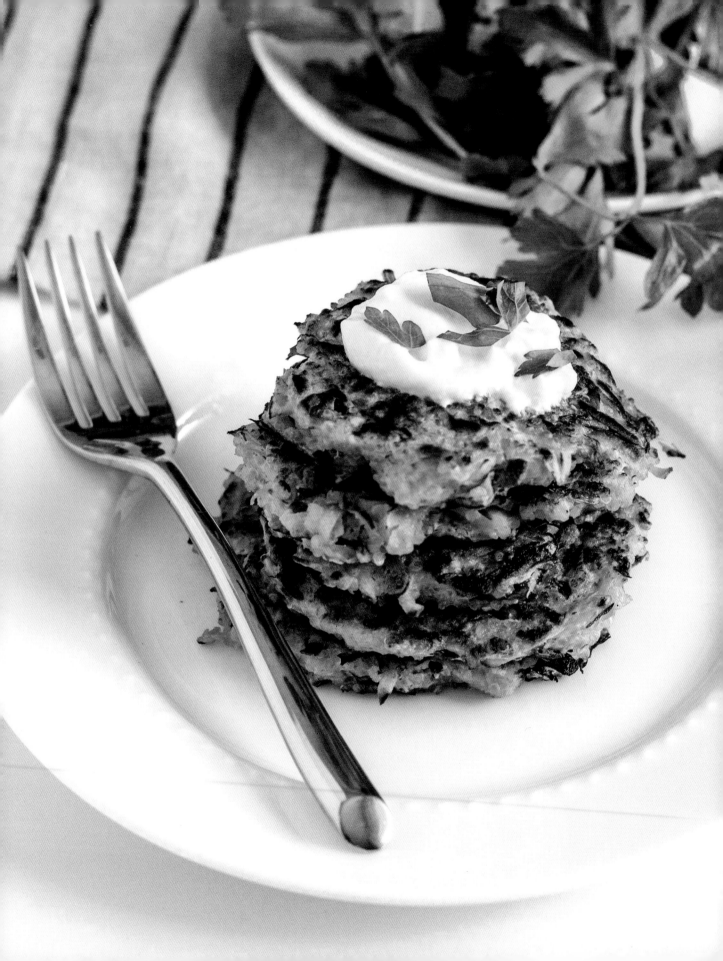

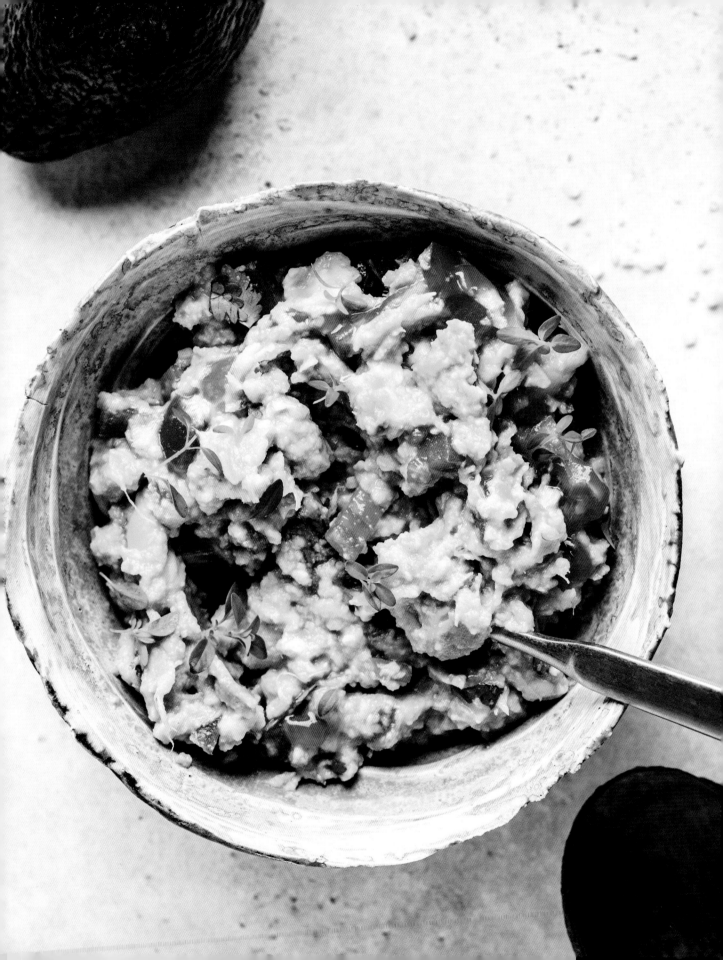

Creamy, Crave-Worthy Guacamole

MAKES: 2½ CUPS   PREP TIME: 10 MINUTES

Hosting a fiesta? This Creamy, Crave-Worthy Guacamole is a must! This is my go-to guac recipe—and, of course, everybody needs to have one to turn to in a pinch. It's like the little black dress of party planning.

No surprise here: Avocado is the star ingredient in this beloved dip. In case you needed another reason to love avocados, this green superfruit (yes, it's actually considered a fruit) is rich in fiber and heart-healthy monounsaturated fats, which help raise good cholesterol and lower bad cholesterol. It's also a great source of potassium; half an avocado has about the same amount as a banana. This power nutrient can help manage blood pressure, among other things.

If you're a hothead like me (in the kitchen, that is), go ahead and add the cayenne. If not, skip the sprinkle and enjoy the more subtle seasonings. The red onion adds flavor and color and the lime helps keep the delish dip tasting bright and looking fresh. Pro tip: If you're making this ahead of time, add a thin layer of water on top, cover tightly with a lid, and refrigerate. The water will prevent the avocado from turning brown. When you're ready to serve, dump the water out, give the guac a good stir, and start dipping.

For an adult-party spin, I sometimes make "Margarita Guacamole" by mixing in 2 tablespoons tequila and serving the guac in a margarita glass complete with a salted rim and surrounded with whole-grain tortilla chips and crunchy carrot sticks. It's a total party pleaser.

3 avocados, 2 mashed and 1 chopped

½ cup finely chopped red onion

½ cup finely chopped tomato

2 tablespoons lime juice

3 to 4 tablespoons minced fresh cilantro

1 jalapeño, seeded and finely chopped

½ teaspoon garlic powder

½ teaspoon ground cumin

¾ teaspoon kosher salt

¼ teaspoon ground cayenne (optional)

1 In a large bowl, combine the avocados, onion, tomato, lime juice, cilantro, jalapeño, garlic powder, cumin, salt, and cayenne, if using.

PER SERVING ¼ CUP **90** CALORIES **2 g** PROTEIN **8 g** FAT (**6.5 g** UNSATURATED FAT, **1.5 g** SATURATED FAT) **0 mg** CHOLESTEROL **6 g** CARBS **5 g** FIBER **1 g** SUGAR (**1 g** NATURAL SUGAR, **0 g** ADDED SUGAR) **150 mg** SODIUM

Black Bean and Basil Ratatouille

MAKES: 7 CUPS   PREP TIME: 10 MINUTES   COOK TIME: 30 MINUTES

This is a dish that looks and sounds fancy—just say "ratatouille" or "herbes de Provence" and it feels like you're in an upscale restaurant in Paris. Yet it's so simple to throw together right in your own kitchen. Plus, the ingredients are all relatively budget-friendly. In addition to the simplicity, I love the versatility. You can serve it as a side or entrée thanks to the protein-rich black beans. You can enjoy it warm or cold right from the fridge as a leftover. You can swap out the herbes de Provence for one of the suggestions below. It's also great for those looking to incorporate more plant-based meals into their diet and/or those who are trying to follow a Mediterranean-style of eating (or both).

1 large eggplant, cut into small pieces (5 to 6 cups)

1 medium yellow onion, finely diced

2 cloves garlic, minced

2 medium zucchini, cut into small pieces (about 2½ cups)

1 (15-ounce) can black beans, rinsed and drained

1 (14.5-ounce) can diced tomatoes flavored with basil, garlic, and oregano, with juice

1 teaspoon herbes de Provence*

¾ teaspoon kosher salt

¼ teaspoon black pepper

¼ cup chopped fresh basil leaves, plus more for garnish

* Or use ½ teaspoon dried thyme, ¼ teaspoon dried rosemary, and ¼ teaspoon dried marjoram

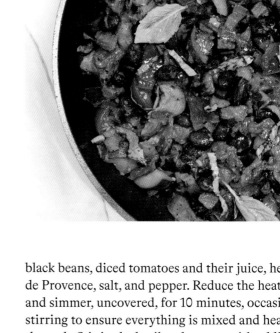

1 Mist a large skillet with nonstick oil spray and warm over medium-high heat. Add the eggplant and cook for about 5 minutes, stirring constantly, adding more oil spray as needed. Remove eggplant from the pan and set aside.

2 Mist the skillet with additional oil spray. Add the onion and cook until softened and translucent, about 5 minutes. Add the garlic and zucchini to the pan and cook, stirring occasionally, for about 6 minutes. Return the eggplant to pan and add the black beans, diced tomatoes and their juice, herbes de Provence, salt, and pepper. Reduce the heat to low and simmer, uncovered, for 10 minutes, occasionally stirring to ensure everything is mixed and heated through. Stir in the basil and season with additional salt and pepper as needed.

PER SERVING 1 CUP **80** CALORIES **5 g** PROTEIN **0 g** FAT **0 mg** CHOLESTEROL **15 g** CARBS **6 g** FIBER **4 g** SUGAR (**4 g** NATURAL SUGAR, **0 g** ADDED SUGAR) **340 mg** SODIUM

Fiery Buffalo Cucumber Boats

MAKES: 2 CUCUMBER BOATS   PREP TIME: 15 MINUTES

This crunchy concoction is filled with spice and refreshing cucumbers. Cukes are comprised of about 96 percent water, making them one of the most hydrating produce picks out there. One eye-grabbing boat offers 12 grams of protein and 4 grams of filling fiber for just 180 calories. Pack your appetite and get on board!

BUFFALO RANCH DRESSING
makes 1 cup

- ½ cup low-fat or nonfat plain Greek yogurt
- 2 tablespoons low-fat mayonnaise
- 1 tablespoon milk (any type)
- 1 tablespoon fresh lemon juice
- ¼ teaspoon kosher salt
- ¼ teaspoon black pepper
- ¾ teaspoon onion powder
- ¼ teaspoon garlic powder
- 1 tablespoon finely chopped fresh chives
- 1 tablespoon finely chopped fresh parsley
- ½ teaspoon finely chopped fresh dill (or ¼ teaspoon dried dill)
- 3 to 4 tablespoons hot sauce, or more to taste

CUCUMBER BOATS AND SALAD

- 2 large cucumbers
- ½ cup crumbled blue cheese
- ½ cup chopped tomato
- 3 scallions, sliced, plus more for garnish
- Chopped fresh parsley for garnish

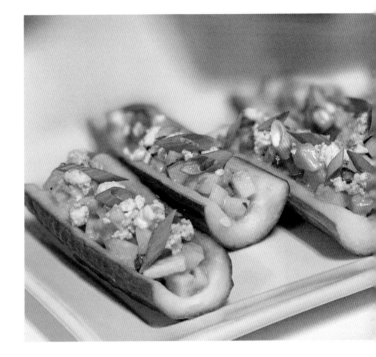

1 FOR THE DRESSING: In a medium bowl, mix all the dressing ingredients. Set aside.

2 FOR THE CUCUMBER BOATS: Cut 1 cucumber in half or in thirds lengthwise. Using a spoon, scoop out the seeds and insides and discard them.

3 FOR THE BUFFALO-CUCUMBER FILLING: Peel the second cucumber and cut it into ¼-inch cubes. You'll have 2 cups. In a medium bowl, mix the cubed cucumbers, blue cheese, scallions, and 2 to 3 tablespoons of the buffalo ranch dressing. (Save leftover dressing in an airtight container for up to 1 week.)

4 Stuff the cucumber boats with the cucumber salad and garnish with extra scallions and parsley.

PER SERVING 1 CUCUMBER BOAT **180** CALORIES **12 g** PROTEIN **10 g** TOTAL FAT (**4 g** UNSATURATED FAT, **6 g** SATURATED FAT) **25 mg** CHOLESTEROL **13 g** CARBS **4 g** FIBER **8 g** TOTAL SUGAR (**8 g** NATURAL SUGAR, **0 g** ADDED SUGAR) **460 mg** SODIUM *ADD 8 CALORIES FOR EACH EXTRA TABLESPOON OF DRESSING.

Pumpkin Seed Hummus

MAKES: 2 CUPS PREP TIME: 10 MINUTES

You're now entering hummus heaven! I'm always experimenting with different variations of the super spread that typically features chickpeas. This one centers on pumpkin seeds, which contain healthy fats and zinc, a mineral that's important for immunity, wound healing, and skin health. Of course, this is a great fall recipe, when pumpkin season is at its peak, but fortunately, pumpkin seeds, like sunflower seeds, are delicious and available year-round.

When my kids were little, we used to go pumpkin-picking every year, then gut the pumpkins and roast the seeds. Now that they're older, I take a shortcut and buy the seeds in bulk from the store. You can do either: roast your own or buy them already roasted. I like eating them with the shell on, but this recipe requires them hulled (shell off). I call for salted pumpkin seeds in the recipe, but you can buy unsalted and simply increase the kosher salt as needed. Don't have garlic cloves or looking to simplify? Throw in ¼ teaspoon garlic powder and gradually increase to taste. I like to garnish with a drizzle of EVOO and a sprinkling of smoked paprika to fancy it up. Hummus has such universal appeal, probably because it has so many wonderful uses. Obviously, it works well as a dip. But I've been known to use it as a sandwich spread, on top of a baked potato, and even on a burger with sliced avocado. Feel free to adjust the cayenne, depending on your heat preference. This will keep in the fridge for about five days.

½ cup roasted, salted shell-off pumpkin seeds, plus more for garnish (optional)

1 (15-ounce) can chickpeas, drained and rinsed

2 to 3 cloves garlic, roughly chopped

2 tablespoons lemon juice

1 teaspoon ground cumin

¼ teaspoon ground cayenne

½ teaspoon sweet paprika

2 tablespoons extra virgin olive oil, plus more for garnish (optional)

¼ teaspoon kosher salt

¼ teaspoon black pepper

Smoked paprika for garnish (optional)

1. In a food processor, combine the pumpkin seeds, chickpeas, garlic, lemon juice, cumin, cayenne, sweet paprika, oil, 3 to 4 tablespoons water, the salt, and pepper and pulse, scraping down the sides as needed, until smooth. If it is too thick, add 1 tablespoon water at a time until you reach your desired consistency.

2. Transfer to a serving bowl and garnish with an optional drizzle of olive oil, a sprinkling of smoked paprika, and toasted pumpkin seeds, if desired.

PER SERVING 2 TABLESPOONS 60 CALORIES 2 g PROTEIN 4 g FAT (3.5 g UNSATURATED FAT, 0.5 g SATURATED FAT) 0 mg CHOLESTEROL 5 g CARBS 1 g FIBER 1 g SUGAR (1 g NATURAL SUGAR, 0 g ADDED SUGAR) 70 mg SODIUM

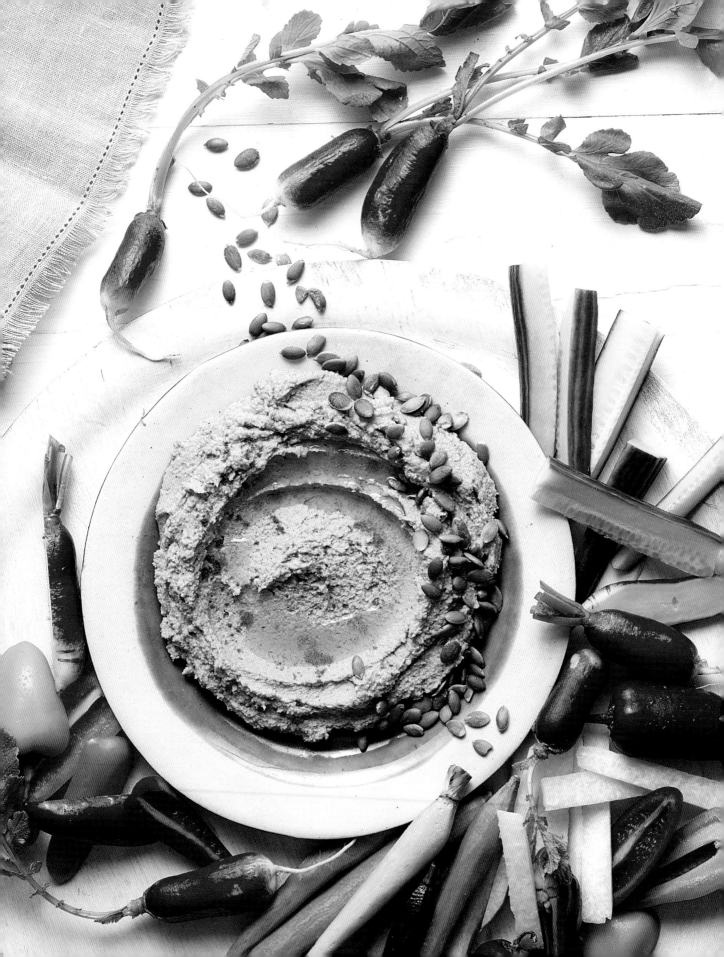

Turmeric Hummus

MAKES: 1¾ CUPS PREP TIME: 5 MINUTES

Because it takes minutes to make, this dish works in a pinch when you have unexpected guests. If you can't find fresh turmeric, use a total of 2 teaspoons ground turmeric for the recipe. In addition to its amazing flavor, you'll love the vibrant color, which makes the spread super-interesting to serve at a party. Note: Wear gloves when handling the turmeric to avoid turning your fingers yellow. (Been there. Done that!)

I love to serve this with fresh veggies, whole grain chips, my Whole Grain Naan with Super Seeds (page 52) or Flaxseed Pita Triangles (page 51).

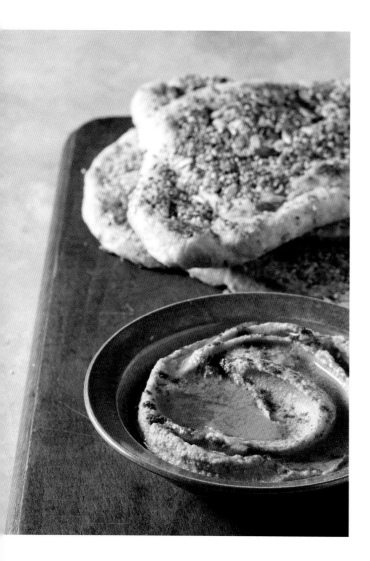

1 (15-ounce) can chickpeas, rinsed and drained

1 large clove garlic, roughly chopped

1 teaspoon finely grated fresh ginger root

1½ teaspoons finely grated fresh turmeric root*

¼ teaspoon ground turmeric

½ teaspoon ground cumin

2 tablespoons lemon juice

2 tablespoons tahini (sesame paste)

¼ teaspoon hot sauce, such as sriracha

½ teaspoon kosher salt, or more to taste

Optional garnishes: sesame seeds (or a mix of seeds), extra virgin olive oil, ground seasonings

*   *If you cannot find fresh turmeric root, you can use a total of 2 teaspoons dry turmeric powder.*

1 In a food processor, combine the chickpeas and garlic, and process. Add the ginger, fresh and ground turmeric, the cumin, lemon juice, tahini, hot sauce, and salt. With the machine running, add warm water, 1 tablespoon at a time, through the feed tube until desired consistency (I usually use 2 to 3 tablespoons total). Transfer to a serving dish and garnish with an optional drizzle of olive oil and sprinkling of ground seasonings (such as turmeric, paprika or cumin) and seeds.

To store leftovers, place in a container, cover, and store in the refrigerator for up to 10 days.

PER SERVING 2 TABLESPOONS **40** CALORIES **2 g** PROTEIN **1.5 g** FAT (**1.5 g** UNSATURATED FAT, **0 g** SATURATED FAT) **0 mg** CHOLESTEROL **4 g** CARBS **1 g** FIBER **1 g** SUGAR **105 mg** SODIUM

Tuscan White Bean and Sun-dried Tomato Baked Hummus

MAKES: 2½ CUPS   PREP TIME: 5 MINUTES   COOK TIME: 25 MINUTES

This recipe is ideal for dip devotees. It's an interesting "baked" spin on classic hummus, incorporating Tuscan flavors and nutritious ingredients, like white beans, sun-dried tomatoes, and extra virgin olive oil. For a vegan version, omit the Parm in the topping and sprinkle on the walnuts halfway through the cooking. Either way, you'll enjoy a potent punch of healthy deliciousness.

TOPPING

¼ cup walnuts

¼ cup grated Parmesan cheese

DIP

2 (15-ounce) cans cannellini beans, drained and rinsed

3 tablespoons lemon juice

½ cup sun-dried tomatoes (12 to 16 pieces)

1 tablespoon extra virgin olive oil*

2 teaspoons dried basil

4 cloves garlic, roughly chopped (or ½ teaspoon garlic powder)

1 teaspoon kosher salt

½ teaspoon black pepper

* *If your sun-dried tomatoes are packed in olive oil, add just 2 teaspoons.*

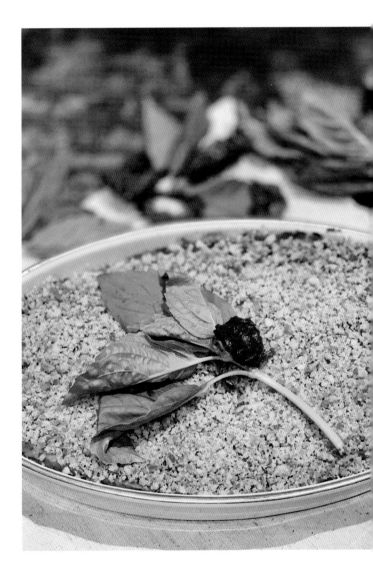

1 Preheat the oven to 350°F.

2 FOR THE TOPPING: In a food processor or high-speed blender, pulse the walnuts a few times, until you get fine crumbs. Pour into a small bowl and stir in the cheese. Set aside.

3 FOR THE DIP: In the same food processor or blender (don't bother cleaning it), combine all the dip ingredients along with 2 tablespoons water and process until smooth. Spoon the mixture into a baking dish and smooth out the top using the back of the spoon. Sprinkle the walnut-Parmesan crumbs evenly over the top and bake for 25 minutes, or until slightly golden and hot.

PER SERVING 2 TABLESPOONS **40** CALORIES **2 g** PROTEIN **1.5 g** FAT (**1.5 g** UNSATURATED FAT, **0 g** SATURATED FAT) **0 mg** CHOLESTEROL **6 g** CARBS **2 g** FIBER **0 g** SUGAR **115 mg** SODIUM

Artichoke Salsa

MAKES: 4 CUPS   PREP TIME: 10 MINUTES   COOK TIME: 5 MINUTES

I combined two stars in this recipe: salsa, a food that everyone loves, and artichoke hearts, one of the highest-fiber veggies out there. Not only are chokes one of the easiest ways to increase your fiber intake, but they're also considered a prebiotic. Prebiotics feed probiotics, which then help to create a gut filled with good bacteria. (Studies suggest a healthy gut promotes better digestion and can aid with weight management.)

Another bonus: They're easy to prepare. Whole artichokes—which are just as terrific, by the way—are a bit fussy. The hearts, on the other hand, come frozen and canned (either works in this dish) and are a breeze to use in recipes. While this serves as a flavorful salsa for dipping, I also use it to top chicken and fish recipes to enhance the flavor and elevate the presentation.

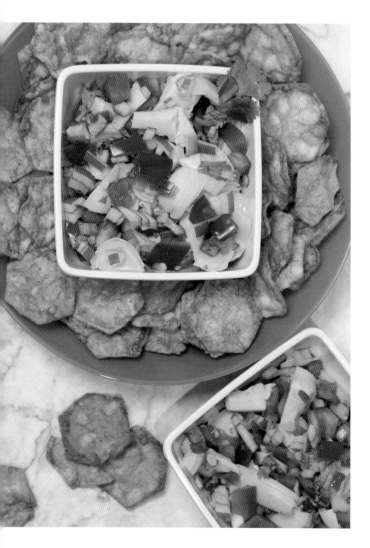

1 (14-ounce) can quartered artichoke hearts, drained, patted dry, and chopped into small pieces

1 tomato, finely chopped

½ to 1 red onion, finely diced

½ to 1 red bell pepper, finely chopped

¼ to ½ teaspoon garlic powder

1 to 2 tablespoons lime juice

½ cup minced fresh basil

¼ cup minced fresh cilantro (optional)

Salt and black pepper

1 In a large bowl, combine the artichoke hearts, tomato, onion, bell pepper, garlic powder, lime juice, basil, and cilantro, if using, and season with salt and black pepper to taste.

PER SERVING ½ CUP **20** CALORIES **1 g** PROTEIN **0 g** FAT **0 mg** CHOLESTEROL **4 g** CARBS **1 g** FIBER **1 g** SUGAR (**1 g** NATURAL SUGAR, **0 g** ADDED SUGAR) **95 mg** SODIUM

Blazin' Buffalo Chicken Dip with Crudités

MAKES: 4 CUPS   PREP TIME: 5 MINUTES   COOK TIME: MINUTES

I had the opportunity to test out this dish on some NFL players live on the *TODAY* show. Touchdown, they loved it! I now regularly get requests to make it for gatherings with family and friends. So why is it worthy of a health cookbook? I snuck in some cauliflower and amplified the protein and calcium with the addition of Greek yogurt. For ease, I use skinless rotisserie chicken, and I grab whatever hot sauce I have on hand. It's fiery good and has become a staple app at my football-watching parties.

1 cup raw cauliflower rice

2 cups cooked shredded chicken*

¾ cup nonfat or lowfat plain Greek yogurt

1 cup light sour cream

½ cup reduced-fat cream cheese, softened

2 tablespoons chopped scallions, plus more for garnish (optional)

¼ cup hot sauce

¼ cup crumbled blue cheese or 2% reduced-fat shredded Mexican cheese blend

¼ teaspoon garlic powder

¼ teaspoon onion powder

Celery sticks, carrot sticks, and whole grain pita chips for serving

*   Add more chicken for a heartier dip.

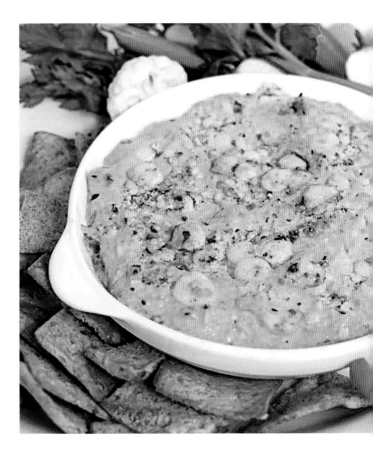

1 Preheat the oven to 350°F.

2 Microwave the cauliflower in a bowl along with a splash of water for about 6 minutes, until soft and mushy. Let cool and drain off as much water as possible by pressing down on the cooked cauliflower with a kitchen towel.

3 Add the chicken, yogurt, sour cream, cream cheese, scallions, hot sauce, blue cheese, garlic powder, and onion powder to the bowl with cauliflower and mix until well combined. Transfer the mixture into a baking dish and cook for 10 to 15 minutes, until the dip is piping hot and the cheese is slightly melted. For an extra cheesy dip, sprinkle more cheese on top and place back in the oven until it melts. Garnish with optional scallions and a drizzle of hot sauce and serve with celery sticks, carrot sticks, and whole grain chips.

PER SERVING ½ CUP **150** CALORIES **18 g** PROTEIN **4.5 g** FAT (**2.5 g** UNSATURATED FAT, **2 g** SATURATED FAT) **40 mg** CHOLES-TEROL **6 g** CARBS **0 g** FIBER **5 g** SUGAR (**5 g** NATURAL SUGAR, **0 g** ADDED SUGAR) **340 mg** SODIUM

Superfood Fries

Rosemary Chickpea Fries with
Creamy Tahini Dipping Sauce 130

Sweet Potato Steak Fries with
Smoky Paprika Dipping Sauce 132

Eggplant Parmesan Fries 135

Bacon-Cheeseburger Carrot Fries
with "Special Sauce" 136

Jicama Fries with Avocado-Lime
Dipping Sauce 139

Cheesy Crispy Zucchini Fries 140

Curried Butternut Squash Fries
with Curry-Lime Ketchup 141

Rosemary Chickpea Fries with Creamy Tahini Dipping Sauce

SERVES: 6   PREP TIME: 10 MINUTES,
PLUS AT LEAST 30 MINUTES IN THE REFRIGERATOR   COOK TIME: 30 MINUTES

This recipe offers a creative spin on fries: It's sort of like polenta, a falafel, and a French fry all in one. The chickpea flour makes them rich in protein and fiber, and they're gluten-free. A few tips to make these perfect: Don't skip the fridge step. You might be looking to save time, but chilling helps firm the batter, which allows you to easily cut into fries. Also, I like a firmer, toastier finished fry texture, but if you like softer, chewier fries, simply take them out of the oven at the 15- to 20-minute mark (and skip the flipping). You can use straight chickpea flour, as I've done here, or swap in a chickpea–fava bean mixture. And while rosemary is my preferred herb in this recipe, but you can certainly use your favorite or experiment with a combo of dried seasonings.

The creamy tahini will remind you of a yummy falafel. It's easy to make and super versatile— you can serve it with my Flaxseed Pita Triangles (page 51), crunchy crudité, or as a topper for my Turkey and Black Bean Burgers (page 181). If you avoid dairy, skip the yogurt or swap in a dairy-free alternative. Trust me, it's just as delish. Another dipping option: Dunk these fries into hummus for a double hit of chickpeas. TGI-Fryday!

FRIES

1½ cups chickpea flour

1 tablespoon chopped fresh rosemary (or 1½ teaspoons dried rosemary)

¾ to 1 teaspoon kosher salt

¼ teaspoon black pepper

CREAMY TAHINI DIP
makes 2¼ cups

1 cup tahini (sesame seed paste), mixed well

¼ cup lemon juice

1 teaspoon ground cumin

1 teaspoon garlic powder

¼ teaspoon kosher salt

¼ cup) nonfat or low-fat plain Greek yogurt

1 to 2 tablespoons chopped fresh herbs, such as parsley, dill, or basil

1 FOR THE FRIES: Mist a baking sheet with nonstick oil spray and line with parchment paper (press down so it sticks to the pan). Set aside.

2 In a medium pot, whisk the chickpea flour with 3 cups water until smooth. The batter will be very thin. Add the rosemary, salt, and pepper and cook over medium-high heat, stirring continuously and scraping the sides and bottom of the pan, until the mixture thickens to the texture of mashed potatoes, about 4 minutes.

3 Spread the batter evenly over the lined baking sheet, smoothing it to create an even layer about ½ inch thick. Place in the fridge to firm for at least 30 minutes.

4 Preheat the oven to 450°F.

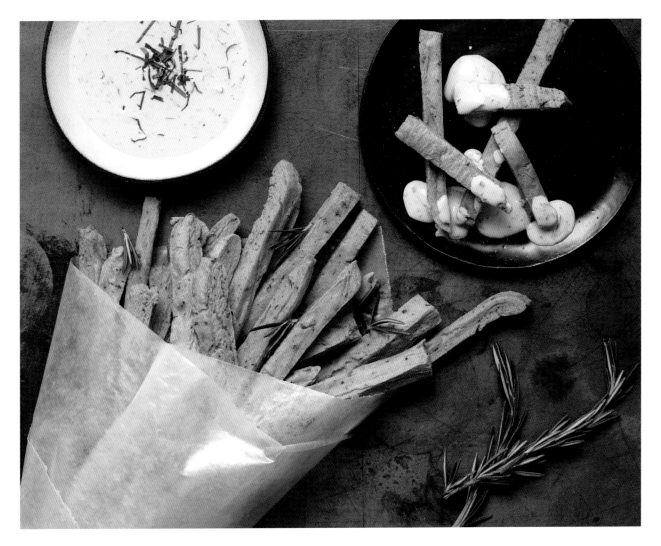

5 Remove the baking sheet from the fridge, carefully lift the parchment paper with the chickpea batter off the sheet, and place on a cutting board. Cut the chickpea layer into quarters, then slice each quarter into 10 (½-inch-wide) fry shapes to yield 40 total.

6 Mist 2 baking sheets with nonstick oil spray. Spread the fries out between the baking sheets, spacing them so they're not touching each other. Lightly mist the tops with oil spray and bake for about 20 minutes. Flip them and bake for another 5 minutes, or until toasty and golden brown.

7 FOR THE DIP: In a medium bowl, stir the tahini with the lemon juice until smooth. The sauce will immediately thicken from the acid. Slowly add ¾ cup warm water, stirring until smooth again. Add the cumin, garlic powder, salt, yogurt, and herbs and stir. Adjust with more warm water, if needed, to your desired consistency.

TO SERVE: Enjoy fries with dip on the side. The dip can be stored in the fridge in a sealed container for up to 3 weeks. Serve the fries with the dip.

PER SERVING 1 SERVING FRIES WITH 2 TABLESPOONS TAHINI DIP **180** CALORIES **8 g** PROTEIN **9 g** FAT (**8 g** UNSATURATED FAT, **1 g** SATURATED FAT) **0 mg** CHOLESTEROL **17 g** CARBS **3 g** FIBER **3 g** SUGAR (**3 g** NATURAL SUGAR, **0 g** ADDED SUGAR) **220 mg** SODIUM

Sweet Potato Steak Fries
with Smoky Paprika Dipping Sauce

SERVES: 4   PREP TIME: 20 MINUTES   COOK TIME: 45 MINUTES

You can choose to make this recipe with white potatoes (equally rich in potassium), but I'm using sweet spuds because they provide the extra bonus of beta-carotene, which can help nurture a radiant, glowing complexion and enhance your immune system. The dipping sauce requires just a few ingredients (including smoked paprika, one of my all-time favorite spices) and it delivers big on taste.

SWEET POTATO FRIES

2 large sweet potatoes (about 1 pound each)

½ teaspoon kosher salt

½ teaspoon garlic powder

½ teaspoon dried thyme

SMOKY PAPRIKA DIPPING SAUCE

¾ cup nonfat or low-fat plain yogurt (traditional, not Greek)

1½ teaspoons tomato paste

½ teaspoon mild smoked paprika

⅛ teaspoon ground cayenne

¼ teaspoon kosher salt

1 teaspoon lemon juice

1 teaspoon honey

1 **FOR THE SWEET POTATOES:** Preheat the oven to 450°F. Mist a baking sheet with oil spray and set aside.

2 Carefully prick the sweet potatoes with a fork and wrap in damp paper towels. Place them on a plate and microwave for 14 minutes, flipping halfway through. At this point, the sweet potatoes should be completely tender. Take them out and let them cool.

3 Cut the ends off of each sweet potato and slice them in half lengthwise. Then, working along the length of each sweet potato half, cut 4 more even wedges. You will have 16 pieces total. Spread the sweet potatoes on the prepared baking sheet in a single layer, liberally mist the tops with oil spray, and sprinkle on the salt, garlic powder, and thyme. Carefully (as they're already cooked and slightly fragile, so you don't want them to fall apart) toss the sweet potatoes around on the sheet to incorporate any loose seasonings. Roast for 30 to 35 minutes, gently flipping halfway through.

4 **FOR THE SMOKY PAPRIKA DIPPING SAUCE:** In a small bowl, stir together all the dipping sauce ingredients until everything is smooth and well combined.

PER SERVING 4 WEDGES WITH 3 TABLESPOONS DIP **160** CALORIES **5 g** PROTEIN **1 g** FAT (**1 g** UNSATURATED FAT, **0 g** SATURATED FAT) **5 mg** CHOLESTEROL **34 g** CARBS **5 g** FIBER **14 g** SUGAR (**13 g** NATURAL SUGAR, **1 g** ADDED SUGAR) **440 mg** SODIUM

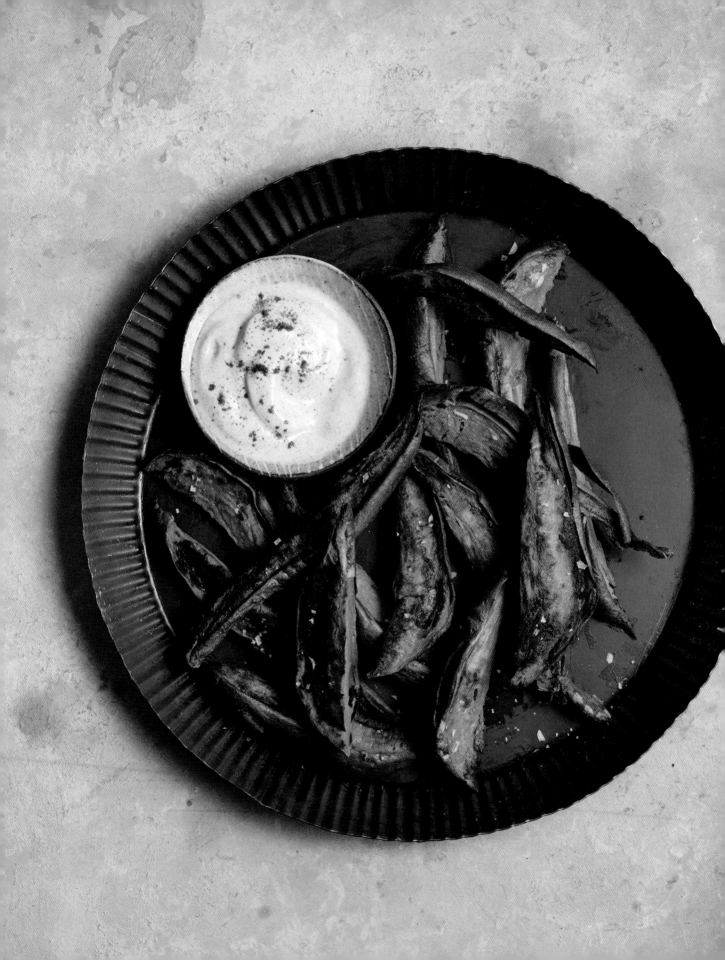

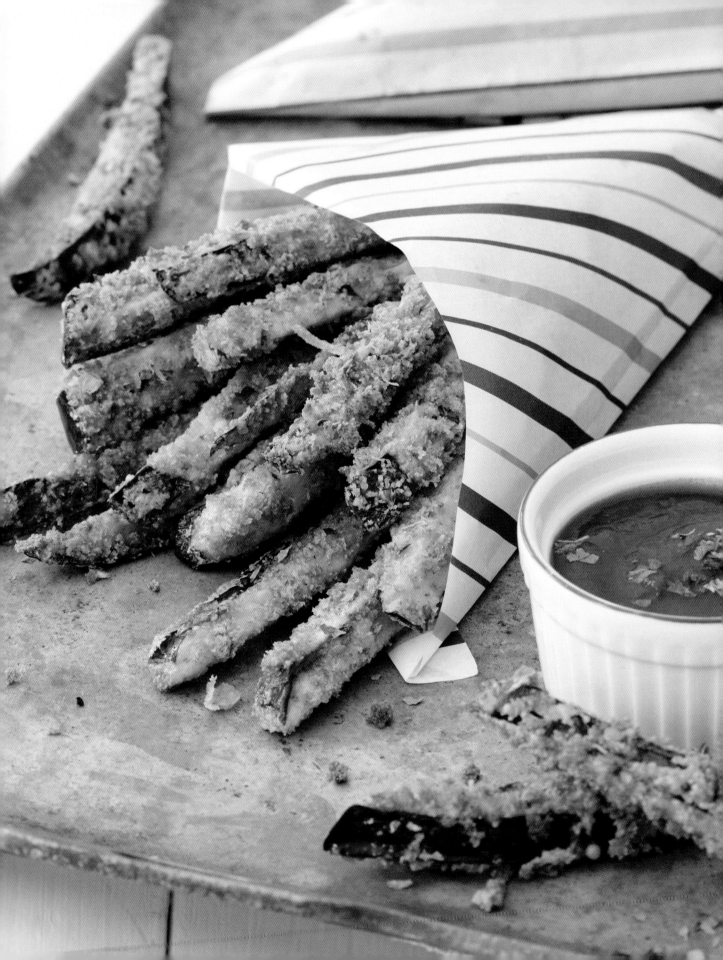

Eggplant Parmesan Fries

SERVES: 6   PREP TIME: 5 MINUTES   COOK TIME: 15 MINUTES

Eggplant makes a fantastic potato replacement for French fries. It breads up easily and softens quickly in the oven. The result: The fries become super crispy on the outside and melt-in-your-mouth soft on the inside. Plus, eggplant is high in fiber and contains beneficial anthocyanins, pigments with antioxidant effects that are responsible for their vibrant hue. One Parmesan-rich serving provides an impressive 12 grams of protein for only 140 calories. Oh, and they're extra finger-licking-good dipped into warm marinara sauce. Follow my lead.

1 medium eggplant

3 large egg whites

1 cup grated Parmesan cheese

½ cup panko bread-crumbs, preferably whole grain*

2 teaspoons garlic powder

2 teaspoons onion powder

2 teaspoons dried oregano

¾ teaspoon kosher salt

½ teaspoon black pepper

Marinara sauce, store-bought or homemade for dipping (optional)

*   *For a lower-carb and gluten-free rendition, swap in almond flour.*

1 Set an oven rack to the top position and preheat the oven to 420°F. Liberally mist 2 baking sheets with nonstick oil spray. Set aside.

2 Cut off both ends of the eggplant, slice in half lengthwise, and cut the entire vegetable into fry-shape sticks that are ¼ to ½ inch thick and about 3 inches long.

3 Place the egg whites in a shallow bowl and whisk. In a separate wide, shallow bowl, combine the cheese, panko, garlic powder, onion powder, oregano, salt, and pepper. Remove half of the mixture to another bowl and use it to refill the breadcrumb bowl as needed; this will help to keep it fresh and dry.

4 One at a time, dunk the eggplant slices in the egg white and then submerge them into the bowl with the breadcrumb topping, pressing to make sure it adheres on all sides. As you finish each fry, place them on the prepared baking sheets, leaving space between each one.

5 Bake for 15 to 20 minutes, until browned and crispy. Use a wide spatula and scrape the bottom of the pan while removing the fries to ensure the coating stays intact. Serve with warm marinara sauce for dunking, if desired.

PER SERVING **140** CALORIES **12 g** PROTEIN **6 g** FAT (**2 g** UNSATURATED FAT, **4 g** SATURATED FAT) **20 mg** CHOLESTEROL **12 g** CARBS **3 g** FIBER **3 g** SUGAR (**3 g** NATURAL SUGAR, **0 g** ADDED SUGAR) **580 mg** SODIUM

Bacon-Cheeseburger Carrot Fries with "Special Sauce"

SERVES: 4   PREP TIME: 10 MINUTES   COOK TIME: 40 MINUTES

These carrot fries are outrageously addictive—truth be told, the first time I made them, Ian and I polished off the entire platter! We devour it two ways: either as a large meaty-cheesy scoop of loaded fries right off the baking sheet, or as a generous mound on a toasted whole grain bun for the full bacon-cheeseburger experience. Either way, it's a win-win.

SPECIAL SAUCE

¼ cup ketchup*

¼ cup low-fat mayonnaise

* *For a spicy sauce, mix 2 tablespoons sriracha with 2 tablespoons of the ketchup.*

FRIES

1 pound carrots (regular or baby), sliced into thin sticks (the thinner they are, the better they will crisp up)

¼ teaspoon kosher salt

BURGERS AND TOPPINGS

8 ounces ground turkey (90 to 93% lean)

1 teaspoon garlic powder

1 teaspoon onion powder

¼ teaspoon kosher salt

¼ teaspoon black pepper

3 strips turkey bacon, cooked and crumbled

¾ cup shredded 2% reduced-fat mild or sharp cheddar cheese

8 pickle chips

OPTIONS FOR SERVING

½ tomato, sliced

½ red onion, thinly sliced

4 whole grain buns, split and toasted

1   FOR THE SAUCE: In a small bowl, combine the ketchup and mayonnaise and set aside.

2   FOR THE FRIES: Preheat the oven to 425°F.

3   Lay the carrots on a baking sheet in a single layer. Liberally coat with nonstick oil spray and sprinkle on the salt. Roast for about 25 minutes, until some of the edges start to burn. Switch on the broiler and finish the fries for 1 to 2 minutes to further crisp them up, watching closely to make sure they don't become overly burnt. (If your carrots don't crisp, this dish is still delicious.)

4   FOR THE BURGER TOPPING: Mist a large skillet with nonstick oil spray. Add the ground turkey, garlic powder, onion powder, salt, and a pinch of black pepper. Cook over medium-high heat, breaking the turkey apart into small crumbles, until it's cooked through and slightly browned. Transfer to a bowl and cover to keep warm.

5   Remove the fries from the oven and top with the crumbled turkey and bacon. Sprinkle the cheese over the top. Place back in the broiler for about 3 minutes, until the cheese is melted, watching closely so it doesn't burn.

6   Remove the fries from the oven, place the pickle chips on top, and garnish with the tomatoes and red onion, if desired. Pipe on the special sauce. Using a spatula, serve on plates or place the loaded fries on toasted buns.

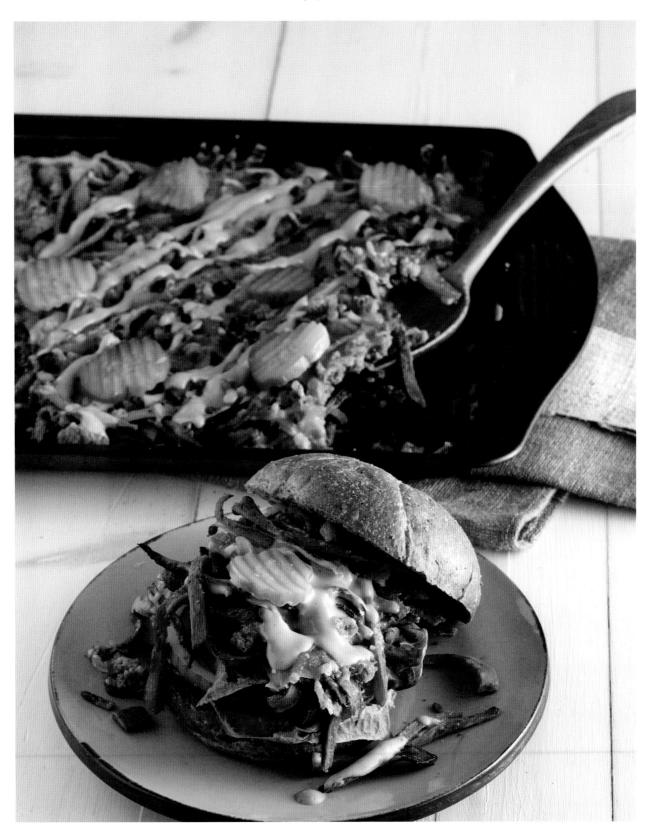

PER SERVING **200** CALORIES **24 g** PROTEIN **7 g** FAT (**4.5 g** UNSATURATED FAT, **2.5 g** SATURATED FAT) **60 mg** CHOLESTEROL **13 g** CARBS **3 g** FIBER **6 g** SUGAR (**6 g** NATURAL SUGAR, **0 g** ADDED SUGAR) **650 mg** SODIUM *ADD 30 CALORIES FOR EACH TABLESPOON OF SPECIAL SAUCE

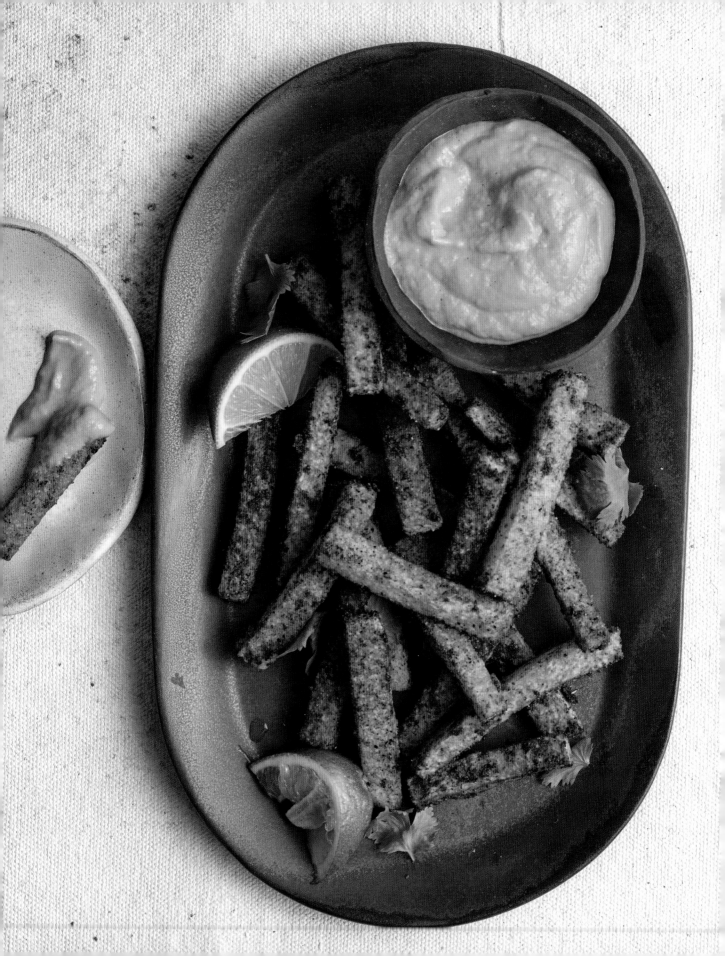

Jicama Fries with Avocado-Lime Dipping Sauce

SERVES: 4   PREP TIME: 10 MINUTES   COOK TIME: 20 MINUTES

Jicama, a root vegetable, brings a natural sweetness to this fry recipe. If you've never tried it before, jicama (pronounced *hick-ama*) has a crisp texture and slightly nutty flavor. It tastes almost like an apple and a potato had a baby.

Jicama is a great source of filling fiber; one serving of these fries provides 9 grams (that's more than one-third of your daily requirement). It also delivers potassium, which helps manage blood pressure and banish bloat. You can serve jicama fries either raw (sliced into fry-like sticks and drizzled with fresh lime juice and a dash of cayenne) or seasoned with flavorful spices and roasted in the oven, as I do here. This version is simply scrumptious and will have you rooting for this root vegetable.

FRIES

1 jicama, skin removed and cut into fry-like pieces (thinner fries will crisp up better)

1 tablespoon olive oil

1 teaspoon smoked paprika

1½ teaspoons garlic powder

1 teaspoon ancho chile powder

1½ teaspoons onion powder

¾ teaspoon kosher salt, plus more to taste

¼ teaspoon black pepper, plus more to taste

1 teaspoon lime zest

1 tablespoon finely chopped fresh cilantro

AVOCADO-LIME DIPPING SAUCE
makes about ¾ cup

1 medium avocado

½ cup roughly chopped fresh cilantro

1 to 2 scallions, roughly chopped

2 tablespoons lime juice

1 tablespoon chopped jalapeño (optional)

½ teaspoon ground cumin

½ teaspoon kosher salt, or more to taste

Ground black pepper

1. **FOR THE FRIES:** Preheat the oven to 425°F. Liberally mist a large baking sheet (or 2 standard-size sheets) with nonstick oil spray and set aside.

2. Place the jicama in a large bowl and toss with the oil. In a small bowl, mix the smoked paprika, garlic powder, ancho chile powder, onion powder, salt, and pepper. Toss with the jicama until the slices are well coated.

3. Spread the fries on the prepared baking sheet in a single layer. Do not overcrowd or overlap or they will not crisp as well. Bake for 20 to 25 minutes, until lightly browned and crisp. Season with extra salt and pepper, if desired.

4. **FOR THE DIPPING SAUCE:** In a food processor or blender, combine the avocado, cilantro, scallion, lime juice, jalapeño, if desired, cumin, salt, and pepper. Process until smooth, scraping the sides and adding 1 to 2 tablespoons water if needed to reach your desired consistency.

TO SERVE: Toss the fries with the lime zest, garnish with cilantro, and serve with dipping sauce.

PER SERVING 110 CALORIES 2 g PROTEIN 4 g FAT (4 g UNSATURATED FAT, 0 g SATURATED FAT) 0 mg CHOLESTEROL 17 g CARBS 9 g FIBER 3 g SUGAR (3 g NATURAL SUGAR, 0 g ADDED SUGAR) 390 mg SODIUM *ADD 25 CALORIES PER TABLESPOON OF DIPPING

Cheesy Crispy Zucchini Fries

SERVES: 5   PREP TIME: 15 MINUTES   COOK TIME: 20 MINUTES

Zucchini makes for a great "fry" foundation. It's sturdy and neutral tasting and, of course, is a fan favorite in fried form. In my oven-roasted rendition, I use a gluten-free breading—a combo of Parm, almond flour, and tasty seasonings that you probably already have in your spice rack. A prep pointer: Use one hand to dunk the fries in the egg and the other hand to cover the fries in the Parm-almond mixture. This helps keep the egg clean (no clumping from the breading) and easier to work with. If you're watching your sodium intake, halve the salt in the breading or omit it completely.

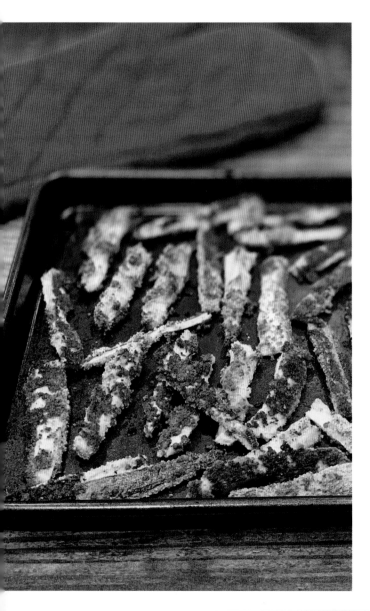

3 small or 2 medium unpeeled zucchini, sliced into fries*

2 large egg whites

¾ cup grated Parmesan cheese

½ cup blanched almond flour

½ teaspoon onion powder

½ teaspoon garlic powder

¼ teaspoon kosher salt

⅛ teaspoon black pepper

*   Slice each zucchini in half horizontally, then slice the halves lengthwise and cut into ¼-inch-thick sticks.

1   Set an oven rack to the middle position and preheat the oven to 450°F. Liberally mist 2 baking sheets with nonstick oil spray.

2   In a shallow bowl, whisk the egg whites. In a separate shallow, wide bowl, combine the cheese, almond flour, onion powder, garlic powder, salt, and pepper.

3   Pat the zucchini dry (this is very important, to ensure that everything adheres). One at a time, dunk the zucchini fries into the egg whites, then press in the cheese mixture to coat all sides. Place "fries" on the baking sheet in a single layer without touching.

4   Bake for 15 minutes, flip (use a spatula to scrape the bottom to keep breading intact), then bake for an additional 3 to 5 minutes.

PER SERVING 140 CALORIES 8 g PROTEIN 9 g FAT (6.5 g UNSATURATED FAT, 2.5 g SATURATED FAT) 10 mg CHOLESTEROL 7 g CARBS 2 g FIBER 2 g SUGAR (2 g NATURAL SUGAR, 0 g ADDED SUGAR) 340 mg SODIUM

Curried Butternut Squash Fries with Curry-Lime Ketchup

SERVES: 6 PREP TIME: 20 MINUTES,
PLUS AT LEAST 30 MINUTES MARINATING COOK TIME: 40 MINUTES

This recipe delivers bold and powerful flavors that are strictly for folks who appreciate the deliciousness and health benefits of Indian-inspired seasonings (my hand is raised high!). I know it can be a pain to cut up butternut squash, so if you can find precut at the store, go for it (crinkle-cut is extra fun). Serve these with my DIY Curry-Lime Ketchup: Simply mix 2 tbsp ketchup + 1 tsp curry powder + ¼ tsp lime juice—it's ridiculously good.

MARINADE AND FRIES

- 5 tablespoons canned lite coconut milk
- 3 tablespoons lime juice
- 2 tablespoons curry powder
- 1 teaspoon ground ginger
- ½ teaspoon ground cinnamon
- 1 to 1¼ pounds butternut squash, peeled and cut into ½-inch-thick sticks

BREADING

- ¾ cup panko breadcrumbs, preferably whole grain
- 3 tablespoons ground flaxseeds
- 2 teaspoons curry powder
- 1 teaspoon ground cinnamon
- 1 teaspoon kosher salt, plus more if needed
- ¼ teaspoon black pepper

1 FOR THE MARINADE: In a large bowl or zip-top bag, combine the coconut milk, lime juice, curry powder, ginger, and cinnamon. Add the squash sticks and toss to fully coat. Cover and place in the fridge for at least 30 minutes or, ideally, overnight.

2 Preheat the oven to 375°F. Line 2 baking sheets with parchment paper and set aside.

3 FOR THE BREADING: In a wide, shallow bowl, combine all the breading ingredients.

4 Remove the squash sticks from the marinade. One at a time, coat the squash with the bread-crumb seasoning (pat it on all sides to help the breading adhere) and place in a single layer on the prepared baking sheets without touching. Mist the tops with nonstick oil spray (ideally coconut oil, but any other oil spray works), sprinkle with additional salt if desired, and bake for about 50 minutes, flipping halfway through. Serve with curry-lime ketchup (see headnote for directions).

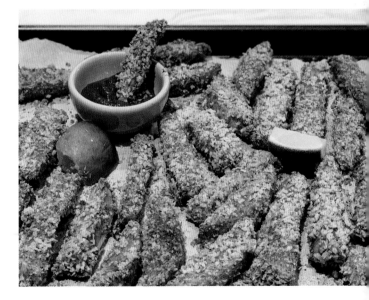

PER SERVING 120 CALORIES 4 g PROTEIN 3 g FAT (2 g UNSATURATED FAT, 1 g SATURATED FAT) 0 mg CHOLESTEROL 22 g CARBS 6 g FIBER 3 g SUGAR (3 g NATURAL SUGAR, 0 g ADDED SUGAR) 340 mg SODIUM

Superfood Pizza and Pasta

Tex-Mex BBQ Chicken Pizza
with Black Bean Crust 145

Pan Pizza with Caramelized Carrots
and Onions 146

Creamy Vegan Penne Alfredo 149

Lavash Thin Crust Salad Pizza
with Balsamic Vinaigrette 150

Spaghetti Squash Mac and Cheese
with Broccoli Breadcrumbs 151

Cauliflower Gnocchi
with Garlicky Marinara 154

No Noodle Cheesy Spinach Lasagna 156

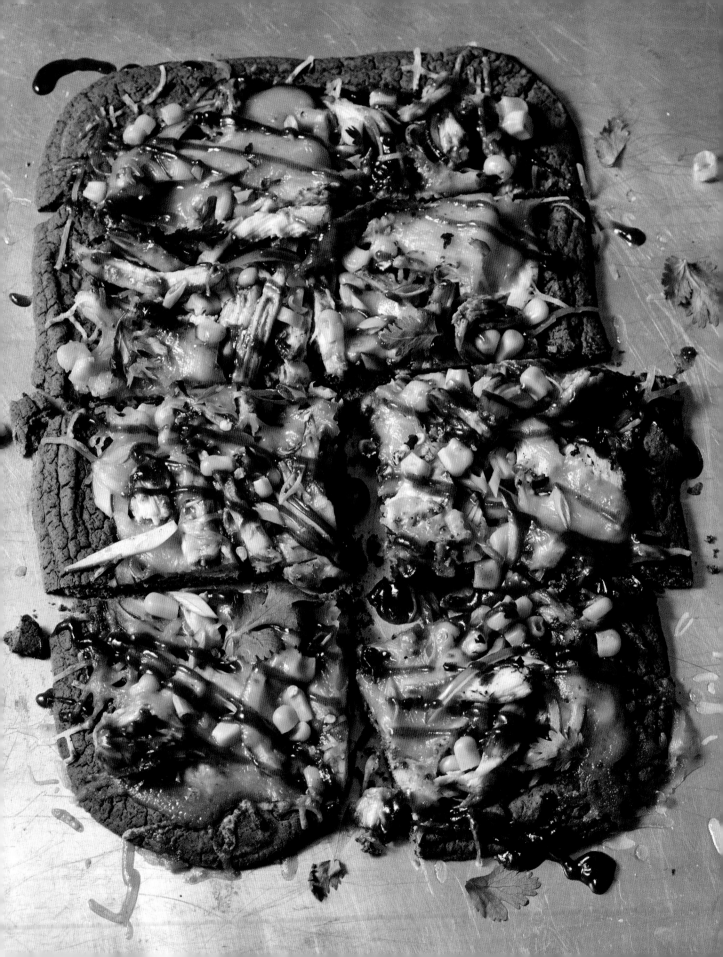

Tex-Mex BBQ Chicken Pizza with Black Bean Crust

MAKES: 18 SLICES   PREP TIME: 10 MINUTES   COOK TIME: 55 MINUTES

Having family and friends in Austin, Texas, we visit frequently, and I'm continuously inspired to make Tex-Mex creations like this one. The gluten-free black bean crust comes together easily—toss everything in the food processor, puree, and you're all set. Then lay it out on a baking sheet and pop it in the oven to crisp up. I use nutritional yeast (a deactivated type of yeast) in the crust because it provides a nice umami flavor along with protein and B vitamins. You can find it in health food stores and most major supermarkets these days. Note on toppings: I like the ones listed below, but you're the boss here, so personalize however you like.

BLACK BEAN CRUST

2 (15-ounce) cans black beans, drained and rinsed

3 tablespoons nutritional yeast

1 tablespoon garlic powder

2 teaspoons ground cumin

1 teaspoon kosher salt

4 egg whites

2 tablespoons olive oil

TOPPINGS

½ cup barbecue sauce, plus more for topping (optional)*

1 cup shredded cooked chicken breast

6 tablespoons shredded 2% reduced-fat Mexican cheese blend

½ cup corn kernels (fresh; frozen and defrosted; or canned, drained and rinsed)

¼ cup thinly sliced red onion

¼ to ½ teaspoon red pepper flakes (optional)

Fresh cilantro, parsley, or scallions for garnish (optional)

*   *Use store-bought or make your own tasty version using my recipe on page 104.*

1 Preheat the oven to 350°F. Line 2 baking sheets with parchment paper and lightly mist with oil spray. Set aside.

2 FOR THE CRUST: In a food processor or a high-speed blender, combine all the black bean crust ingredients and process until smooth, scraping down the sides halfway through to ensure all the ingredients are well incorporated. Divide the black bean puree between the prepared baking sheets (about 1½ cups per sheet) and evenly spread it out into a 10 by 7-inch rectangle, about ¼ inch thick. Bake for 15 minutes, rotate the pans, and bake for another 15 minutes. Then carefully flip the crusts and bake 15 more minutes, for a total of 45 minutes. (To flip the crusts, you'll need a second baking sheet or cutting board. Let the crusts slightly cool. Once cooled, cover each crust with a fresh additional sheet of parchment paper and top it with either another baking sheet or a cutting board and carefully flip. Then slide the parchment paper and crust back to a baking sheet and into the oven.)

3 TO ASSEMBLE THE PIZZAS: Remove the crusts from the oven and top with barbecue sauce, shredded chicken, cheese, corn, red onion, and red pepper flakes, if using. Place back in the oven and bake for 10 to 15 minutes, until the cheese is melted. Cut into squares and garnish with herbs and extra barbecue sauce, if desired.

PER SERVING 2 SLICES 170 CALORIES 15 g PROTEIN 3.5 g FAT (2 g UNSATURATED FAT, 1.5 g SATURATED FAT) 25 mg CHOLESTEROL 19 g CARBS 7 g FIBER 2 g SUGAR (2 g NATURAL SUGAR, 0 g ADDED SUGAR) 470 mg SODIU

Pan Pizza with Caramelized Carrots and Onions

MAKES: ONE 12-INCH PIZZA (8 SLICES)   PREP TIME: 10 MINUTES
COOK TIME: 1 HOUR AND 35 MINUTES

In my house, the announcement "Pizza for dinner" is usually welcomed with a chorus of "hoorays!" and "woohoos!" followed by satisfied silence as we devour whatever fun spin I've come up with. This creation features a nutrient-packed dough (the same recipe I use for my bagel bites, page 37) that's rich in protein and fiber, thanks to the Greek yogurt, whole grain flour, and chia seeds. It's thick and chewy, almost like a Sicilian slice or focaccia bread. I top it with part-skim ricotta mixed with feta for a tangy creaminess and a thick balsamic glaze, which takes this over the top. If you don't have a bottle of balsamic glaze on hand, follow the simple instructions for making your own using balsamic vinegar. The carrots and red onion are caramelized to perfection, bringing not only amazing flavor but extra nutrition to your meal.

PIZZA TOPPING

½ cup part-skim ricotta cheese

½ cup crumbled feta cheese, plus 3 tablespoons to scatter on top

¼ cup balsamic glaze*

2 tablespoons coarsely chopped fresh parsley

* *If using a standard balsamic vinegar, pour ½ cup into a small saucepan and bring to a gentle boil. Reduce the heat and simmer for 7 to 10 minutes to create a thickened balsamic glaze.*

CARAMELIZED CARROTS AND ONIONS

5 carrots, sliced in half lengthwise

1 large red onion, sliced

1 tablespoon olive oil

2 teaspoons ground cumin

¼ teaspoon kosher salt

⅛ teaspoon black pepper

¼ to ½ teaspoon red pepper flakes (optional)

PIZZA CRUST

2 cups whole wheat flour†

2 tablespoons chia seeds

1½ teaspoons kosher salt

1 tablespoon baking powder

2 cups nonfat plain Greek yogurt

† *For a slightly softer chew, use white whole wheat flour.*

1 Set an oven rack to the middle position and preheat the oven to 350°F. Line a baking sheet with parchment paper. Set aside.

2 FOR THE TOPPING: In a small bowl, mix the ricotta and feta cheeses and stash in the fridge until you're ready to assemble.

3 FOR THE CARAMELIZED CARROTS AND ONIONS: Combine the carrots and onions in a large bowl and toss with the oil. Add the cumin, salt, black pepper, and red pepper flakes, if using, and toss to coat the veggies. Place them on the baking sheet in a single layer (don't worry if there's some overlap) and bake for about 1 hour, tossing halfway through, until they're soft and caramelized. Remove from the oven and set aside. Leave the oven on.

4 FOR THE DOUGH: While the carrots are cooking, make the dough: In a large bowl, combine the flour, chia seeds, salt, and baking powder. Add the yogurt and stir until all of the flour is incorporated to make a batter. Use your hands to fold and press until the dough comes together. At first it will seem dry and piecey, but keep working it and it will soon form a dough ball (it will take about 1 to 2 minutes). If at any point it gets sticky, add a sprinkle of flour to the bowl or your hands.

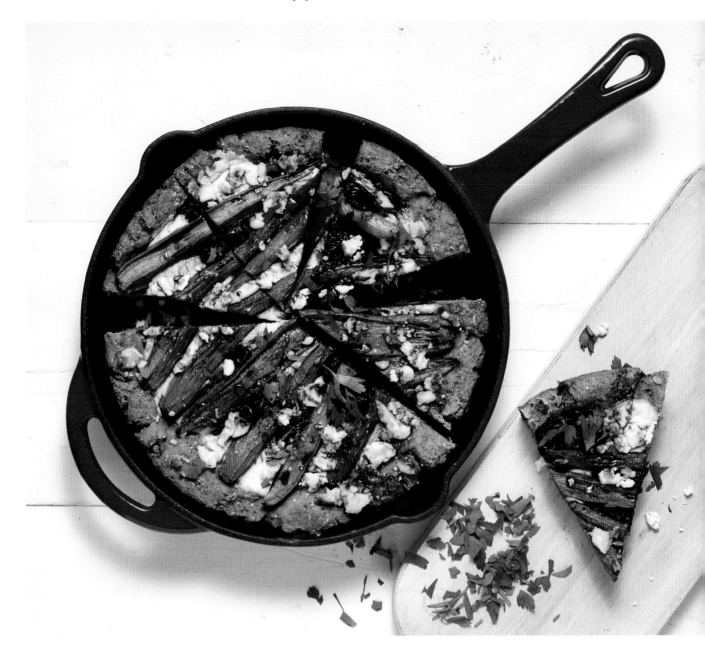

5 Liberally mist a large skillet with olive oil spray. Place the dough into the skillet and spread it out across the bottom of the pan by pressing and pushing until the entire skillet is evenly covered and the dough creeps up the sides. Spread 3 tablespoons of the cheese mixture over the dough and arrange the onions and carrots on top. Add the remaining cheese in small decorative dollops over the top and place in the oven and bake for 35 to 45 minutes, until the crust is golden brown on the edges and it has a soft and chewy consistency on the inside.

6 Remove from the oven, drizzle with the balsamic glaze, and garnish with the parsley. Cut into 8 slices while it's still in the skillet and serve family-style straight from the pan.

PER SERVING 1 SLICE 250 CALORIES 15 g PROTEIN 8 g FAT (5 g UNSATURATED FAT, 3 g SATURATED FAT) 20 mg CHOLESTEROL 34 g CARBS 6 g FIBER 6 g SUGAR (6 g NATURAL SUGAR, 0 g ADDED SUGAR) 660 mg SODIUM

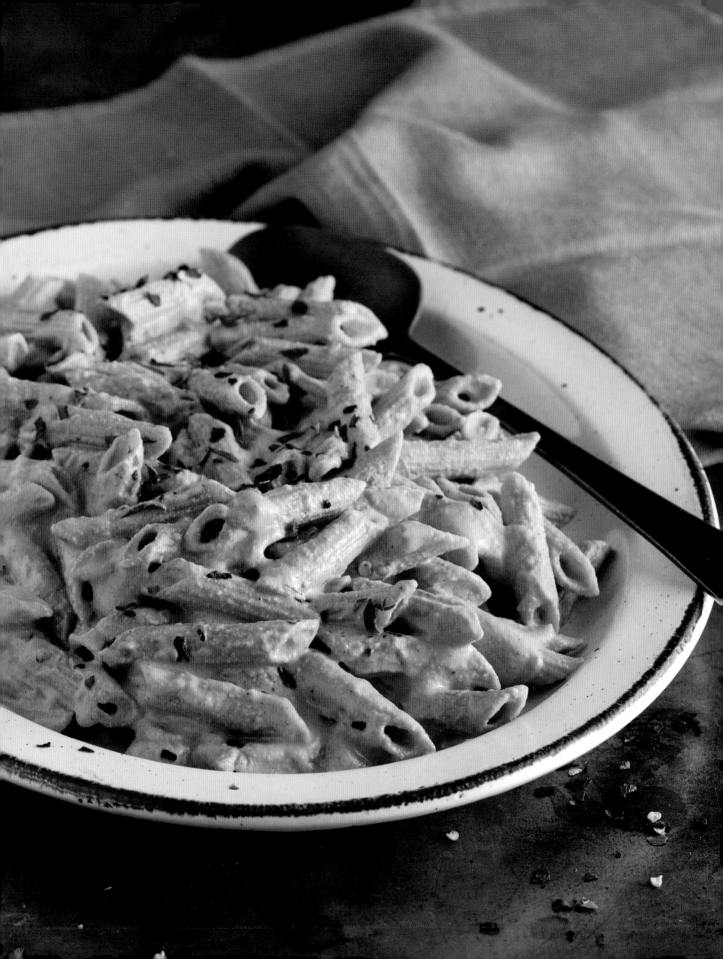

Creamy Vegan Penne Alfredo

MAKES: 8 CUPS   PREP TIME: 20 MINUTES   COOK TIME: 45 MINUTES

Here is a silky and indulgent cream sauce without any dairy. My secret: cashews! I soak the soft, buttery nuts and then toss them in the blender with roasted garlic, red peppers, and smoked paprika. OMG—it's insanely delicious. The roasted garlic adds a complex smoky, sweet flavor, but if you're short on time, you can easily substitute 2 cloves of roughly chopped fresh garlic; just toss it in the blender with the other ingredients. It will still be amazing.

1 head garlic*

1 cup raw cashews

⅓ cup jarred roasted red peppers, drained

¾ teaspoon kosher salt

¼ teaspoon black pepper

¼ teaspoon smoked paprika

1 pound whole grain pasta, cooked

Red pepper flakes for garnish (optional)

Chopped fresh parsley for garnish (optional)

* *If you're short on time, swap in 2 roughly chopped garlic cloves.*

1 Preheat the oven to 400°F.

2 Carefully cut off the top quarter of the garlic head, exposing the cloves but leaving the root end intact. Mist the cut side of the garlic with olive oil spray and loosely wrap in aluminum foil. Place the garlic directly on the oven rack and roast for 45 minutes to 1 hour, until the garlic is fragrant, golden brown, and tender. Set aside to cool, then gently squeeze out the garlic cloves and discard the papery skins. You should have about ¼ cup roasted garlic cloves.

3 While the garlic is in the oven, put the cashews in a small bowl and add boiling water. Cover the bowl and set aside for about 20 minutes to soak. Then drain.

4 In a high-speed blender or food processor, combine the drained cashews, ¾ cup boiling water, the roasted garlic cloves, roasted red peppers, salt, pepper, and smoked paprika and pulse for 30 to 60 seconds, scraping down the sides of the blender if necessary. If the sauce is too thick, add more boiling water 1 tablespoon at a time until you reach your preferred consistency. Toss the sauce with the cooked pasta and garnish with red pepper flakes and parsley, if desired.

PER SERVING 1 CUP PASTA WITH ¼ CUP SAUCE **270** CALORIES **12 g** PROTEIN **8 g** FAT (**7 g** UNSATURATED FAT, **1 g** SATURATED FAT) **0 mg** CHOLESTEROL **46 g** CARBS **6 g** FIBER **5 g** SUGAR (**5 g** NATURAL SUGAR, **0 g** ADDED SUGAR) **500 mg** SODIUM

Lavash Thin Crust Salad Pizza with Balsamic Vinaigrette

SERVES: 2   PREP TIME: 10 MINUTES   COOK TIME: 6 MINUTES

Lavash is a delicious Middle Eastern flatbread that transforms into a super-thin, cracker-like crust when toasted in the oven. Topped with a bright and savory salad, this is a fresh and flavorful treat for your taste buds. Feel free to use any other base, like a toasted whole grain tortilla or pita, and you can also swap in a favorite salad dressing. The options are endless.

DRESSING
makes ¾ cup

½ cup balsamic vinegar

3 tablespoons extra virgin olive oil

1 tablespoon Dijon mustard

1 teaspoon honey

1 teaspoon garlic powder

¼ teaspoon kosher salt

⅛ teaspoon black pepper

SALAD

3 loosely packed cups arugula

½ cucumber, sliced into half moons

½ cup artichoke hearts, quartered and sliced

½ cup grape tomatoes, halved

¼ cup pitted kalamata olives (about 10 olives), halved and patted dry

2 tablespoons toasted pine nuts

1 ounce shaved Pecorino Romano cheese (optional)

CRUST

2 whole grain lavash breads

2 to 3 teaspoons olive oil

½ to 1 teaspoon garlic powder

Kosher salt and ground black pepper (optional)

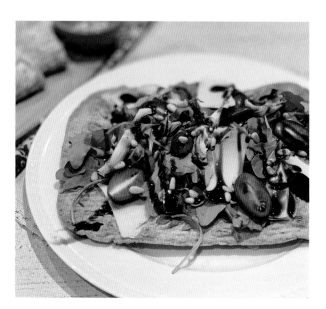

1 Preheat the oven to 400°F and mist a baking sheet with olive oil spray. Set aside.

2 FOR THE DRESSING: In a small bowl, add all of the dressing ingredients and stir until everything is well combined.

3 FOR THE SALAD: In a large bowl, combine all of the salad ingredients and gently toss with 1 to 2 tablespoons of the dressing.

4 FOR THE CRUST: Place the lavash on the prepared baking sheet. Brush each piece with oil and sprinkle with garlic powder. Bake for 6 to 8 minutes, until the lavash is crisp and browned on the edges. Cool slightly, then top with the salad and sprinkle with salt and pepper, if desired. Serve with extra dressing on the side to drizzle on top.

PER SERVING 1 PIZZA **290** CALORIES **14 g** PROTEIN **13 g** FAT (**12 g** UNSATURATED FAT, **1 g** SATURATED FAT) **0 mg** CHOLESTEROL **29 g** CARBS **8 g** FIBER **4 g** SUGAR (**4 g** NATURAL SUGAR, **0 g** ADDED SUGAR) **710 mg** SODIUM *ADD 35 CALORIES FOR EACH ADDITIONAL TABLESPOON OF DRESSING.

Spaghetti Squash Mac and Cheese with Broccoli Breadcrumbs

SERVES: 2   PREP TIME: 15 MINUTES   COOK TIME: 50 MINUTES

Here's a confession: My family adores mac and cheese, especially my youngest daughter, Ayden Jane, who considers herself somewhat of an aficionado. I'm constantly experimenting with new and creative ways to health-ify the beloved comfort food, and Ayden often volunteers to serve as my ultimate judge, helping decide which versions make the cut and which go to the chopping block (full disclosure, not all my creations pass muster).

This version was declared a winner. It's a super-low-carb spin, because it doesn't require pasta. Instead I swap in spaghetti squash, which produces delicious noodle-like strands when cooked and pulled apart with a fork. The creamy cheese sauce is lighter than restaurant or boxed versions, but it's packed with flavor, thanks to a handful of scrumptious spices and seasonings. And to top if all off, I add a "breadcrumb" topping made from a surprisingly healthy ingredient: broccoli. And because presentation counts, I serve it up in the spaghetti squash shells. It's mac and cheese magnificence—creamy, cheesy, and indulgent—but it's also wholesome, light, and nutritious. And the best part: It's Ayden Jane–approved!

SQUASH

1 medium spaghetti squash

Kosher salt and ground black pepper

CHEESE SAUCE

¾ cup nonfat or low-fat milk, divided

¼ teaspoon reduced-sodium soy sauce

¼ teaspoon ground cayenne

⅛ to ¼ teaspoon ground nutmeg

¼ teaspoon dry mustard

¼ teaspoon onion powder

1 tablespoon cornstarch or tapioca flour

1 cup shredded reduced-fat sharp cheddar cheese

1 tablespoon whipped butter

BROCCOLI BREADCRUMBS

1 cup fresh broccoli florets (or ¾ cup fresh riced broccoli)

2 tablespoons grated Parmesan cheese

1 FOR THE SQUASH: Preheat the oven to 375°F.

2 Microwave the squash for about 4 minutes to soften. (This makes cutting it in half easier and safer.)

3 Cool slightly, then slice the squash in half lengthwise. Scoop out the seeds and pulp and discard. Place the squash cut-side up on a baking sheet, mist with oil spray, and season with a sprinkling of salt and black pepper. Flip over the squash (so it is now cut-side down) and bake for about 20 minutes. (Remember, it has been slightly precooked in the microwave, so it's a shorter oven time than usual.)

RECIPE CONTINUES

4 Remove from the oven and cool, then use a fork to scrape out the spaghetti-like strands into a large bowl. Pat the strands with paper towels to remove as much moisture as possible, so they're somewhat dry before adding the cheese sauce. Save your squash shells, as they will become your mac and cheese "bowls."

5 FOR THE CHEESE SAUCE: In a small saucepan, combine ½ cup of the milk, the soy sauce, cayenne, nutmeg, mustard, and onion powder and bring to a simmer over medium heat.

6 In a small bowl, whisk the cornstarch or tapioca flour into the remaining ¼ cup milk. Add the mixture to the saucepan and stir well. Continue to stir over medium heat for a few minutes, until the sauce starts to thicken slightly. Turn off the heat. Add the cheddar cheese and mix until melted. Add the butter and stir to melt.

7 Pour the cheese sauce over the spaghetti squash noodles and mix until well combined. Season with salt and black pepper to taste. Spoon evenly into the two squash shells.

8 FOR THE "BREADCRUMBS": To make riced broccoli, mince the broccoli florets by hand using a sharp knife (discard large stems before chopping) or pulse the florets in a food processor for about 10 seconds (be careful not to over-pulse, or they'll wind up pureed). Mix the broccoli pieces with the Parmesan cheese and sprinkle on top of your stuffed squash halves. Bake for about 25 minutes, until the tops are toasty and slightly browned.

PER SERVING 1 STUFFED SHELL **390** CALORIES **28 g** PROTEIN **19 g** FAT (**7 g** UNSATURATED FAT, **12 g** SATURATED FAT) **55 mg** CHOLESTEROL **32 g** CARBS **5 g** FIBER **13 g** SUGAR (**13 g** NATURAL SUGAR, **0 g** ADDED SUGAR) **790 mg** SODIUM

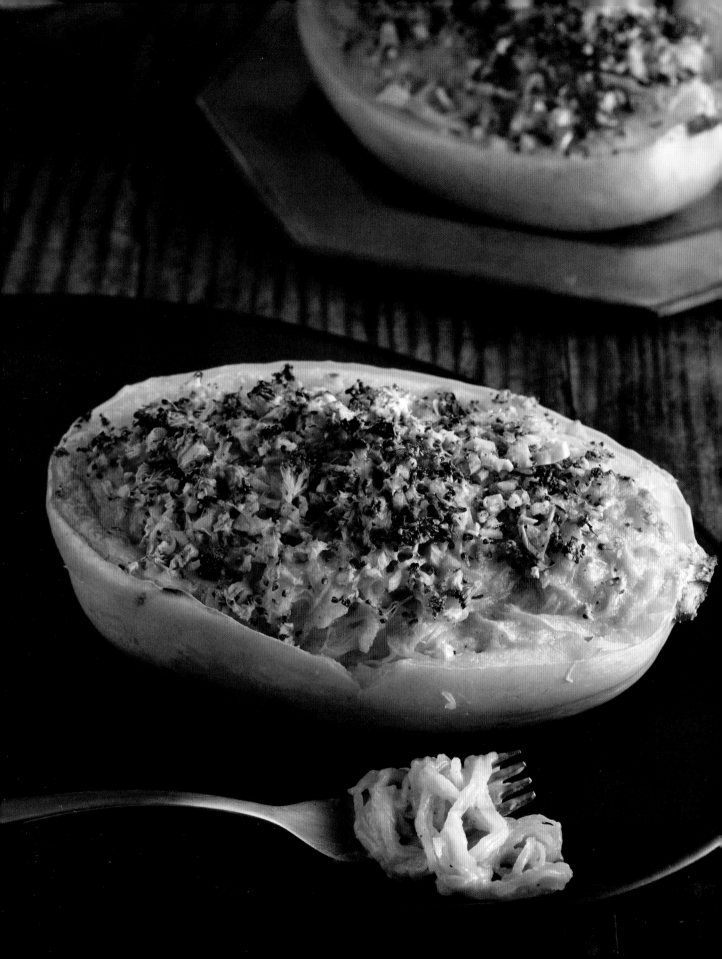

Cauliflower Gnocchi
with Garlicky Marinara

MAKES: ABOUT 9 CUPS   PREP TIME: 40 MINUTES   COOK TIME: 20 MINUTES

I'm a regular at Trader Joe's (some women crave purses or shoes; for me, it's groceries, haha). From my frequent visits, I happen to know that one of the chain's most popular items is their cauliflower gnocchi. So of course, I had to take on the challenge of creating my own version. I even titled my quest "Mission Cauli Gnocchi." I tried countless renditions and even hosted tasting parties until I got a thumbs-up from all my guests. I experimented with omitting flour and going gluten-free, but while I loved the idea of a no-flour gnocchi, it came out too gummy and inauthentic. This recipe, by far, wins the gold. It's delish topped with garlicky marinara, but you can also go green and toss with pleasing pesto.

12 heaping cups cauliflower florets (2 medium heads)

1 cup white whole wheat flour*

1 teaspoon kosher salt, plus more for sprinkling

1 jar marinara sauce

Grated Parmesan cheese for topping (optional)

* If you can't find white whole wheat flour, use 1 cup standard whole wheat and 1 cup all-purpose.

1 Place the cauliflower in a large pot, cover with water (make sure veggies are submerged), and bring to a boil. Reduce heat to low, cover, and simmer for about 20 minutes, until the cauliflower is very soft. Drain and set aside to cool. Once cooled, put ⅓ to ½ of the cauliflower in a dish towel or layered paper towels, squeeze out as much excess water as possible and place in a large bowl. Repeat with the remaining cauliflower until all of it is well-drained and squashed.

2 Add the flour and salt into the bowl with the mashed cauliflower and mix with a fork at first, then using your hands to fold and squeeze everything together into a sticky dough. Place the bowl in the freezer for 20 to 30 minutes to firm (this will make it easier to form the gnocchi).

3 Line 2 baking sheets with parchment paper and set them near your workstation. Remove the dough from the freezer. One at a time, roll a handful of dough into a ½-inch-thick rope and set on the prepared baking sheets. Continue until all the dough is used up. Then, make classic gnocchi ridges by gently pressing the back of a fork along each of the ropes repeatedly. Next, cut each rope into 1-inch-long (gnocchi-like) pieces, slightly nudging the pieces apart so they're not touching. You should get about 160 pieces total. If at any point the dough becomes too sticky to work with, dampen your hands with cold water.

4 Liberally mist a large skillet with nonstick oil spray and warm over medium heat. Using a spatula, carefully lift the gnocchi off the baking sheets, one row at a time, and place them on the hot skillet (if the pieces stick together, just slice them apart in the skillet using the spatula). Do not over-crowd the pan; you'll need to cook the gnocchi in several batches. Let the gnocchi sit in the hot pan undisturbed for two minutes, then gently flip using a spoon or tongs, being careful not to squish them. Sprinkle salt over the tops and continue to cook for another two to four minutes or until desired doneness. Serve topped with warm marinara sauce and optional grated cheese.

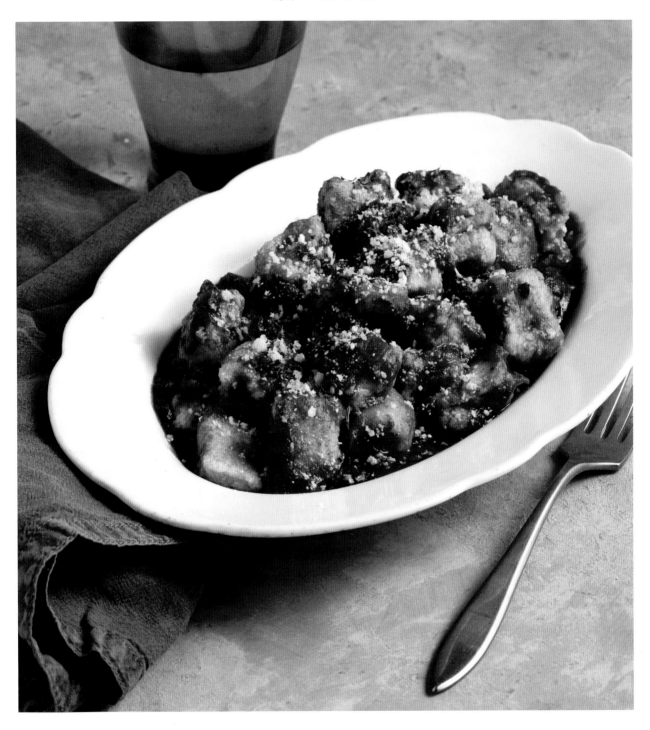

TO FREEZE: Allow your gnocchi to completely cool, then transfer to a sealed container and store in the freezer for up to a month.

PER SERVING 1 CUP GNOCCHI AND ½ CUP SAUCE PER SERVING **340** CALORIES **17 g** PROTEIN **3 g** FAT (**3 g** UNSATURATED FAT, **0 g** SATURATED FAT) **0 mg** CHOLESTEROL **71 g** CARBS **14 g** FIBER **13 g** SUGAR (**13 g** NATURAL SUGAR, **0 g** ADDED SUGAR) **800 mg** SODIUM

No Noodle Cheesy Spinach Lasagna

SERVES: 6   PREP TIME: 15 MINUTES   COOK TIME: 1 HOUR

I could probably survive for months on lasagna alone. I never get bored of eating it. For me, this dish is the end all, be all—creamy, cheesy ecstasy in a pan. Every bite makes me excited for the next. And while I love noodles as much as the next person, I felt the need to create a lower-carb, lower-calorie, noodle-free rendition. Lasagna without noodles . . . how is that even possible? I promise, one bite of this veggie, flavor-filled masterpiece will answer that question. Roasted eggplant, zucchini, spinach, and tomatoes are smothered in warm ricotta, melted mozzarella cheese, and fresh aromatic basil. Drooling yet? Just one warning: It's not as stable or firm as traditional lasagna, but it's every bit as delicious. Enjoy it with a side salad for a full meal.

Pro tip: Because there are no noodles to absorb any excess moisture, you want to make sure to squeeze out as much of the liquid from the thawed spinach as possible. I typically microwave the great greens for a quick defrost, and then press with a kitchen towel to remove the water. Also, the longer the lasagna rests, the easier it'll be to cut into portions, so be patient. No easy task, I know!

1 medium eggplant (about 1½ pounds), cut in half widthwise and sliced ¼ inch thick lengthwise

3 medium zucchini, cut in half widthwise and sliced ¼ inch thick lengthwise

¼ teaspoon kosher salt

¾ teaspoon ground black pepper, divided

1 (15-ounce) container part-skim ricotta cheese

1 (10-ounce) pack frozen chopped spinach, defrosted and well-drained of excess water

2 large egg whites, beaten

¼ cup chopped fresh basil, plus additional whole leaves for topping

3 cloves garlic, minced (or ½ teaspoon garlic powder)

¼ cup plus 2 tablespoons grated Parmesan cheese, divided

3 cups marinara sauce (store-bought or homemade), divided

1½ cups part-skim shredded mozzarella cheese, divided

¾ cup grape tomatoes, cut in half lengthwise

¼ to ½ teaspoon red pepper flakes (optional)

1 Preheat the oven to 400°F. Mist a 9 by 13-inch baking dish or lasagna pan with nonstick oil spray. Set aside.

2 Mist 2 baking sheets with nonstick oil spray and arrange the eggplant and zucchini in a single layer. Mist the veggies with additional oil spray and sprinkle the salt and ½ teaspoon of the black pepper over the tops. Place in the oven and bake for 20 to 25 minutes, until the vegetables become tender and slightly browned. Remove from the oven and reduce the oven temperature to 350°F.

3 While the veggies are roasting, in a large bowl, combine the ricotta cheese, drained spinach, egg whites, basil, garlic, ¼ cup of the Parmesan cheese, and the remaining ¼ teaspoon black pepper. Set aside until you're ready to assemble.

4 TO ASSEMBLE THE LASAGNA: Spread 1 cup of the marinara sauce on the bottom of the prepared baking dish or lasagna pan. Next, add an even layer of roasted eggplant and spread another 1 cup of the sauce across the top, followed by half of the ricotta-spinach mixture (about 1½ cups), ¾ cup of the mozzarella cheese, all of the roasted zucchini (and any leftover eggplant slices), the remaining 1 cup sauce, the remaining ricotta-spinach mixture, and the remaining ¾ cup mozzarella cheese.

5 Arrange the grape tomatoes and a few whole basil leaves on the top of the lasagna and sprinkle on the remaining 2 tablespoons Parmesan cheese and the red pepper flakes, if using. Place the lasagna in the oven and bake for 40 minutes. Remove from the oven and allow the lasagna to cool for about 10 minutes before serving.

TO FREEZE: Allow the lasagna to cool completely, then cut into individual portions and freeze in airtight containers.

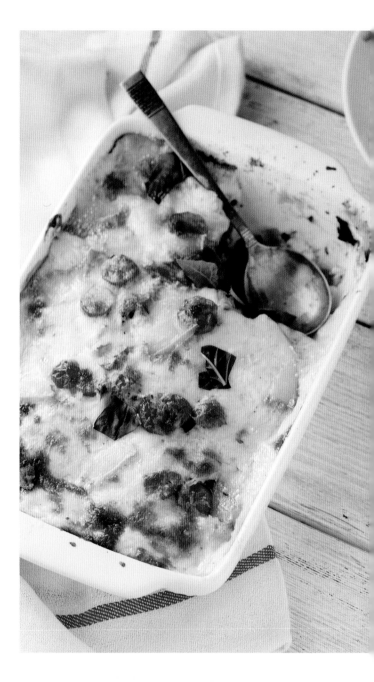

PER SERVING **300** CALORIES **26 g** PROTEIN **14 g** FAT (**8 g** UNSATURATED FAT, **6 g** UNSATURATED FAT) **50 mg** CHOLESTEROL **28 g** CARBS **6 g** FIBER **16 g** SUGAR (**16 g** NATURAL SUGAR, **0 g** ADDED SUGAR) **850 mg** SODIUM

One-Pot Wonders

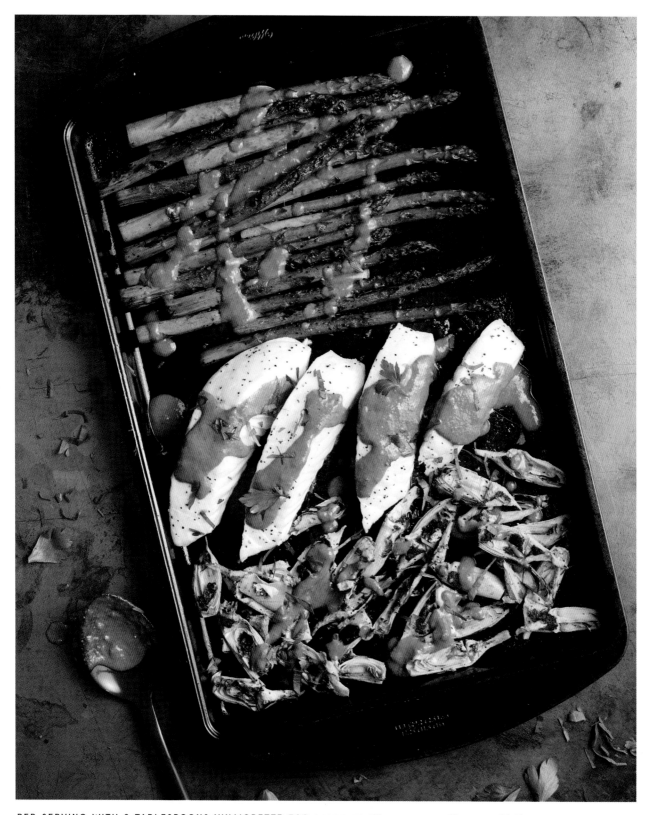

PER SERVING WITH 2 TABLESPOONS VINAIGRETTE **300** CALORIES **37 g** PROTEIN **12 g** FAT (**10.5 g** UNSATURATED FAT, **1.5 g** SATURATED FAT) **85 mg** CHOLESTEROL **11 g** CARBS **9 g** FIBER **2 g** SUGAR (**2 g** NATURAL SUGAR, **0 g** ADDED SUGAR) **530 mg** SODIUM *ADD 45 CALORIES FOR EACH ADDITIONAL TABLESPOON OF VINAIGRETTE.

Roasted Fish Fillets
with Smoky Apple Cider Vinaigrette

SERVES: 4   PREP TIME: 10 MINUTES   COOK TIME: 30 MINUTES

This dish has so many outstanding components. First, there's the fish, which lends lean protein and has a mild taste and a tender texture. Then asparagus, which, among its many benefits, contains quercetin, a flavonoid that has been shown to help boost immune function and may even help tame seasonal allergies. The artichoke hearts also deliver big, providing a hearty hit of fiber as well as a meaty, satisfying texture. Finally, the apple cider vinaigrette infuses an out-of-this world flavor for the ultimate finishing touch.

SMOKY PAPRIKA VINAIGRETTE
makes ¾ cup

- 3 tablespoons apple cider vinegar
- 1 tablespoon Dijon mustard
- 1 small shallot, roughly chopped (about 1 tablespoon)
- 2 teaspoons smoked paprika
- ⅛ teaspoon kosher salt
- ⅛ teaspoon black pepper
- 4 tablespoons extra virgin olive oil, divided

FISH AND VEGGIES

- 14 ounces quartered artichoke hearts (fresh, canned, or frozen)*
- ½ to 1 teaspoon kosher salt
- Ground black pepper
- 1 large clove garlic, minced
- 2 bunches fresh asparagus, tough ends cut off
- 4 (6-ounce) fish fillets

* If using canned artichoke hearts, rinse, drain, and pat dry. If using frozen, thaw before seasoning.

1 Preheat the oven to 425°F. Lightly mist a large baking sheet with nonstick oil spray.

2 FOR THE DRESSING: In a small blender or food processor, combine the vinegar, 3 tablespoons water, the mustard, shallot, and paprika and blend until smooth. Add the salt, pepper, and 2 tablespoons of the oil and blend again until the mixture emulsifies and lightens in color. Add the remaining 2 tablespoons oil and blend until the dressing is smooth and deep orange in color.

3 FOR THE FISH AND VEGGIES: Place the artichoke hearts in a medium bowl and mist with oil spray, season with a pinch of salt and pepper, and add the garlic. Toss well and place on one side of the prepared baking sheet. Roast for about 10 minutes, until they start to brown. Use a spatula or tongs to flip them.

4 Remove the baking sheet from the oven and add the asparagus spears to the other side. Mist with oil spray, season with ¼ teaspoon salt and pepper, place the sheet back in the oven, and roast for another 10 minutes.

5 While the veggies are cooking, season the fish fillets on both sides with ¼ teaspoon salt and pepper. Remove the sheet from the oven. Clear a spot for the fish to nestle into the vegetables, place back in the oven, and roast until the fish is cooked through and the vegetables are browned, 8 to 10 minutes. NOTE: Timing will depend on the thickness of your fish; the general rule is 7 minutes per 1-inch thickness.

TO SERVE: Plate the asparagus on a serving tray, top with the fish, and scatter the artichoke hearts around the fish. Generously spoon the vinaigrette over the fish and veggies and serve the remaining dressing on the side.

Layered Chicken and Eggplant Parmesan

SERVES: 4 PREP TIME: 10 MINUTES COOK TIME: 12 MINUTES

My signature "chickplant Parm" combines the best of both of the southern Italian staples, lightens them up, and fuses them into one singular masterpiece. Instead of frying, I bake slices of fiber-rich eggplant and protein-packed chicken cutlets with immunity-boosting and blood pressure–lowering garlic and bright, citrusy fresh thyme leaves.

To assemble the dish, the eggplant and chicken cutlets are layered one on top of the other, like a culinary Leaning Tower of Pisa. Before finishing the stacks off in the oven, they are topped with marinara sauce and juicy grape tomatoes—both teeming with lycopene—and an indulgent mixture of cheeses.

1 medium to large unpeeled eggplant, sliced into 8 rounds (each ¾ to 1 inch thick)

1 to 1¼ pounds boneless, skinless chicken thighs or breasts (4 to 8 pieces)

3 to 4 cloves garlic, minced

1 to 1½ tablespoons chopped fresh thyme (or 1 teaspoon dried thyme)

½ teaspoon kosher salt

Ground black pepper

12 to 16 grape or cherry tomatoes

2 cups marinara sauce

½ cup grated Parmesan cheese

½ cup shredded part-skim mozzarella cheese (or 4 slices reduced-fat provolone cheese)

Torn fresh basil leaves or chopped fresh parsley for garnish

1 Place an oven rack on the second highest position and preheat the broiler.

2 Mist 2 baking sheets with nonstick oil spray. Place the eggplant slices on one sheet and the chicken pieces on the other. Mist all of the tops with oil spray and sprinkle on the garlic, thyme, salt, and some pepper.

3 Place in the oven and broil for 12 to 15 minutes, flipping the eggplant halfway through using a spatula or tongs. If using thin-cut chicken breast, it will be done before the thighs, so prepare to remove them at about the 10-minute mark (I recommend using a thermometer and removing when it hits 165°F to ensure you don't overcook it).

4 Remove the sheets from the broiler and adjust the oven temperature to 400°F.

5 TO ASSEMBLE THE STACKS: Rearrange the roasted eggplant slices so there's an empty row of space in the middle of the baking sheet. Add 2 tablespoons tomato sauce to the cleared opening and cover with one eggplant slice. Next, layer on 1 piece of chicken, 1 tablespoon tomato sauce, ½ tablespoon Parmesan cheese, and a second slice of roasted eggplant. Add a final 1 tablespoon tomato sauce, 2 or 3 grape tomatoes, 1 tablespoon of the mozzarella cheese (or a slice of provolone), and a sprinkling of Parmesan cheese. Repeat with the remaining ingredients to make 4 stacks. Place back in the oven and bake for about 10 minutes, until the cheese is melted and bubbling. Garnish with basil or parsley before serving.

PER SERVING 310 CALORIES 33 g PROTEIN 11 g FAT (8 g UNSATURATED FAT, 3 g SATURATED FAT) 110 mg CHOLESTEROL 22 g CARBS 6 g FIBER 6 g SUGAR (6 g NATURAL SUGAR, 0 g ADDED SUGAR) 840 mg SODIUM

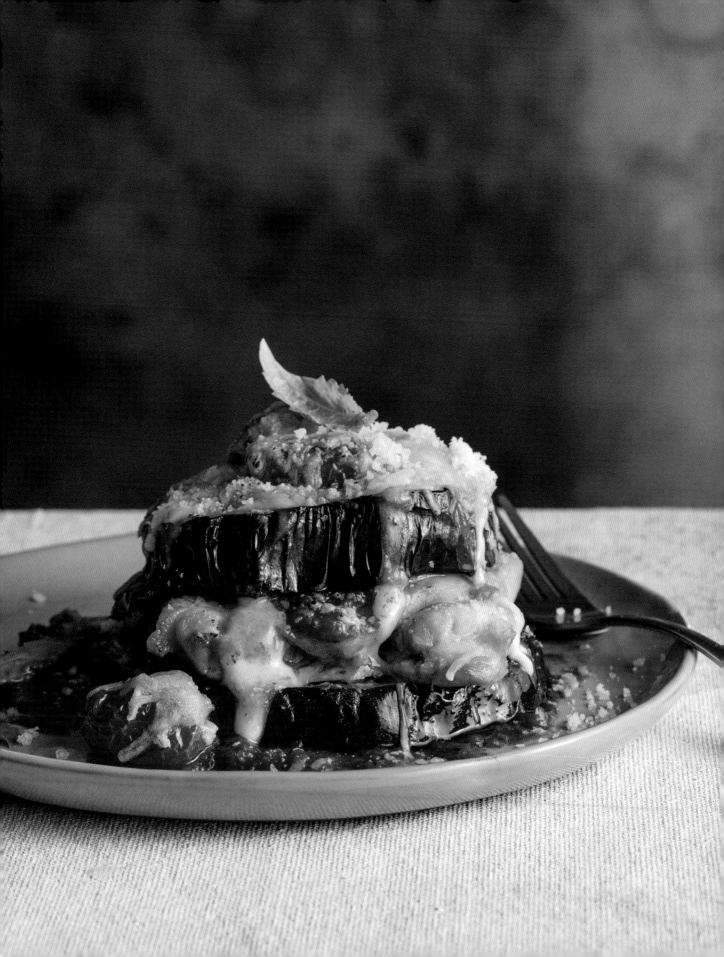

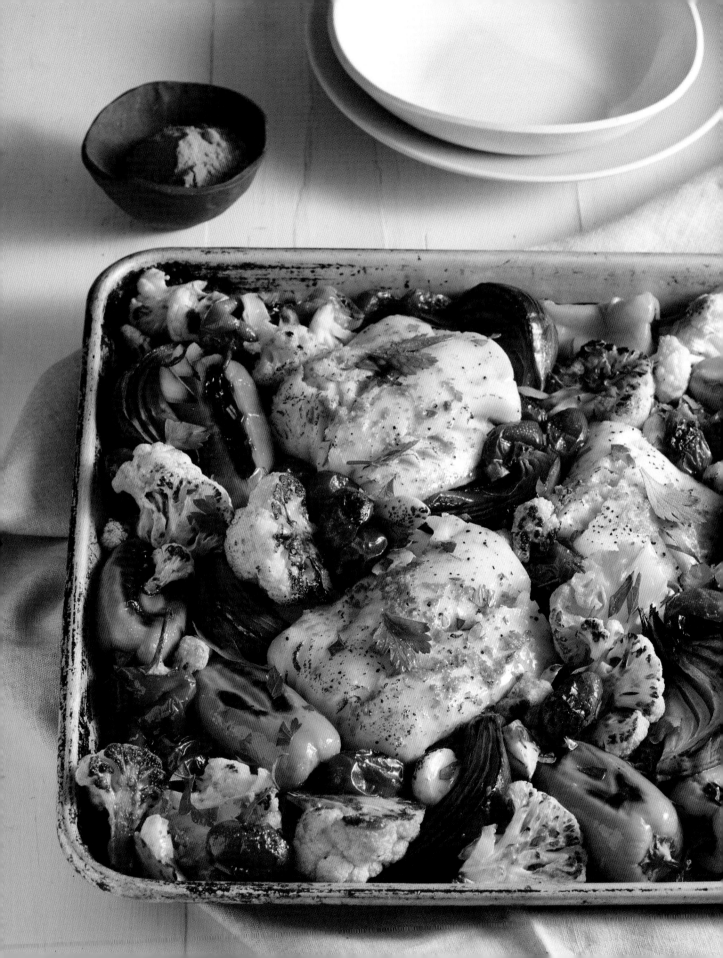

Roasted Cod and Blistered Tomatoes with Turmeric Wine Sauce

SERVES: 4   PREP TIME: 10 MINUTES   COOK TIME: 25 MINUTES

Cod is a clean-tasting fish that requires minimal prep and fuss-free cooking. In this recipe, I dress it up with a unique sauce that boasts anti-inflammatory properties, courtesy of the turmeric. I toss in some vitamin C–rich bell peppers and tomatoes, packed with lycopene (which becomes more bioavailable when cooked). The result: You end up with a complete meal that comes together easily on one baking sheet.

¼ cup white wine

1 tablespoon grated fresh turmeric root (or 1½ teaspoons dried turmeric)

¼ cup reduced-sodium vegetable or chicken broth

1 medium head cauliflower, cut into florets (4 to 5 cups)

12 mini red, orange, and yellow bell peppers

1 large red onion, peeled and cut into 8 wedges, still attached at the core

3 cloves garlic, minced

1 tablespoon olive oil

½ teaspoon kosher salt, divided, plus more to taste

4 (5- to 6-ounce) wild-caught cod fillets

Ground black pepper

1 pint grape tomatoes

¼ cup roughly chopped fresh flat-leaf parsley (optional)

1 Preheat the oven to 420°F and place a baking sheet in the oven to heat.

2 In a small bowl, whisk together the wine, turmeric, and broth. Set aside.

3 In a large bowl, combine the cauliflower, bell peppers, onion, and garlic. Add the oil and ¼ teaspoon of the salt and gently toss.

4 Remove the hot sheet from the oven and mist it with nonstick oil spray. Add the vegetables and spread them out in a single layer, placing the cut sides of the cauliflower flat on the pan. Roast in the oven for 15 minutes.

5 While the veggies are roasting, season the cod on both sides with the remaining ¼ teaspoon salt and a sprinkle of black pepper.

6 Remove the baking sheet from the oven and carefully flip the onion wedges and cauliflower. Scatter the tomatoes onto the sheet and nestle the cod into open spots. Spoon half of the sauce over the cod and veggies. Place the sheet back in the oven and roast for another 10 minutes, or until the fish is cooked through and flakes.

7 Remove the sheet from the oven, immediately spoon the remaining sauce over the fish and vegetables, and let the heat of the food and pan warm the seasoning liquid. (This will also help to release any stuck bits from the sheet). Transfer to a serving tray, season with extra salt and pepper, if needed, and garnish with the parsley, if desired.

PER SERVING 240 CALORIES 29 g PROTEIN 5 g FAT (4 g UNSATURATED FAT, 1 g SATURATED FAT) 60 mg CHOLESTEROL 18 g CARBS 5 g FIBER 9 g SUGAR (9 g NATURAL SUGAR, 0 g ADDED SUGAR) 370 mg SODIUM

One-Skillet Enchiladas

SERVES: 6   PREP TIME: 20 MINUTES   COOK TIME: 40 MINUTES

With traditional enchiladas, the tortillas are rolled up, placed in a baking dish, and finished off in the oven. With these, I layer everything in the same skillet, then I top it off with plenty of shredded cheese, and the single pan goes straight into the oven to cook. (Note on the tortillas: Any whole grain variety will work great here.) If you're a double cheese lover (count me in), you can sneak a little extra in between the tortilla layers for additional gooey richness. If you don't have Mexican cheese blend, no problem—whatever is in your fridge will work just fine. Try these topped with chopped avocado and fresh cilantro, or salsa, pico de gallo, guacamole, and light sour cream or Greek yogurt.

1 red or orange bell pepper, diced (about 1 cup)

1 onion, diced (about 1½ cups)

1 pound ground turkey (90 to 93% lean)

½ teaspoon kosher salt, or more to taste

⅛ teaspoon black pepper, or more to taste

1 teaspoon ground cumin

1½ teaspoons chili powder

1 teaspoon paprika

½ teaspoon dried oregano

1 to 2 cloves garlic, minced

2¼ cups canned crushed tomatoes (plain or fire-roasted)

1 (15-ounce) can black beans, drained and rinsed

1 cup) chopped (½-inch pieces) butternut squash

6 (10-inch) whole grain tortillas

1 cup 2% reduced-fat shredded Mexican cheese blend

OPTIONAL TOPPERS

Diced avocado, nonfat or low-fat plain Greek yogurt, chopped fresh cilantro

1. Preheat the oven to 400°F.

2. Liberally mist a 12-inch skillet with nonstick oil spray and warm over medium-high heat. Add the bell pepper and onion and cook, stirring occasionally, for about 6 minutes, until the vegetables soften.

3. Add the turkey, salt, and pepper and cook for 6 to 7 minutes, using a spatula or large spoon to break up the meat as it cooks. Stir in the cumin, chili powder, paprika, oregano, and garlic and cook until fragrant, about 1 minute.

4. Stir in the tomatoes, beans, and butternut squash, scraping the bottom of the pan to incorporate all the browned bits and seasonings, and bring to a low simmer. Cover, reduce the heat to medium-low, and cook for 12 to 15 minutes, until the squash is tender.

5. Remove half of the mixture (about 2½ cups) and set aside. Evenly spread out what's left in the skillet to coat the bottom. Top with 3 tortillas, tearing one or two apart to cover as much surface as possible. Top with the remaining turkey mixture and tortillas. Sprinkle the cheese over the top and transfer the skillet to the oven for 10 to 14 minutes, until the cheese is melted and the edges of the tortillas become golden. Remove from the oven and allow to set for 5 minutes before serving with your choice of toppings.

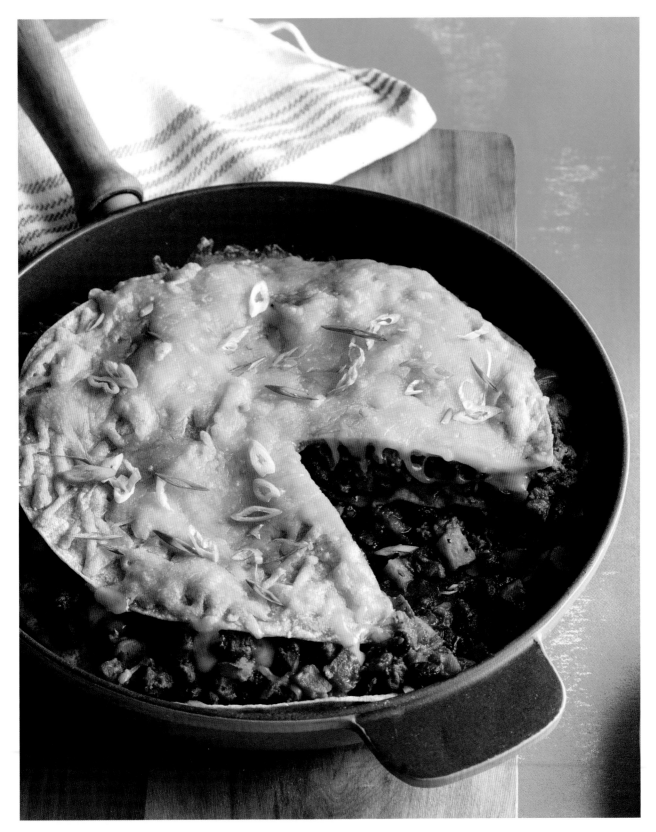

PER SERVING **320** CALORIES **32 g** PROTEIN **13 g** FAT (**10 g** UNSATURATED FAT, **3 g** SATURATED FAT) **45 mg** CHOLESTEROL **34 g** CARBS **8 g** FIBER **6 g** SUGAR (**6 g** NATURAL SUGAR, **0 g** ADDED SUGAR) **750 mg** SODIUM

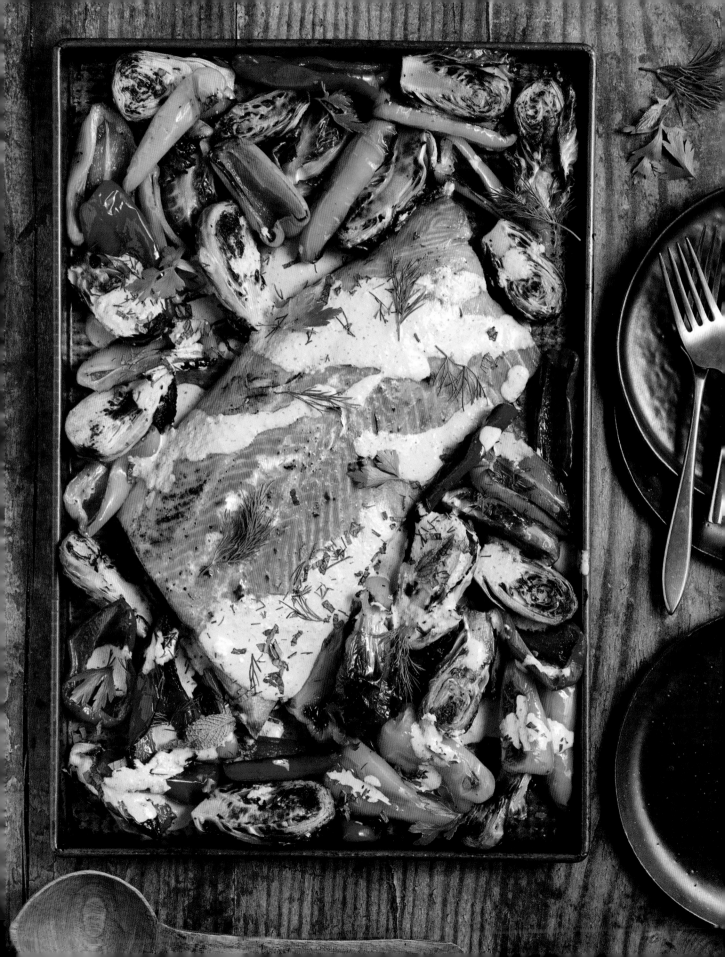

One-Sheet Salmon with Herb-Infused Green Sauce

SERVES: 4   PREP TIME: 20 MINUTES   COOK TIME: 30 MINUTES

I'm always looking to create new ways to enjoy salmon, which features omega-3 fats, shown to help with a variety of ailments, from depression and anxiety to heart disease, cancer, and Alzheimer's. This recipe appeals because cleanup is a cinch, you can use a variety of vegetables, and the herb-infused green sauce elevates every delectable bite you take.

SAUCE
makes 1½ cups

- ½ cup packed fresh flat-leaf parsley
- ¼ cup fresh dill
- ¼ cup fresh cilantro
- ¼ cup fresh mint leaves
- 2 scallions, white and green parts, trimmed
- 1 tablespoon dried tarragon
- 1 small shallot, sliced
- 1 tablespoon apple cider vinegar
- 1 cup nonfat or low-fat plain Greek yogurt
- ¼ teaspoon kosher salt
- Ground black pepper

SALMON

- 12 multicolored baby bell peppers, halved lengthwise and seeded
- 12 ounces Brussels sprouts, halved (saving any loose outer leaves)
- 1 tablespoon olive oil
- ½ teaspoon kosher salt, divided
- 4 (6-ounce) skin-on wild-caught salmon fillets, or 1 large fillet (1½ pounds)
- Ground black pepper

1 **FOR THE SAUCE:** Remove the stems from the parsley, dill, and cilantro. Add all the sauce ingredients to a food processor or high-speed blender and process until smooth. Set aside to serve at room temperature or chill in the refrigerator (it's delicious both ways).

2 **FOR THE SALMON:** Preheat the oven to 400°F. Place a baking sheet in the oven to heat.

3 In a large bowl, combine the bell peppers and Brussels sprouts (with any loose outer leaves) and toss with the oil and ¼ teaspoon of the salt. Remove the hot sheet from the oven and place the bell peppers and Brussels sprouts on it. Place back in the oven and roast for 15 minutes.

4 Remove the sheet from the oven, flip the vegetables with a spatula, and push them to the outer sides of the sheet. Place the salmon fillet(s), skin-side down, in the center of the sheet. Mist with olive oil spray and season with the remaining ¼ teaspoon salt and some black pepper. Place back in the oven and roast for 10 to 15 minutes, depending on the thickness of the fillets, until the salmon feels firm, resisting your finger when pushed at the thickest part, about 7 minutes per inch of thickness. Switch the oven to broil and cook for 1 to 2 minutes to brown the top. Remove from the oven. **TO SERVE:** Slide a long, wide spatula between the skin and the flesh of the fish and lift it cleanly from the sheet to the plate, leaving the skin behind.* Toss the vegetables, transfer to the plate around the salmon, and top the fillet(s) with a dollop of the green sauce or serve on the side.

* If you're a fan of crispy salmon skin, turn off the oven and place the sheet (with the skin still on it) back in the oven for a few minutes to crisp it up. Remove it from the sheet and enjoy it as a treat during cleanup!

PER SERVING **320** CALORIES **36 g** PROTEIN **13 g** FAT (**11 g** UNSATURATED FAT, **2 g** SATURATED FAT) **80 mg** CHOLESTEROL **14 g** CARBS **5 g** FIBER **6 g** SUGAR (**6 g** NATURAL SUGAR, **0 g** ADDED SUGAR) **640 mg** SODIUM

Chicken Stir-Fry with Sweet Dates and Bell Peppers

SERVES: 4   PREP TIME: 5 MINUTES   COOK TIME: 10 MINUTES

If you love Chinese takeout as much as my family does, this recipe is for you. There's one layer of flavor after the next here: dates for natural sweetness without adding in sugar, toasted sesame seeds for crunch, and so much more. Bell peppers provide a crispy texture, and you'll notice I've opted for the sweeter varieties like red, yellow, and orange, but hey—if you prefer the fourth bell pepper hue, then, as they say, go green!

If you're cooking for more than 3 people, my advice is to make a double batch—it goes fast and people always want seconds. With a stir-fry, though, it's important that all elements are exposed to the surface of the pan or wok evenly; too crowded and they'll lose the pan-fried effect that makes stir-fries so tasty. So, if you end up doubling the recipe, sear the chicken in separate batches, one after the other. It's the best way to guarantee a mouthwatering outcome.

2 tablespoons rice vinegar

2 tablespoons reduced-sodium soy sauce

½ teaspoon red pepper flakes

½ medium onion, finely chopped (about 1 cup)

1 pound boneless, skinless chicken breasts, cut into 1-inch pieces

2 medium bell peppers (red, yellow, or orange), cut into ½-inch pieces (about 2 cups)

½ cup pitted dried dates, thinly sliced

1 scallion, thinly sliced (optional)

1 to 2 teaspoons toasted sesame seeds (optional)

1. In a small bowl, stir together the vinegar, soy sauce, and red pepper flakes. Set aside.

2. Liberally mist the bottom of a large pan with nonstick oil spray and warm over medium-high heat. Add the onion to the pan and cook, stirring constantly, for about 30 seconds. Reduce the heat to medium, add the chicken, spread it out so all the pieces are touching the bottom of the pan, and cook, undisturbed, for 1 minute. Stir-fry for another 1 minute, adding more oil spray if the pan gets too dry.

3. Add the bell peppers and dates and cook, stirring, for 1 minute. Reduce the heat to low, add the vinegar–soy sauce mixture, and stir-fry for 4 to 5 more minutes, until the chicken is cooked through. Garnish with scallions and sesame seeds, if desired, and serve.

PER SERVING ABOUT 1¼ CUPS 230 CALORIES 27 g PROTEIN 3 g FAT (2.5 g UNSATURATED FAT, 0.5 g SATURATED FAT) 85 mg CHOLESTEROL 22 g CARBS 4 g FIBER 14 g SUGAR (14 g NATURAL SUGAR, 0 g ADDED SUGAR) 340 mg SODIUM

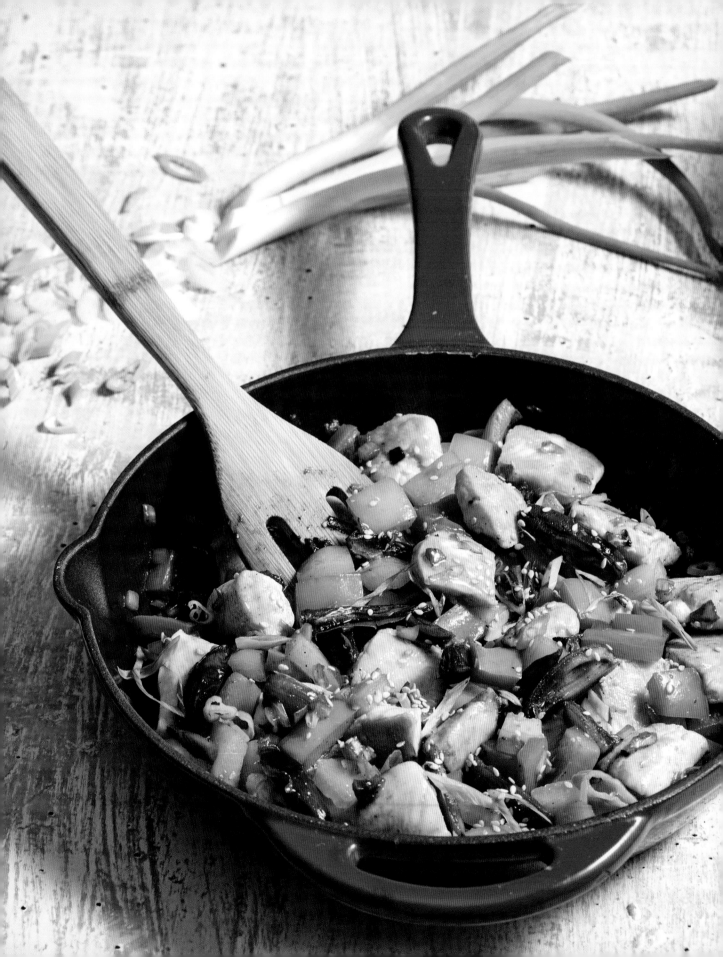

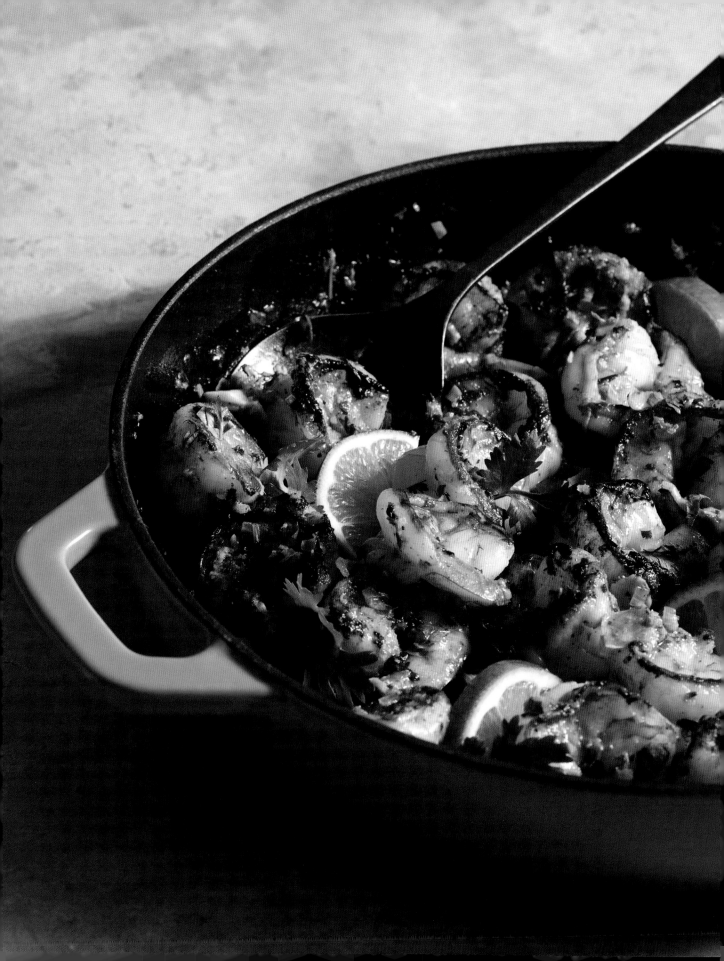

One-Skillet Lime Cilantro Shrimp

SERVES: 6 PREP TIME: 10 MINUTES COOK TIME: 5 MINUTES

People always ask me what's in my fridge or freezer. Here's one thing you'll always find: frozen shrimp. It's budget-friendly, easy to cook with, and a great source of lean protein. It's a no-fail solution for hectic weeknights when you don't know what to cook and don't have a ton of time. I typically take a shortcut and buy peeled and deveined, sometimes tail on and sometimes tail off. This shrimp recipe is always a crowd favorite. The marinade is full of flavor and really jazzes up the shrimp. If you don't like cilantro, you can swap it for parsley. Both herbs add flavor, freshness, and an element of elegance.

1 tablespoon extra virgin olive oil

2 tablespoons lime juice

1 shallot, minced

2 cloves garlic, minced (or ¼ teaspoon garlic powder)

¼ teaspoon kosher salt, plus more to taste

¼ cup minced fresh cilantro, plus more for garnish

2 pounds raw shrimp, peeled and deveined, tail off

Ground black pepper

Lime slices for serving

1 In a large bowl, combine the oil, lime juice, shallot, garlic, salt, and cilantro. Add the shrimp and toss to coat.

2 Liberally mist a large skillet with olive oil spray and warm over medium-high heat. Add half of the shrimp to the skillet and cook, undisturbed, for 2 minutes. (It's important to add only half the shrimp, so as not to overcrowd the pan and allow the shrimp to sear.) Flip and cook for another 2 minutes, or until the shrimp is cooked through. Transfer to a plate and cover to keep warm. Reapply oil spray and repeat with the remaining shrimp. Transfer to a serving plate, season with additional salt and pepper, and garnish with cilantro and lime slices.

PER SERVING **150** CALORIES **31 g** PROTEIN **3 g** FAT (**3 g** UNSATURATED FAT, **0 g** SATURATED FAT) **245 mg** CHOLESTEROL **1 g** CARBS **0 g** FIBER **0 g** SUGAR **260 mg** SODIUM

Creamy Farro Risotto with Riced Broccoli and Parm

SERVES: 7   PREP TIME: 10 MINUTES   COOK TIME: 50 MINUTES

What would life be without risotto? Even dietitians—in fact, *especially* dietitians—have a healthy respect for the importance of indulging from time to time, and rich, decadent risotto hits the spot for me. That said, there are some clever swaps I've made to introduce an array of health benefits. For instance, I use farro—a grain that overflows with protein, fiber, and nutrients including zinc and magnesium—instead of rice. Farro delivers its distinct texture and nutty flavor, lending extra dimension to the dish.

Another modification I've made is the introduction of riced broccoli (finely chopped broccoli florets also work fine), which is rich in vitamins C and K. I pair it with a full cup of grated Parmesan, and the combo is like feasting on a grown-up version of mac and cheese.

- 1 tablespoon butter or olive oil, plus more if needed
- 1 large white or yellow onion, finely chopped (about 2 cups)
- 1 teaspoon kosher salt, plus more to taste
- 1 teaspoon black pepper, plus more to taste
- 3 cloves garlic, minced
- ½ teaspoon dried thyme
- 2 cups dry farro, preferably semi-pearled
- ¾ cup white wine, such as pinot grigio or chardonnay
- 6 cups reduced-sodium vegetable or chicken broth
- 1 cup grated Parmesan cheese
- 2 cups finely chopped fresh broccoli florets or riced broccoli

1 Preheat the oven to 400°F.

2 Warm a Dutch oven or other oven-safe pot over medium heat and melt the butter or heat the oil in it. Add the onion, salt, and pepper and cook for 2 minutes, or until translucent, stirring occasionally. Add the garlic and thyme and cook for 1 minute, or until the garlic is fragrant, stirring so the garlic doesn't burn. Add the dry farro and cook for 2 minutes to toast the grains. If the pot becomes dry, mist with olive oil spray or add a bit more butter or oil.

3 Add the wine to the pot and cook, stirring occasionally, until most of the liquid is absorbed, about 4 minutes. Add the broth, increase the heat to high, and bring to a boil. Give it one more good stir, cover, and carefully transfer the pot to the oven. Cook for 35 minutes, or until the farro is tender and a good amount of the liquid is absorbed (you'll still have some liquid in the pan).

4 Remove the covered pot from the oven and return it to the stovetop over medium heat. Remove the lid and stir constantly for a full 3 minutes; the remaining liquid will slowly be absorbed and the farro will become creamier. Reduce the heat to low, add the cheese and broccoli, and stir continuously for 2 more minutes. Season with additional salt and pepper.

PER SERVING 1 CUP **280** CALORIES **11 g** PROTEIN **5 g** FAT (**2 g** UNSATURATED FAT, **3 g** SATURATED FAT) **15 mg** CHOLESTEROL **44 g** CARBS **6 g** FIBER **3 g** SUGAR (**3 g** NATURAL SUGAR, **0 g** ADDED SUGAR) **800 mg** SODIUM

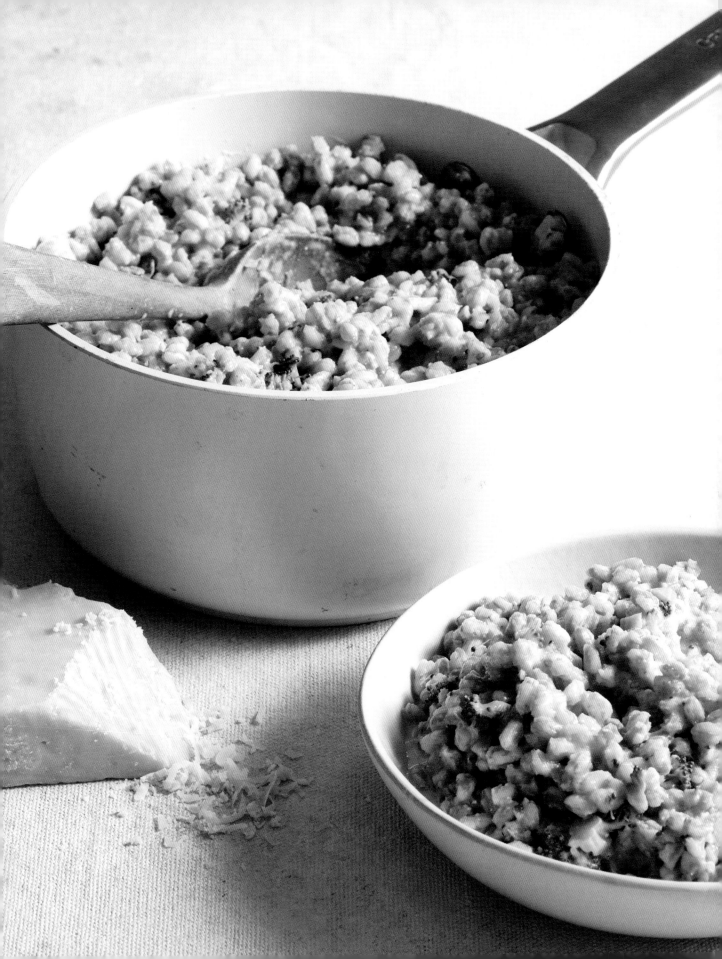

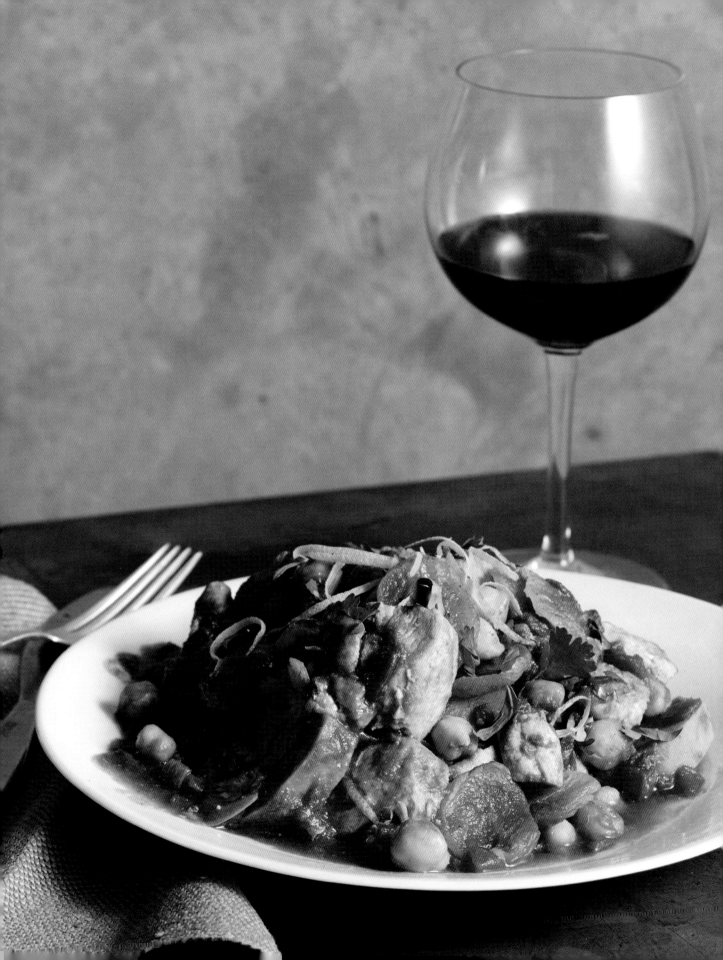

Moroccan-Spiced Chicken Stew

SERVES: 7   PREP TIME: 10 MINUTES   COOK TIME: 40 MINUTES

Morocco—surrounded by the Mediterranean Sea to the north, the Atlantic to the west, and the rugged, mountainous Maghreb region of North Africa to the east—is home to an exotic and lively cuisine. This stew, a definite one-pot wonder, brings Morocco's bold flavors straight to your doorstep. I caramelize sweet onions and fragrant garlic, then add a bouquet of spices: ginger, coriander, cumin, and cinnamon. Once I've crafted the base of the stew, I add chicken and broth, plus tomato paste and canned tomatoes—the latter two are chock-full of vitamin C and lycopene, which offer protection against cancer and contribute to skin health—and encourage the soup's flavors to meld over a low simmer. Sweet potatoes, chickpeas, and dried apricots blossom and absorb the stew's seasonings to create a truly transcendent dish. I love how recipes like this one allow us to have adventures through food and bring the big, delicious world right to our tables.

1 large yellow onion, finely diced (about 2 cups)

2 teaspoons kosher salt

2 cloves garlic, minced (or ¼ teaspoon garlic powder)

1 tablespoon minced fresh ginger root (or 1 teaspoon ground ginger)

2 tablespoons ground cumin

1 tablespoon ground coriander

1 tablespoon ground cinnamon

2 tablespoons tomato paste

2 to 2½ pounds boneless, skinless chicken breast, cut into 1-inch chunks

1 (14.5-ounce) can no-salt-added diced tomatoes, with juice (or 2 cups chopped fresh tomatoes)

1 cup reduced-sodium chicken broth

1 (15-ounce) can chickpeas, drained and rinsed

1 medium sweet potato, peeled and cut in half lengthwise and then into 1-inch pieces widthwise (about 2½ cups)

¾ cup dried apricots

½ cup roughly chopped fresh cilantro or parsley (optional)

1¼ teaspoons lemon zest (optional)

1 Liberally mist the inside of a medium pot with nonstick oil spray and warm over medium heat. Add the onions and salt and cook for 5 to 7 minutes, stirring occasionally. Add the garlic, ginger, cumin, coriander, cinnamon, and tomato paste and cook, stirring, for 1 minute, or until the spices are slightly toasted and fragrant. Mist with additional oil spray so the spices don't burn.

2 Add the chicken and cook for another 2 minutes. Then add the diced tomatoes and chicken broth and, using a spatula or wooden spoon, gently scrape up any browned bits from the bottom of the pan. Add the chickpeas, sweet potatoes, and dried apricots.

3 Increase the heat to high and bring the stew to a boil, then reduce the heat to low, cover, and simmer for 30 minutes. Stir in the cilantro and lemon zest, if desired, and serve.

PER SERVING 330 CALORIES 35 g PROTEIN 5 g FAT (4 g UNSATURATED FAT, 1 g SATURATED FAT) 95 mg CHOLESTEROL 36 g CARBS 9 g FIBER 13 g SUGAR (13 g NATURAL SUGAR, 0 g ADDED SUGAR) 800 mg SODIUM

Enticing
Entrées

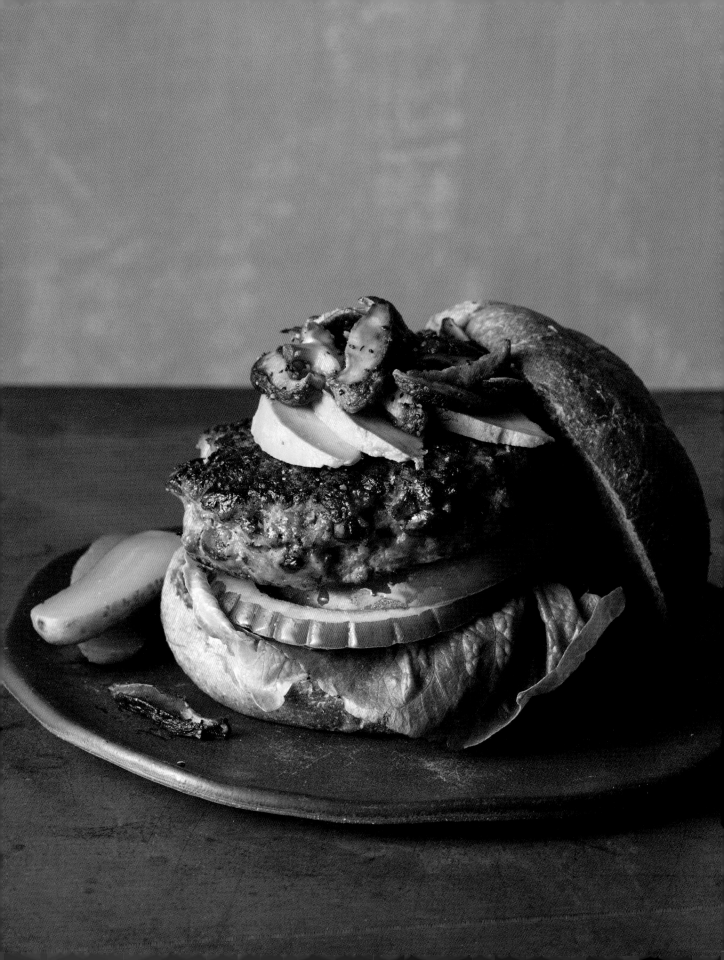

Turkey and Black Bean Burgers

MAKES: 6 BURGERS   PREP TIME: 10 MINUTES   COOK TIME: 10 MINUTES

If you love beefy burgers but are looking for a better-for-you swap without going totally vegetarian, look no further. In this recipe, I've replaced the fatty ground beef with seasoned lean ground turkey and fiber-rich black beans. (If you're a true red meat lover, you can also go for grass-fed, lean beef or ground sirloin.) This is a recipe I turn to over and over again, and my kids are always happy to see it on the dinner table.

I've never had any problem forming the mixture into patties, but if you find yours to be too wet or fussy, add a few tablespoons of rolled oats to help the batter firm up. Another option: Place the entire meat mixture bowl (covered) in the fridge for about 30 minutes. This will also make it a little easier to handle.

I like to serve these as nice, hearty burgers for dinner or as smaller sliders on little whole-grain buns to pass around as party apps. Sometimes, I serve sliders with just a bottom bun and skewer a toothpick through it with a piece of avocado, roasted red pepper, and some feta on top. Another idea: Serve the patty in lettuce wraps to go super low-carb.

1 (15-ounce) can black beans, rinsed and drained

1 large egg, lightly beaten

1 tablespoon reduced-sodium soy sauce

1 tablespoon Worcestershire sauce

1 teaspoon garlic powder

1 teaspoon onion powder

1 pound ground turkey (90 to 93% lean)

Kosher salt for sprinkling

1. In a large bowl, mash the beans by hand using a potato masher or the back of a large fork (mash them as much as you can, but it's okay to leave chunks throughout). Add the egg, soy sauce, Worcestershire sauce, garlic powder, and onion powder and mix to combine. Add the ground turkey and gently combine using your hands or a spatula. Form the mixture into 6 large patties.

2. Liberally coat a large skillet with nonstick oil spray and warm over medium-high heat. Place 3 or 4 patties in the skillet. Mist the tops with oil spray and sprinkle them with salt. Cook for 4 to 5 minutes, then carefully flip, scraping the bottom to keep them intact. Next, lightly sprinkle the browned tops with salt and cook for another 4 to 5 minutes, until the internal temperature reaches 165°F. Reapply oil spray to the skillet and repeat with the remaining burgers.

Serve the burgers on toasted whole grain hamburger buns with your choice of toppings.

PER SERVING 1 BURGER **180** CALORIES **21 g** PROTEIN **6 g** FAT (**5 g** UNSATURATED FAT, **1 g** SATURATED FAT) **60 mg** CHOLESTEROL **14 g** CARBS **5 g** FIBER **1 g** SUGAR (**1 g** NATURAL SUGAR, **0 g** ADDED SUGAR) **280 mg** SODIUM

Loaded Bell Pepper Nachos

SERVES: 6 PREP TIME: 15 MINUTES COOK TIME: 15 MINUTES

Think the gang will miss those crunchy nachos? Prepare to be surprised. Everyone seems to enjoy the sweet, crispy bell pepper base and appreciate the color, nutrition, and flavor that they bring to the table. It's low-carb love! And this dish is incredibly versatile: If you're serving a vegan crowd, skip the meat, cheese, and sour cream and double up on the beans, corn, and salsa. Dairy-free? Omit the cheese and sour cream. It's a cinch to adjust, it's ridiculously easy to toss together, and you can warm leftovers in the oven or microwave when you're ready to eat.

6 large red, yellow, or orange bell peppers

1 pound ground turkey (90 to 93% lean)

1 taco seasoning packet

¾ cup canned black beans, rinsed and drained

¾ cup canned or frozen sweet yellow corn, drained (thawed if frozen)

¼ cup sliced jalapeños (optional)

½ to 1 cup reduced-fat shredded Mexican cheese blend

OPTIONAL TOPPERS

Mild or spicy salsa, ¼ cup light sour cream or nonfat plain Greek yogurt, chopped scallions

1 Preheat the oven to 375°F. Coat a large baking sheet (or 2 standard sheets) with nonstick oil spray and set aside.

2 Remove the stems and seeds from the bell pepper and cut each into quarters. Lay the bell pepper "chips" on the prepared baking sheet(s) in a single layer with their insides facing up.

3 In a large heated skillet, stir the ground turkey until it's cooked through and crumbled. Add the taco seasoning along with about ⅔ cup water and stir. Add the black beans, corn, and jalapeños, if using. Mix until well combined and heated through.

4 Spoon the turkey-bean mixture over the bell pepper pieces. Sprinkle on the cheese and bake for about 10 minutes, until the cheese is melted.

5 Remove the baking sheet from the oven and, if desired, top with the salsa, pipe on swirls of the yogurt or sour cream, and garnish with scallions.

PER SERVING 4 QUARTERS **220** CALORIES **20 g** PROTEIN **7 g** FAT (**6 g** UNSATURATED FAT, **1 g** SATURATED FAT) **50 mg** CHOLESTEROL **19 g** CARBS **5 g** FIBER **6 g** SUGAR (**6 g** NATURAL SUGAR, **0 g** ADDED SUGAR) **310 mg** SODIUM

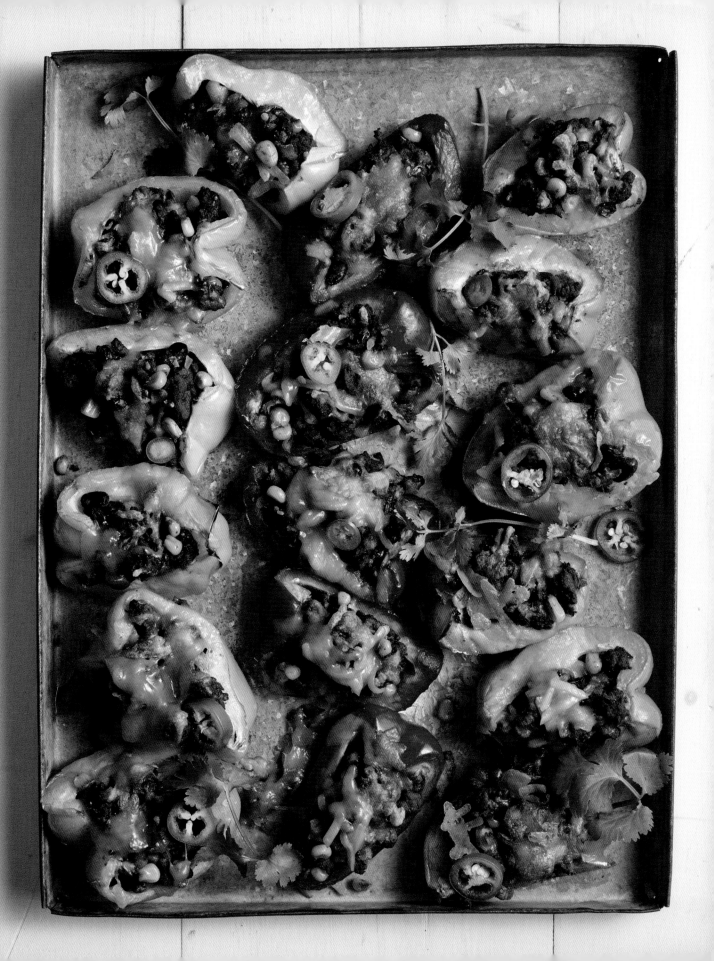

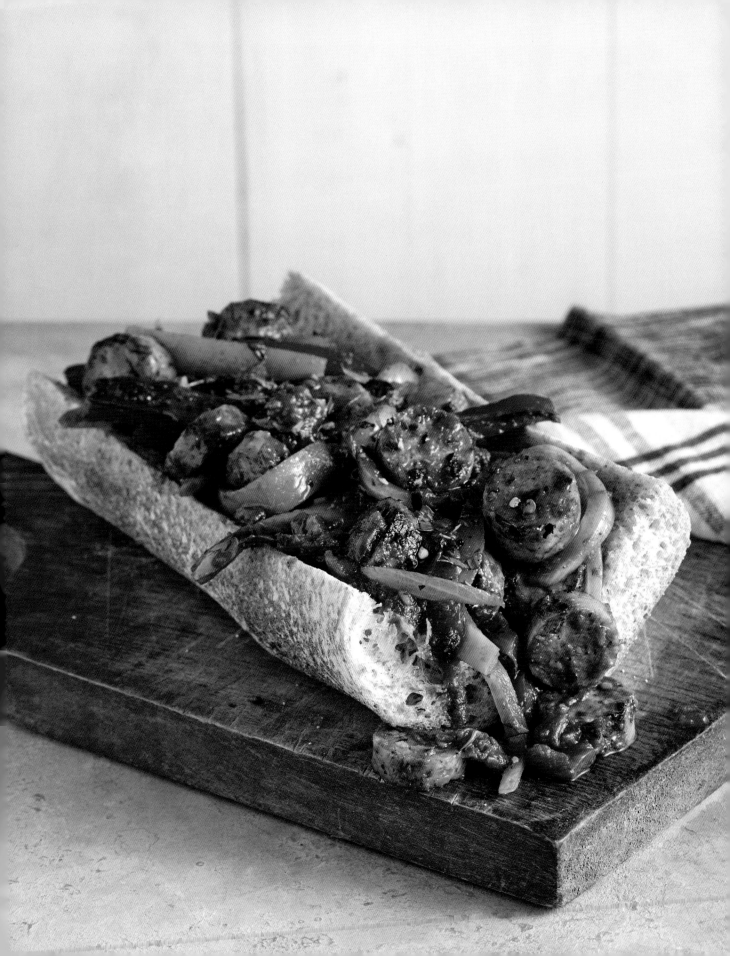

Italian-Style Sausage, Peppers, and Onions

SERVES: 4   PREP TIME: 10 MINUTES   COOK TIME: 40 MINUTES

Every Bauer family party requires a hearty and saucy comfort food dish. This recipe is one that my crew always looks forward to when we gather to celebrate a birthday, anniversary, or other significant milestone. I like to put it out in a big skillet on the table and let everyone help themselves. It's organized chaos while everyone digs into the Italian classic (sometimes to make a heaping hero sandwich, as shown). As they fill their stomachs and the yummy skillet quickly empties, my heart fills with joy.

You can use whatever lean poultry sausages you like, and with so many outstanding options available, you're sure to find a winner. You can also speed up the process by opting for already cooked sausages, so they just have to be warmed. After the sausages are initially cooked and cut into slices, I like to quickly sear the small, bite-size pieces on the hot pan to sop up the mouthwatering flavors and intensify the overall taste. Then you're ready to build the rest.

The dish (without the bun) is low-carb and packed with protein and fiber, which makes it especially good for people looking to manage their blood sugar or cut carbs.

1 pound Italian turkey or chicken sausage

3 red, yellow, or orange bell peppers, sliced

2 large yellow onions, sliced

½ teaspoon Italian seasoning or dried oregano

¼ to ½ cup chopped fresh basil leaves

½ teaspoon garlic powder

½ cup reduced-sodium chicken broth

2 tablespoons tomato paste

1 (14.5-ounce) can diced tomatoes with liquid

Salt and black pepper

Red pepper flakes (optional)

Chopped fresh parsley for garnish (optional)

1 Liberally coat a large and wide skillet with nonstick oil spray and warm over medium-high heat. Add the sausage and cook until browned on all sides and firm enough to slice but not fully cooked through. Remove from the pan and slice the sausages into ¼-inch rounds. Add back to the pan and cook for another minute or so to sear the insides. Transfer to a plate, cover, and set aside.

2 Reapply oil spray to the skillet and add the bell peppers and onions. Cook for 8 to 10 minutes, until they're slightly browned and starting to caramelize. Add the Italian seasoning (or oregano), basil, and garlic and cook, stirring, for another minute.

3 Add the broth, tomato paste, and diced tomatoes with their liquid. Bring to a boil, then reduce the heat to low and add the sausage. Simmer for about 15 minutes, until the sauce thickens. Season with salt, black pepper, and red pepper flakes to taste. Transfer to a serving plate and garnish with parsley, if desired.

PER SERVING **160** CALORIES **13 g** PROTEIN **5 g** FAT (**3.5 g** UNSATURATED FAT, **1.5 g** UNSATURATED FAT) **60 mg** CHOLESTEROL **12 g** CARBS **3 g** FIBER **6 g** SUGAR **770 mg** SODIUM

Lemon Thyme Chicken Paillard with Citrus Vinaigrette

SERVES: 5   PREP TIME: 5 MINUTES   COOK TIME: 10 MINUTES

Chicken Paillard will flatten any notions you have about chicken being boring. In case it's new to you, the French classic calls for chicken that's been pounded thin and seared until it develops a beautiful, crispy browned exterior. Be sure to keep an eye on it once you start cooking—it's thin, so it will sear in a flash (just a few minutes on each side).

I usually pile on heaps of fresh chopped greens when serving this dish; arugula is my go-to, but other salad mixes work just as well. Mound the greens on top of the chicken, and then drizzle on my homemade dressing. The lemony vinaigrette brings all the flavors together, highlighting the fresh thyme that I use to dress up the chicken. (Dressing tip: Make extra and stash it in your fridge. It's amazing with sliced avocado and cucumbers, crudités, or any salad.)

I love how simple, yet sophisticated this recipe is. You can throw it together on busy weeknights—but, served with that yummy dressing and a glass of white wine, it also makes for an elegant dinner for guests.

CHICKEN AND GREENS

3 tablespoons olive oil

½ teaspoon lemon zest

3 tablespoons lemon juice

1 to 2 tablespoons fresh thyme leaves

1 to 2 tablespoons chopped fresh parsley

¼ teaspoon black pepper

1¼ pounds boneless, skinless thin chicken breasts*

Kosher salt

4 to 8 cups leafy greens

* *You can purchase thinly sliced chicken breast or butterfly larger chicken breasts and place them between parchment paper and pound with your fist or a can until they are super thin.*

LEMON VINAIGRETTE
makes ½ cup

2 tablespoons extra virgin olive oil

1½ teaspoons lemon zest

3 tablespoons lemon juice

1 tablespoon rice vinegar

1 teaspoon Dijon mustard

⅛ teaspoon salt

⅛ teaspoon black pepper

1 FOR THE CHICKEN: Whisk the oil, lemon zest, lemon juice, thyme, parsley, and pepper in a large bowl. Add the chicken and coat in the marinade.

2 Warm a large skillet over medium-high heat. Add the chicken and top each piece with a sprinkling of salt. (Work in batches, being careful not to overcrowd the pan.) Cook for about 3 minutes per side (because they are so thin, they will cook fast), seasoning with an additional sprinkling of salt after you flip them, if desired.

3 FOR THE DRESSING: Place all of the dressing ingredients in a small bowl and whisk until well combined.

TO SERVE: Top each chicken paillard with mixed greens and a drizzle of lemon vinaigrette.

PER SERVING 280 CALORIES 26 g PROTEIN 18 g FAT (15.5 g UNSATURATED FAT, 2.5 g SATURATED FAT) 40 mg CHOLESTEROL 2 g CARBS 0 g FIBER 1 g SUGAR (1 g NATURAL SUGAR, 0 g ADDED SUGAR) 330 mg SODIUM

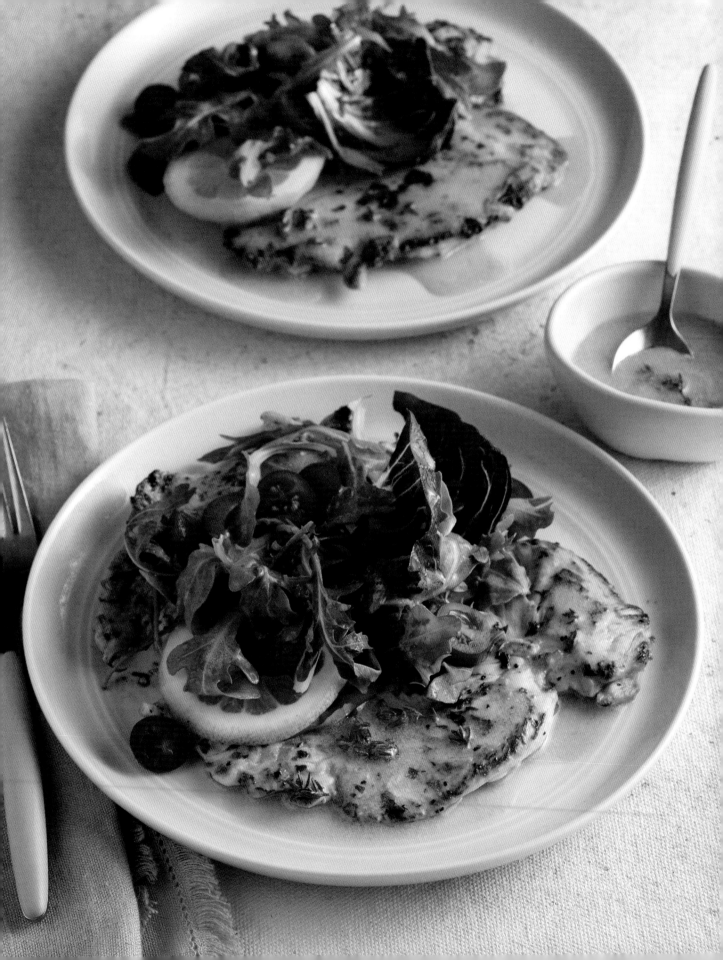

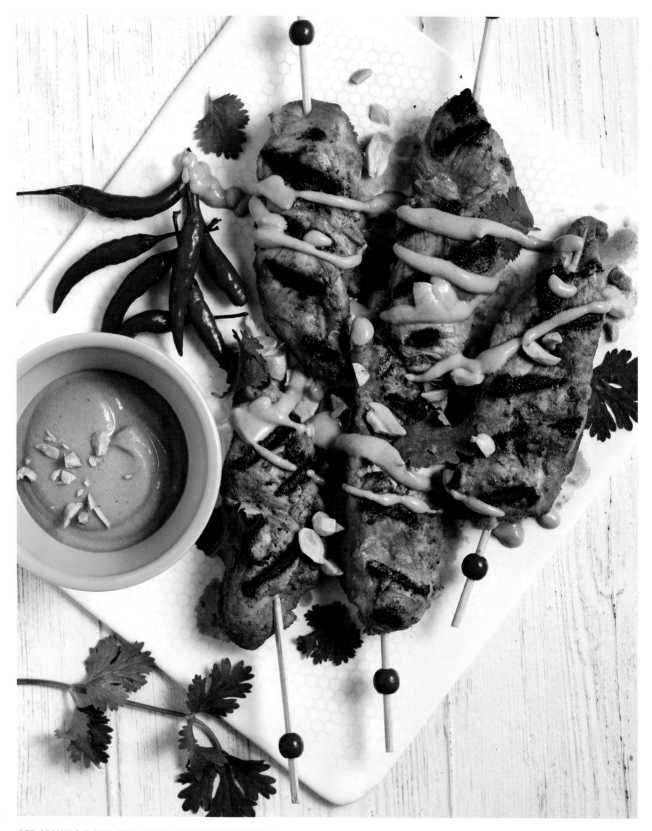

PER SERVING 3 SKEWERS AND ¼ CUP PEANUT SAUCE **300** CALORIES **34 g** PROTEIN **12 g** FAT (**9.5 g** UNSATURATED FAT, **2.5 g** SATURATED FAT) **100 mg** CHOLESTEROL **12 g** CARBS **2 g** FIBER **5 g** SUGAR (**1 g** NATURAL SUGAR, **4 g** ADDED SUGAR) **720 mg** SODIUM

Chicken Satay with Creamy Peanut Sauce

SERVES: 5   PREP TIME: 10 MINUTES, PLUS 30 MINUTES MARINATING
COOK TIME: 10 MINUTES

This dish is delicious together, but the marinade and peanut sauce can easily stand on their own. You can use the marinade for all sorts of chicken dishes, including drumsticks and paillard. And the peanut sauce, which is made with peanut butter and chickpeas, is also fantastic stirred into whole grain pasta (think cold sesame noodles!). In fact, I usually double the sauce recipe so I have leftovers; it keeps for up to two weeks in the fridge.

Pro tip: If you don't have skewers, you can cook the tenders directly on the grill—they're equally delicious.

CHICKEN SKEWERS

- 3 tablespoons canned lite coconut milk
- 2 cloves garlic, minced (or ¼ teaspoon garlic powder)
- 1 tablespoon minced fresh ginger root (or 1½ teaspoons ground ginger)
- 2 tablespoons reduced-sodium soy sauce
- 1 tablespoon honey
- 1 tablespoon toasted sesame oil
- 1½ teaspoons curry powder
- 1½ teaspoons ground turmeric
- 1½ teaspoons ground coriander
- 1½ teaspoons ground cumin
- ½ teaspoon kosher salt
- Zest and juice of 1 lime

- 1½ pounds chicken tenders (about 10)
- 10 bamboo skewers (6 to 8 inches long)
- 2 or 3 scallions, sliced (optional)
- Chopped roasted peanuts for garnish (optional)

PEANUT SAUCE
makes about 1½ cups

- ¾ cup canned chickpeas, rinsed and drained
- ¼ cup peanut butter
- ¼ teaspoon garlic powder
- 3 tablespoons reduced-sodium soy sauce
- 1 tablespoon rice vinegar
- 1 tablespoon toasted sesame oil
- 1½ teaspoons ground ginger
- 1 teaspoon honey
- 1½ to 2 teaspoons sriracha

1   FOR THE CHICKEN: In a large bowl, whisk together the coconut milk, garlic, ginger, soy sauce, honey, oil, curry powder, turmeric, coriander, cumin, salt, lime zest, and lime juice. Add the chicken, stir to fully coat, and marinate in the fridge for at least 30 minutes.

2   While the chicken is marinating, soak the bamboo skewers in water for about 30 minutes.

3   FOR THE SAUCE: Place the chickpeas in a food processor and pulse to break them down. Add the peanut butter, garlic, soy sauce, vinegar, oil, ginger, honey, and sriracha and process to a thick paste. If needed, add warm water, 2 tablespoons at a time, until the sauce is smooth and your desired consistency.

4   Heat an outdoor grill (or indoor grill pan) over medium heat. One at a time, thread each piece of chicken through a skewer, winding it around as needed, or simply push the stick through the middle of the meat. Place them back in the marinade bowl until all the skewers are completed.

5   Mist the skewered meat with nonstick oil spray. Place on the grill and cook undisturbed for 3 to 5 minutes, until the bottom is seared. Mist again with oil spray, flip, and cook for 3 to 4 minutes on the second side, until the chicken is cooked through. Garnish with scallions and peanuts, if desired, and serve with peanut sauce on the side.

Oven-Braised Pork Tenderloin with Tangy Apple Chutney

SERVES: 3   PREP TIME: 10 MINUTES,
PLUS AT LEAST 30 MINUTES IN THE REFRIGERATOR   COOK TIME: 1 HOUR

In one of my all-time favorite scenes from *The Brady Bunch*, Peter Brady does his very best impression of Humphrey Bogart as he repeats the refrain "pork chops and applesauce" to describe that night's dinner. Way back in the day (ahem), my siblings and I would have fun mimicking Peter and Humphrey and basically drive my parents crazy, haha. Needless to say, this was a fun recipe for me to create.

First, I opted for a chunky apple chutney instead of applesauce. Tart Granny Smith apples are combined with a touch of honey for sweetness, cinnamon for warmth, and a kick of ginger and red pepper flakes for delicate heat. Raisins add additional texture and sweetness. (You may choose to omit the honey and use red apples to maximize sweetness.)

For the meat, I use a lean cut that shares a similar nutritional profile to that of chicken breast—pork tenderloin. Its delicate flavor soaks up the vibrant cumin and fennel seeds in my homemade spice rub. While five minutes of marinating time is fine, half an hour is better, and overnight is ideal—the longer, the better. In fact, I always prep the meat the night before, because it saves me a lot of time when I start to cook the dish.

Braising the tenderloin is key. The two-step process—first, searing the meat on the stovetop and then finishing it in the oven—seals in moisture and enables the flavors to really harmonize. Once you've transferred it to the oven, just set your timer and let the dish do the rest. The Bradys—and Humphrey—would be proud!

PORK

1 pound pork tenderloin (cut into 2 pieces if it doesn't fit into your pot)

1 teaspoon kosher salt

½ teaspoon ground cumin

¼ teaspoon black pepper

¼ teaspoon fennel seeds, roughly chopped

Parsley or cilantro for garnish (optional)

APPLE CHUTNEY
makes about 2¼ cups

1 small yellow onion, chopped (about ¾ cup)

1 tablespoon minced fresh ginger root (or 1 teaspoon ground ginger)

¾ teaspoon kosher salt

¼ teaspoon ground mustard seeds

1 teaspoon ground cinnamon

⅛ teaspoon red pepper flakes, or more to taste

¼ cup orange juice

2 tablespoons apple cider vinegar

4 cups peeled, cored, and chopped Granny Smith apples (about 3 apples)

¼ cup raisins

2 teaspoons honey (optional)

1 Preheat the oven to 350°F.

2 Pat the pork dry with paper towels and season with the salt, cumin, pepper, and fennel seeds. Cover and place in the fridge for at least 30 minutes, or ideally overnight.

3 Liberally coat the bottom of a Dutch oven or other oven-safe pot (make sure you have a lid that fits) with nonstick oil spray and warm over medium heat. Add the tenderloin and sear on all sides for a total of 6 to 7 minutes. Remove from the pot and set aside. Reapply oil spray, add the onion, ginger, and salt, and cook for 1 to 2 minutes. Add the ground mustard, cinnamon, and red pepper flakes and cook, stirring constantly, for 1 to 2 more minutes. Add the orange juice and vinegar and stir, gently scraping up any bits from the bottom of the pot. Add the apples, raisins, and honey, if using, and stir to combine.

4 Add the tenderloin back to the pot with the apple mixture, cover, and transfer to the oven to cook for 20 to 25 minutes, flipping it halfway through, until the pork reaches an internal temperature of 145°F. If the pan becomes dry at the halfway mark, add a splash of water, broth, or additional orange juice.

If you prefer your chutney on the smoother side, mash the larger apple chunks with a spoon or spatula before serving. Garnish with parsley or cilantro, if desired.

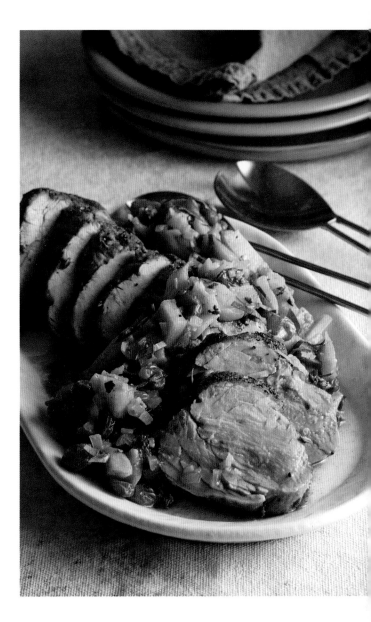

PER SERVING **240** CALORIES **25 g** PROTEIN **3 g** FAT (**2 g** UNSATURATED FAT, **1 g** SATURATED FAT) **75 mg** CHOLESTEROL **28 g** CARBS **5 g** FIBER **18 g** SUGAR (**18 g** NATURAL SUGAR, **0 g** ADDED SUGAR) **900 mg** SODIUM

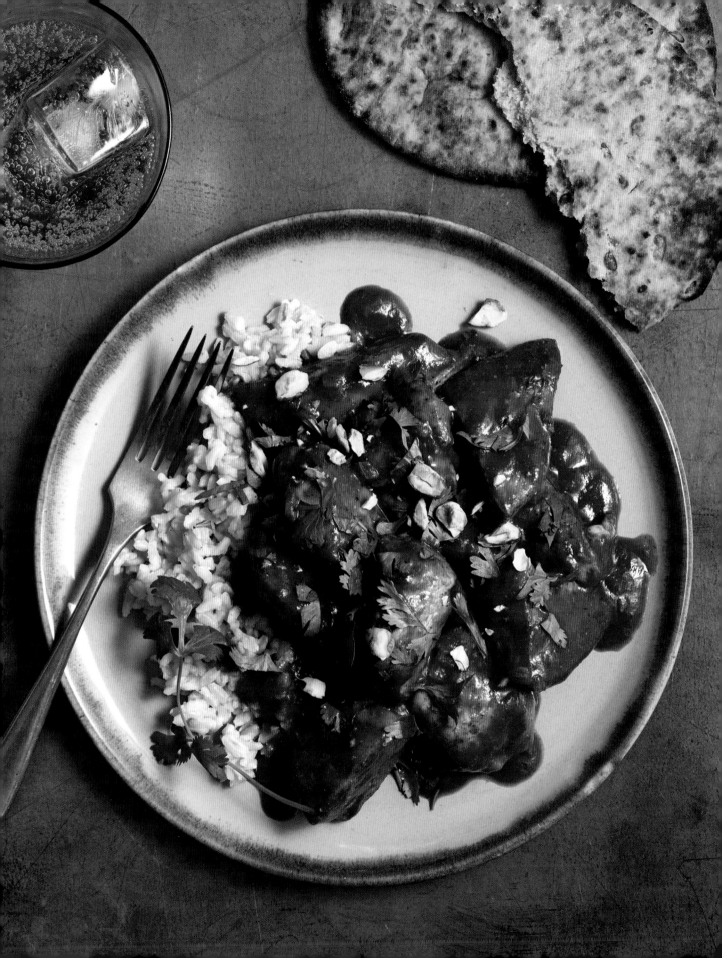

Indian Butter Chicken

SERVES: 4   PREP TIME: 10 MINUTES   COOK TIME: 30 MINUTES

My son Cole shares my affinity for Indian food and its bright, bold signature flavors. We savor the well-rounded spices and the vibrant spirit that permeates each dish. Cole requested I share this recipe in the book, and I hope you love it as much as we do. One of the key ingredients is garam masala, an Indian seasoning blend that, in Hindi, translates to "hot spices." It's not so much that garam masala is super spicy, per se, but these are full-bodied flavors that don't shy away from making a statement. You can purchase a premade garam masala mix, as I've done here, which traditionally includes ingredients like cumin, coriander, bay leaves, black and white peppercorns, cinnamon, cloves, and cardamom.

I serve the dish over brown basmati rice (or sometimes cauliflower rice), drizzling it liberally with extra sauce. It's an awesome—and yummy—journey to New Delhi or Bombay!

CHICKEN

- 1½ pounds chicken breast, cut into large chunks
- ¼ teaspoon kosher salt
- 1 teaspoon garam masala

BUTTER SAUCE

- ½ yellow onion, finely diced
- 3 cloves garlic, minced (or ½ teaspoon garlic powder)
- 2 tablespoons butter
- 1 tablespoon plus 1 teaspoon garam masala
- 1 teaspoon ground cumin
- 1 teaspoon ground ginger
- 1 to 2 tablespoons lemon juice
- 1 (6-ounce) can tomato paste
- 1 (14-ounce) can lite coconut milk
- ⅛ teaspoon ground cayenne (skip if you're sensitive to heat)
- ½ teaspoon kosher salt, or more to taste
- Minced fresh cilantro or parsley for garnish (optional)
- Toasted pistachios for garnish (optional)

1 FOR THE CHICKEN: Liberally mist a large skillet with nonstick oil spray and warm over medium-high heat. Add the chicken to the pan, mist the top with oil spray, and sprinkle on the salt and garam masala. Cook for 5 to 7 minutes on each side, until browned on the outside but not completely cooked through. Transfer to a plate, cover, and set aside.

2 FOR THE SAUCE: Mist the same skillet with oil spray and warm over medium heat. Add the onion and cook until softened and slightly browned, 3 to 4 minutes. Add the garlic and cook for 30 to 60 seconds. Reduce the heat to low and add the butter, garam masala, cumin, ginger, lemon juice, tomato paste, coconut milk, cayenne, and salt. Stir to combine, deglazing the pan, and simmer, uncovered, stirring occasionally, for about 10 minutes to allow the sauce to thicken. Taste and season with extra salt, a dash of cayenne, and lemon juice, if desired.

3 Add the chicken back to the skillet with the sauce, mix well, and simmer, uncovered, for another 5 to 10 minutes, until everything is hot. Transfer to a serving plate and garnish with cilantro or parsley and pistachios, if desired.

PER SERVING 350 CALORIES 41 g PROTEIN 13 g FAT (5 g UNSATURATED FAT, 8 g SATURATED FAT) 115 mg CHOLESTEROL 17 g CARBS 3 g FIBER 8 g SUGAR (8 g NATURAL SUGAR, 0 g ADDED SUGAR) 690 mg SODIUM

Middle Eastern Kofta with Roasted Garlic Tahini

SERVES: 6   PREP TIME: 20 MINUTES   COOK TIME: 45 MINUTES

Kofta—meat kebabs popular throughout India, the Middle East, and parts of Central Asia—is a dish often served with a fiery harissa sauce that involves Tunisian chili paste. Here, I've diversified the delicious classic by using lean ground poultry mixed with grated zucchini and a bouquet of seasonings like parsley, mint, scallions, cumin, coriander, and paprika. You can grill 'em—indoors or outdoors—or bake them in the oven. Oh, and don't forget the "special sauce," a creamy and garlicky tahini made for dipping, drizzling, and devouring. The combo is addictively good!

ROASTED GARLIC TAHINI SAUCE

- 4 to 6 medium unpeeled cloves garlic, stem ends sliced off
- 2 teaspoons extra virgin olive oil, divided
- 3 tablespoons tahini (sesame paste)
- ⅓ cup fresh parsley leaves
- ¼ cup fresh mint leaves
- 2 tablespoons lemon juice
- ¼ teaspoon kosher salt, or more to taste
- ⅛ teaspoon black pepper, or more to taste

KOFTAS

- 2 pounds ground turkey (90 to 93% lean)
- 1 medium unpeeled zucchini, grated and drained of excess moisture
- ¼ cup fresh parsley leaves
- ¼ cup fresh mint leaves
- 4 scallions, chopped
- 2 cloves garlic, peeled
- ⅓ cup uncooked old-fashioned oats (or whole grain breadcrumbs)
- ½ teaspoon ground cumin
- 1 teaspoon ground coriander
- ½ teaspoon smoked paprika
- ½ teaspoon kosher salt, or more to taste
- ¼ teaspoon black pepper, or more to taste
- 1 tablespoon olive oil

1 Preheat the oven to 400°F. Mist a baking sheet with nonstick oil spray and set aside. If grilling, soak the bamboo skewers in water for about 30 minutes while you prep the dish. If using the oven roasting method, there's no need to soak (you'll skewer the koftas after they're cooked).

2 FOR THE SAUCE: Place the garlic cloves on a piece of foil and drizzle with 1 teaspoon of the oil. Make a small pouch with the foil around the garlic and roast until cloves are lightly browned and tender, about 30 minutes. Allow to cool slightly, then gently squeeze so the cloves release from their shells. Set aside to slightly cool. Leave the oven on if you are roasting your koftas.

3 In the bowl of a food processor or high-speed blender, combine the roasted garlic, tahini, 3 tablespoons warm water, the parsley, mint, lemon juice, salt, and pepper. Process until smooth, adding an additional 1 to 2 tablespoons warm water if it is too thick. Set aside until koftas are ready.

4 FOR THE KOFTAS: Place the ground turkey in a large bowl. Put the grated zucchini in a bunch of paper towels or a kitchen towel and ring out any extra liquid. Add the grated and drained zucchini to the turkey. Set aside.

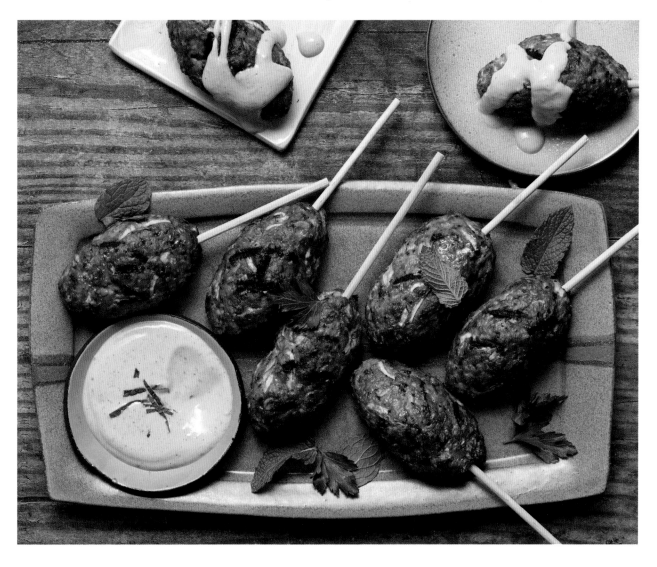

5 In the bowl of a food processor, combine the parsley, mint, scallions, garlic, oats, cumin, coriander, paprika, salt, pepper, and oil. Pulse until finely chopped. Add the mixture to the bowl with turkey and zucchini and mix until everything is well incorporated.

6 Using a ¼-cup measure, form about 18 piles of meat on your prepared baking sheet. Using wet hands (this will prevent the batter from sticking), form each portion into an oval-shaped log. If you are grilling, one at a time, thread a skewer through the length of each kofta log. Skip this step if you

are roasting in the oven. Liberally mist the tops with oil spray.

7 Grill (indoors or outdoors) over medium-high heat for 6 to 8 minutes per side. Or, alternatively, roast in the oven on the baking sheet for about 20 minutes, and then broil for a final 2 to 4 minutes to brown the tops, watching closely so they do not burn. When they come out of the oven you can decide to skewer the cooked meat for a pretty presentation or leave as is. Serve the koftas with the tahini sauce on the side.

PER SERVING 3 KOFTAS WITH SAUCE 320 CALORIES 35 g PROTEIN 19 g FAT (16 g UNSATURATED FAT, 3 g SATURATED FAT) 65 mg CHOLESTEROL 10 g CARBS 2 g FIBER 1 g SUGAR (1 g NATURAL SUGAR, 0 g ADDED SUGAR) 350 mg SODIUM

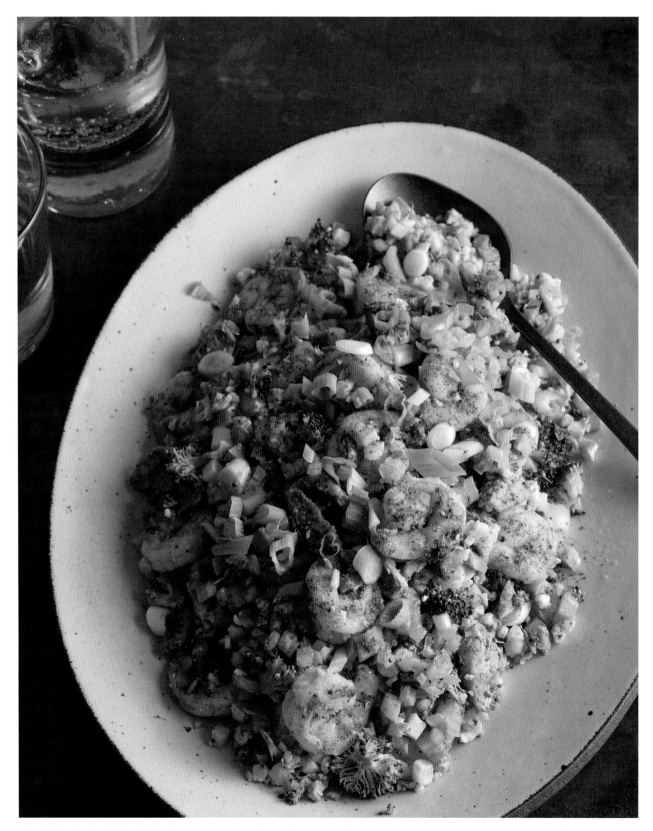

PER SERVING ABOUT 2 CUPS **270** CALORIES **34 g** PROTEIN **9 g** FAT (**7 g** UNSATURATED FAT, **2 g** SATURATED FAT) **185 mg** CHOLES-TEROL **15 g** CARBS **5 g** FIBER **5 g** SUGAR (**5 g** NATURAL SUGAR, **0 g** ADDED SUGAR) **860 mg** SODIUM

Louisiana Dirty Rice with Sausage and Shrimp

SERVES: 5   PREP TIME: 10 MINUTES   COOK TIME: 20 MINUTES

Boy, are your taste buds in for a spicy surprise . . . this dish is HOT. It gets its "dirty" title from two dirty little secrets: First, the rice is a medley of veggies in disguise. And second, it's fiery hot in the best possible way. (If you can't stand heat, just omit the cayenne and it'll turn out perfect.) Feel free to use any 6-cup combo of riced veggies—anything goes.

FYI: The Cajun spice blend is salt-free—no sodium . . . zero, zilch! So you can make a big batch and stash it in your pantry for a go-to seasoning blend.

CAJUN SPICE BLEND

1 tablespoon paprika

1½ teaspoons onion powder

1½ teaspoons garlic powder

1½ teaspoons ground black pepper

½ teaspoon dried oregano

½ teaspoon dried thyme

¼ to ½ teaspoon ground cayenne (depending on your heat preference)

RICED VEGGIES*

2 cups riced broccoli

2 cups riced cauliflower

2 cups riced carrot

¼ teaspoon kosher salt

*   If you can't find "riced" veggies, you can hand-chop veggies into small rice-like pieces or pulse florets and carrot chunks in a food processor in small batches, being careful not to puree.

SHRIMP AND SAUSAGE

1 large yellow onion, finely diced (about 2 cups)

1 large red bell pepper, finely diced

3 cloves garlic, minced (or ½ teaspoon garlic powder)

1 pound precooked poultry sausage, cut into small pieces (andouille-style if possible)

1 pound raw shrimp, peeled, deveined, and tail off

6 scallions, sliced

¼ cup chopped fresh parsley

1 FOR THE CAJUN SEASONING: In a bowl, combine all the spice blend ingredients. Set aside.

2 FOR THE RICED VEGGIES: Set an oven rack to the middle position and preheat the oven to 425°F. Liberally coat 2 baking sheets with oil spray. Spread the riced veggies on the baking sheets in a single layer. Mist the tops with additional oil spray and sprinkle salt over the tops. Roast for 15 minutes.

3 FOR THE SHRIMP AND SAUSAGE: While the riced veggies cook, mist a large skillet with oil spray and warm over medium-high heat. Add the onion, bell pepper, and garlic and cook for about 5 minutes, stirring occasionally, until the veggies are softened and slightly browned. Add the sausage and cook for about 3 minutes to brown all sides. Mist the pan with additional oil spray if it becomes dry. Add the shrimp and Cajun seasoning blend (it will look like a lot, but it will get incorporated as the shrimp cooks). Continue to stir until the shrimp is cooked through, about 5 minutes (depending on the size of your shrimp), scraping the bottom of the pan to incorporate the tasty browned bits.

TO SERVE: Remove the riced veggies from the oven and toss into the skillet with the shrimp and sausage, or place the veggies on a platter and layer the sausage and shrimp on top. Garnish with scallions and parsley.

Mexican Meatballs in Chipotle Tomato Sauce

SERVES: 6 PREP TIME: 15 MINUTES COOK TIME: 30 MINUTES

Whenever I serve these—as an app with toothpicks or loaded on a dinner platter smothered with melty cheese and tasty toppings—I get the same reaction: "Mmmm, meatballs!" These gems are loaded with ingredients that to deliver big on flavor and health. Fire-roasted tomatoes provide the antioxidant lycopene, shown to help protect against certain cancers. Black beans are rich in magnesium and potassium, minerals to help enhance heart health. And then there's the oats, chili peppers, and countless other superstar extras. Cue the fiesta!

MEATBALLS

¼ cup rolled oats

¼ cup milk

1¼ pounds ground turkey (90 to 93% lean)

1 egg white

1 canned chipotle chile, seeded and minced

1½ tablespoons adobo sauce from the chipotle can

½ teaspoon kosher salt

¼ teaspoon black pepper

1 teaspoon ground cumin

½ teaspoon cumin seeds

1 teaspoon garlic powder

1 teaspoon onion powder

½ (15-ounce) can black beans (¾ cup), rinsed, drained, and mashed with a fork

1 teaspoon dried oregano

1 medium carrot, shredded

3 scallions, chopped

SAUCE

1 medium red onion, finely chopped

2 canned chipotle chiles in adobo sauce

1 teaspoon garlic powder

1 tablespoon ground cumin

½ teaspoon kosher salt

½ (15-ounce) can black beans (¾ cup), rinsed and drained

1 (28-ounce) can fire-roasted crushed tomatoes

OPTIONAL TOPPERS

Shredded Mexican cheese or other preferred cheese, cilantro, diced avocado, corn

1 FOR THE MEATBALLS: Preheat the oven to 350°F. Line a baking sheet with parchment paper. Set aside.

2 In a small bowl, combine the oats and milk. Let sit while you assemble the rest of the ingredients.

3 In a large bowl, combine the ground turkey, egg white, chipotle chile, adobo sauce, salt, pepper, ground cumin, cumin seeds, garlic powder, and onion powder. Add the oat mixture, beans, oregano, carrot, and scallions and stir together. Using a small ice cream scoop or your hands, form into 1½-inch meatballs and place onto the prepared baking sheet. If they seem too soft or wet, put the sheet in the freezer for about 20 minutes. You'll then be able to roll them between wet palms to give them a smooth surface. Transfer to the oven and bake for 20 to 25 minutes.

4 FOR THE SAUCE: Mist a medium pot with oil spray. Add the onion and cook until softened, 7 minutes or so. Add the chipotle chile, garlic, cumin, salt, beans, and. tomatoes and bring to a boil. Reduce the heat and simmer for 5 to 8 minutes, stirring occasionally. Add a little water if it is too thick. Place the meatballs in the sauce, gently stir, and let them simmer for 15 to 20 minutes. TO SERVE: Place the saucy meatballs on a serving plate and top with cheese, cilantro, avocado, and corn, if desired.

PER SERVING 5 MEATBALLS WITH SAUCE 260 CALORIES 28 g PROTEIN 8 g FAT (6.5 g UNSATURATED FAT, 1.5 g SATURATED FAT) 40 mg CHOLESTEROL 24 g CARBS 7 g FIBER 5 g SUGAR (5 g NATURAL SUGAR, 0 g ADDED SUGAR) 810 mg SODIUM

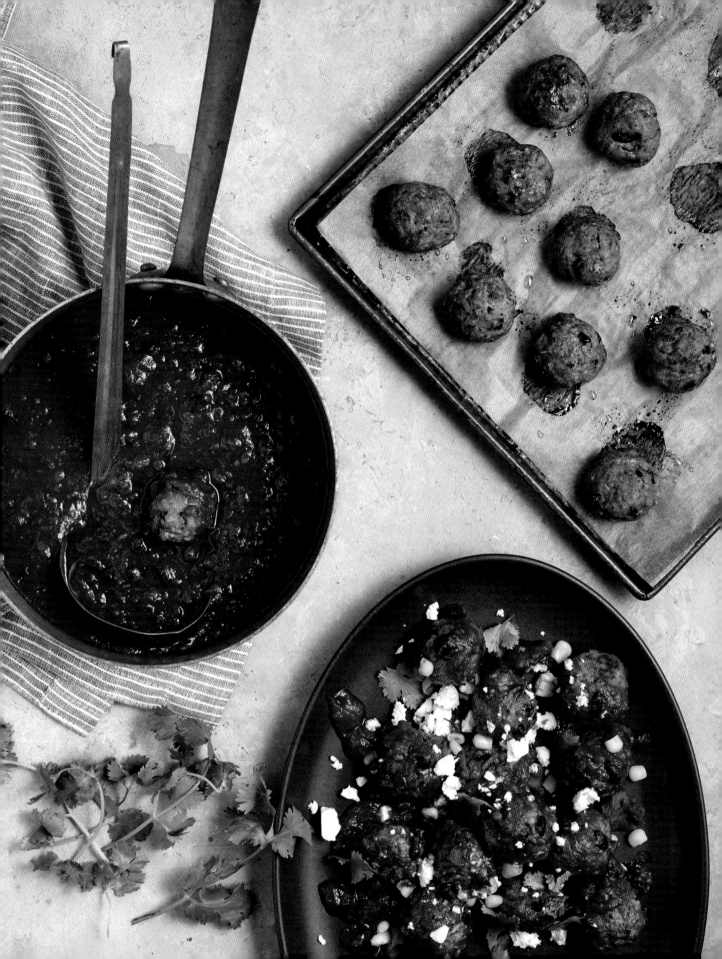

Roast Beef Tenderloin
with White Wine Mushroom Sauce

SERVES: 12   PREP TIME: 20 MINUTES   TOTAL TIME: 1 HOUR

I created this holiday roast with my foodie friend Tieghan, the brain behind *Half Baked Harvest*. Tieghan is an uber-talented chef, and we had a ball cooking up this winner dinner for an NBC special series. Roasts are terrific because they're fairly fuss-free, feed a large crowd, and are irresistible. When it comes to the meat selection, I choose beef tenderloin, because it's a super-lean yet tender cut. However, it can also be *very* pricey, so definitely look for sales, and save this dish for special family gatherings. Also, ask your butcher to tie it up at the market to save yourself a step; this helps to maintain its shape and allows it to cook more evenly in the oven.

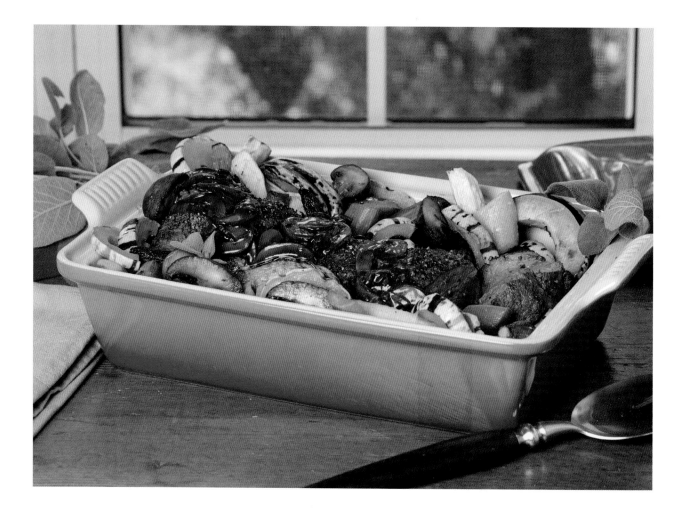

BEEF TENDERLOIN

16 ounces cremini mushrooms halved

1 tablespoon kosher salt, divided

⅛ teaspoon black pepper

1 whole beef tenderloin (4 to 5 pounds), tied with string

2 tablespoons Dijon mustard

3 tablespoons peppercorns crushed, or fresh black pepper

1 to 2 tablespoons butter, melted (optional)

1 medium Delicata squash, seeded and cut into ¾-inch rings

1 pound carrots, cut into 1-inch) chunks

3 parsnips, peeled and cut into 1-inch chunks

1 to 2 red onions, cut into small wedges

3 to 4 fresh thyme sprigs

MUSHROOM SAUCE

2 tablespoons extra virgin olive oil

1 shallot, minced

1 pound mushrooms, roughly sliced (any type)

½ teaspoon kosher salt

¼ teaspoon black pepper

2 tablespoons fresh thyme leaves

1 tablespoon fresh chopped sage

3 tablespoons balsamic vinegar

¼ to ½ cup dry white wine (or broth)

1 **FOR THE BEEF TENDERLOIN:** Preheat the oven to 425°F. Liberally mist a large skillet with nonstick olive oil spray and warm over medium-high heat. Add the cremini and cook 5 minutes or until just tender. Transfer to the bottom of a roasting pan and sprinkle on ⅛ teaspoon salt and pepper.

2 Add the beef on top of the mushrooms in the roasting pan, and rub with mustard, crushed peppercorns, and 2 teaspoons salt. Drizzle the optional melted butter over the top of the beef.

3 Toss the squash, carrots, parsnips, and onions into the pan evenly around the beef, mist them generously with olive oil spray, season with a sprinkling of salt and pepper and nestle in thyme sprigs. Roast in the oven for 15 minutes. Then, adjust temperature to 375°F, give the veggies a good stir, and cook for an additional 30 to 45 minutes (or until the beef reaches an internal temperature of 145°F). If you like your steak rare, while its not recommended for safety reasons, remove when the thickest part hits 125°F. It's always best to use a meat thermometer.

4 Transfer the beef and veggies to a serving plate and cover with foil for at least 10 minutes before slicing to lock in the juices.

5 **FOR THE MUSHROOM SAUCE:** Heat the olive oil in a large skillet over medium heat. Add the shallot and cook until fragrant, 1 to 2 minutes. Add the mushrooms and cook 8 to 10 minutes, stirring only occasionally to allow the mushrooms to become golden and caramelized. Add the thyme, sage, salt, and pepper. Cook, stirring occasionally, about 5 more minutes. Add the balsamic vinegar and wine. Cook for 2 final minutes, deglazing the pan. If you prefer more liquid, add a splash of additional wine or broth. Season with extra salt and pepper to taste. Remove from the heat and serve on top of the roast or on the side.

For a smooth gravy, transfer the finished sauce to a blender or food processor with 1 cup additional reduced-sodium broth and puree until smooth.

PER SERVING **320** CALORIES **37 g** PROTEIN **11 g** FAT (**7.5 g** UNSATURATED FAT, **3.5 g** SATURATED FAT) **95 mg** CHOLESTEROL **20 g** CARBS **4 g** FIBER **7 g** SUGAR (**7 g** NATURAL SUGAR, **0 g** ADDED SUGAR) **650 mg** SODIUM

Asian Shiitake Meatloaf with General Tso's Glaze

SERVES: 6   PREP TIME: 15 MINUTES   COOK TIME: 1½ HOURS

In the comfort food constellation, classic meatloaf and Chinese takeout are two of the brightest stars. In this recipe, they've collided into each other and left a supernova of flavor in their wake. The result is a tender, super-moist meatloaf, teeming with Asian flavors. What makes this dish really stand out is my homemade General Tso's thick, sweet sauce. It has zero added sugar—instead, I optimize sweetness by reducing pineapple juice and mixing it with soy sauce and rice vinegar. (I'm telling you, I was like an excited chemist developing this recipe.)

2 cups pineapple juice

2 tablespoons rice vinegar

¼ cup plus 2 tablespoons reduced-sodium soy sauce, divided

¼ cup uncooked old-fashioned oats

1 tablespoon plus 1 teaspoon arrowroot flour or cornstarch

1½ cups shredded coleslaw mix (or cabbage)

1 cup grated carrot (1 to 2 medium carrots)

2 cups sliced shiitake mushroom caps (3.5-ounce package)

1 cup sliced scallions (7 to 8 scallions)

2 tablespoons ground flaxseeds

1 large egg, lightly beaten

1½ teaspoons ground ginger

1½ teaspoons garlic powder

¼ teaspoon red pepper flakes

1 pound ground turkey (90 to 93% lean)

1 to 2 tablespoons sesame seeds

1 Place the pineapple juice in a small saucepan and bring to a boil. Adjust the heat to low and simmer until the liquid is reduced to roughly 1 cup, about 30 minutes. Remove from the heat and stir in the vinegar and ¼ cup of the soy sauce. Transfer ¼ cup of this mixture into a small bowl, stir in the oats, and set aside. (This will be added to your meat mixture later.)

2 In a small cup, stir together the arrowroot or cornstarch and 2 tablespoons water until the starch is completely dissolved. Add to the pan with the remaining pineapple juice mixture, stir, and bring to a boil over medium-high heat, stirring constantly. Turn off the heat, cover, and set aside. The sauce will thicken while you prepare the meatloaf.

3 Preheat the oven to 375°F. Mist an 8½ by 4½-inch loaf pan with nonstick oil spray. Set aside.

4 In a large bowl, combine the shredded cabbage, carrot, mushrooms, scallions, flaxseeds, egg, ginger, garlic powder, and red pepper flakes. Then add the ground turkey, soaked oats, and remaining 2 tablespoons soy sauce, and stir to combine. Transfer the mixture into the prepared loaf pan. Tent loosely with foil or lay a piece of parchment paper on top and bake for 30 minutes.

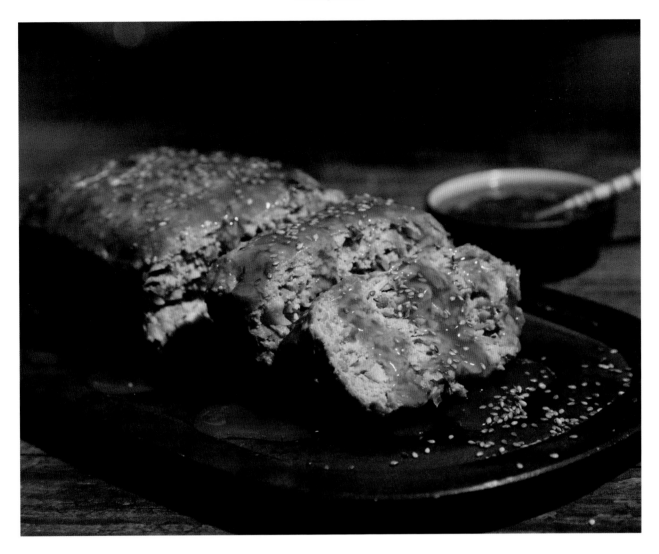

5 Remove the foil (or parchment paper) and pat the top to remove any extra liquid that has accumulated (don't worry about liquid on the sides; just let it be). Spread about ¼ cup of the thickened pineapple sauce on top and sprinkle on some sesame seeds. Place back in the oven and bake uncovered for another 30 minutes, or until the top starts to brown and an internal thermometer reads 160°F when inserted in the center of the loaf.

6 Remove from the oven and let sit for 10 minutes before slicing (this will allow the liquid generated from the veggies to be reabsorbed for extra moistness). Warm the remaining sauce and spoon over the top or serve it on the side.

PER SERVING 220 CALORIES **19 g** PROTEIN **8 g** FAT (**6.5 g** UNSATURATED FAT, **1.5 g** SATURATED FAT) **60 mg** CHOLESTEROL **21 g** CARBS **2 g** FIBER **12 g** SUGAR (**12 g** NATURAL SUGAR, **0 g** ADDED SUGAR) **270 mg** SODIUM

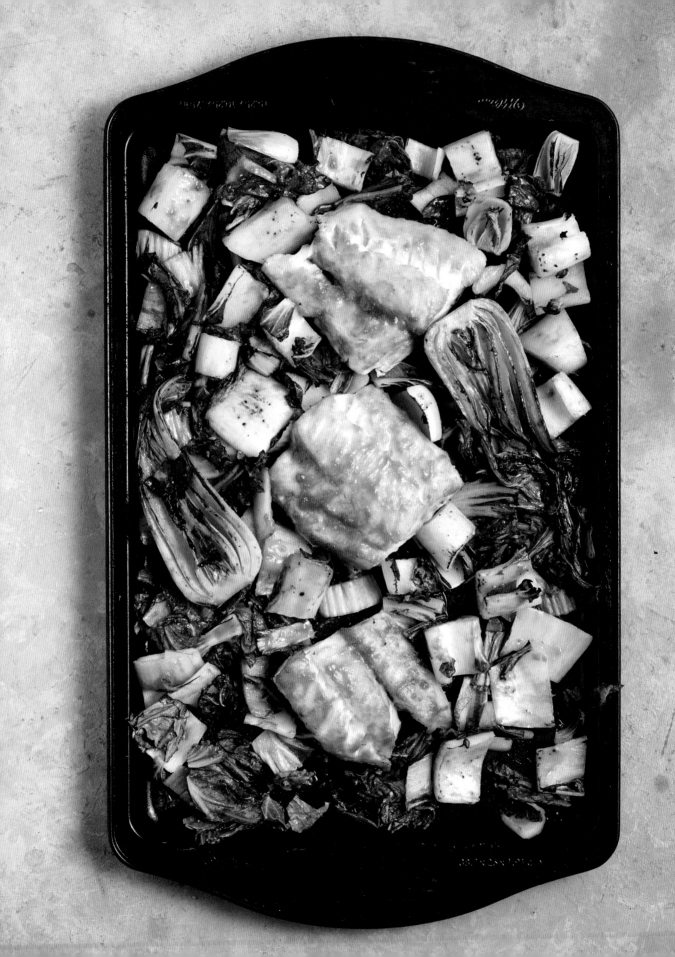

Oven-Roasted Miso Cod with Saucy Bok Choy

SERVES: 3   PREP TIME: 5 MINUTES   COOK TIME: 10 MINUTES

This dish marries tender, flaky cod with crisp bok choy, and then douses the power couple in a sweet-and-savory miso glaze. Bok choy is one of those veggies my family adores. It's part of the "cruciferous" clan of vegetables. It boasts a firm texture and tender green leaves, which are wellsprings of nutrients like vitamins A, C, and K; beta-carotene; folate; and more.

Some advice for the cod: Position the fish close to the broiler, about two to three inches away from the heat, to develop a caramelized crust on the surface of the fillets, helping to intensifying the miso taste. It's a swimmingly flavorful dish that provides serious health perks.

2 tablespoons miso paste

1 tablespoon reduced-sodium soy sauce

1 tablespoon rice vinegar

2 tablespoons honey

10 cups chopped (1- to 2-inch pieces) bok choy (from 1 large bunch)

1 tablespoon olive oil

1¼ pounds cod fillets, patted dry

Toasted sesame seeds for garnish (optional)

1 Set an oven rack to the highest position and another to the middle. Preheat the broiler. Liberally mist 2 baking sheets with oil spray and set aside.

2 In a small bowl, whisk together the miso, soy sauce, vinegar, and honey. Set aside.

3 In large bowl, toss the bok choy with the oil to coat. Add ¼ cup of the prepared miso sauce mixture and toss gently to evenly coat the leaves. Spread the bok choy on one of the baking sheets and set aside.

4 Place the cod fillets in a single layer on the second baking sheet and spoon or brush the remaining miso sauce mixture on top.

5 Place the cod in the oven on the highest rack and the bok choy on the middle rack and cook for 8 minutes, or until the miso sauce starts to get golden and caramelized on the fillets (when ready, the cod will flake with a fork). Remove the cod from the oven, then move the bok choy to the highest rack and cook for 1 to 2 minutes, until slightly crispy at the edges.

TO SERVE: Transfer veggies and fish to a plate and garnish with extra toasted sesame seeds, if desired.

PER SERVING 290 CALORIES 38 g PROTEIN 6 g FAT (5 g UNSATURATED FAT, 1 g SATURATED FAT) 80 mg CHOLESTEROL 21 g CARBS 3 g FIBER 15 g SUGAR (5 g NATURAL SUGAR, 10 g ADDED SUGAR) 800 mg SODIUM

Coconut-Crusted Shrimp with Asian Dipping Sauce

SERVES: 4   PREP TIME: 15 MINUTES   COOK TIME: 10 MINUTES

Coconut + shrimp is a match made in culinary heaven. I rely on almond flour to turn this into a grain-free dish, which complements the coconut flavor beautifully. If you're gluten-free, use gluten-free soy sauce or tamari. Substituting with coconut aminos, a salty-sweet sauce that you can swap for soy sauce, makes the recipe paleo-friendly. If you have coconut oil spray on hand, it's ideal for misting the shrimp's tops, but really any oil spray will work well.

A few quick tips: I like to use the shrimp tail as a handle when dredging so I can keep my other hand dry and clean, and to use for pressing the coconut topping around each shrimp. And while I typically place the shrimp directly on a baking sheet, a wire rack (if you have one) will create a crispier finish, since it allows the heat to circulate around the bottom of the shrimp as they cook. Just mist the rack beforehand with oil spray so your beauties don't stick. Also, you must whip up the Spicy Asian Dipping Sauce—it's non-negotiable!

SHRIMP

2 large egg whites

1 teaspoon reduced-sodium soy sauce

½ cup unsweetened shredded coconut

½ cup blanched almond flour (or other preferred flour)

1 teaspoon garlic powder

½ teaspoon black pepper

1 to 1½ pounds large raw shrimp, peeled and deveined, tail on, patted dry

DIPPING SAUCE

¼ cup reduced-sodium soy sauce

¼ cup rice vinegar

2 teaspoons toasted sesame oil

¼ to ½ teaspoon red pepper flakes, or more to taste

1 scallion, thinly sliced

1 FOR THE SHRIMP: Set an oven rack to the middle position and preheat the oven to 450°F. Mist a baking sheet with nonstick oil spray. Set aside.

2 In a small bowl, whisk the egg whites and soy sauce. In a second shallow, wide bowl, combine the coconut, almond flour, garlic powder, and black pepper.

3 Using one hand to hold the tail of the shrimp, dip each shrimp into the egg mixture, then use your other hand to fully coat and press on the coconut topping. Transfer to the prepared baking sheet and repeat with the remaining shrimp.

4 Lightly mist the tops of the shrimp with oil spray and bake for 5 minutes. Flip the shrimp using the tail as a handle, being careful not to disturb the coconut coating. Bake for another 3 to 5 minutes, until the coating is slightly golden and the shrimp are completely cooked through.

5 FOR THE DIPPING SAUCE: While the shrimp are cooking, whisk together all of the sauce ingredients. Serve the shrimp with the dipping sauce on the side.

PER SERVING: SHRIMP WITH 1 TABLESPOON DIPPING SAUCE **250** CALORIES **22 g** PROTEIN **16 g** FAT (**9 g** UNSATURATED FAT, **7 g** SATURATED FAT) **145 mg** CHOLESTEROL **9 g** CARBS **3 g** FIBER **1 g** SUGAR (**1 g** NATURAL SUGAR, **0 g** ADDED SUGAR) **850 mg** SODIUM

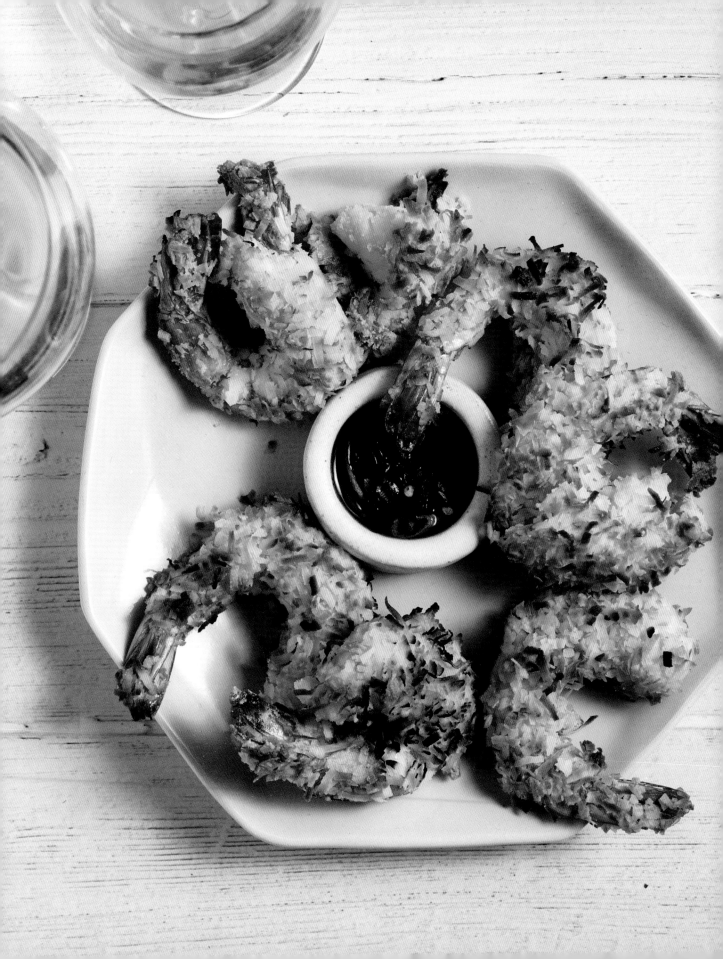

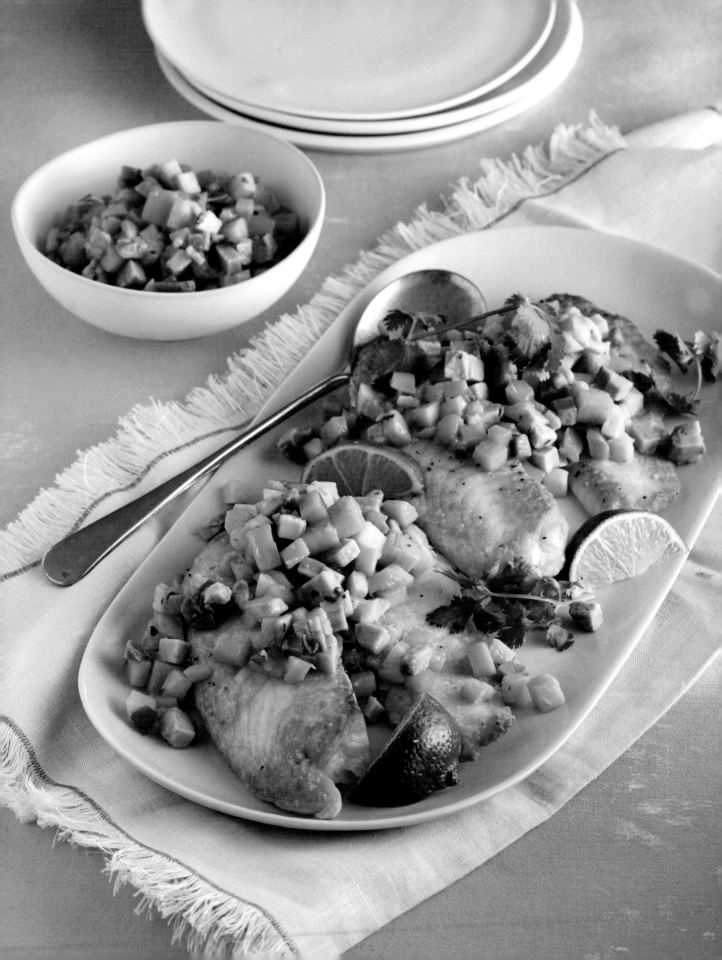

Tilapia with Mango-Avocado Salsa

SERVES: 4 PREP TIME: 10 MINUTES COOK TIME: 10 MINUTES

This elegant entrée is a breeze to prepare, but it's filled with flavor and has a beautiful, vibrant color. Tilapia is a super source of lean protein and is low in contaminants like mercury. (For the most eco-friendly pick, look for tilapia farmed worldwide in indoor recirculating tanks, Ecuador in ponds, and Peru in raceways; avoid those from China and Taiwan.) It's also mild-flavored, making it a smart choice for people who don't necessarily love "fishy" fish. In this recipe, I sauté it with just a basic salt and pepper seasoning, but the salsa topping (which also acts as a marinade as the hot fish absorbs the yummy juices) takes this to a whole other level.

SALSA
makes 2 cups

- 1 cup diced mango (from 1 fresh mango)
- 1 cup diced avocado (from 1 large avocado)
- 3 tablespoons lime juice
- 1 to 2 tablespoons minced jalapeño*
- ½ teaspoon salt, or more to taste
- ½ cup roughly chopped fresh cilantro

* *If you're heat sensitive, remove the seeds and ribs.*

TILAPIA

- 4 tilapia fillets (about 20 ounces total)
- ½ teaspoon kosher salt
- ⅛ teaspoon black pepper

1 FOR THE SALSA: Place all of the salsa ingredients in a large bowl and gently stir to combine. Season with extra salt and pepper, if desired. Set aside.

2 FOR THE FISH: Mist a large skillet with nonstick oil spray and warm over medium heat. Add the tilapia to the skillet and sprinkle with salt and pepper. (Do not overcrowd the skillet; cook in two batches if needed.) Cook fish for 4 to 5 minutes, then flip and cook for an additional 2 to 3 minutes or until fish is cooked through.

TO SERVE: Place the hot fish on a plate and top with the mango-avocado salsa.

PER SERVING **260** CALORIES **36 g** PROTEIN **9 g** FAT (**7 g** UNSATURATED FAT, **2 g** SATURATED FAT) **85 mg** CHOLESTEROL **11 g** CARBS **5 g** FIBER **6 g** SUGAR (**6 g** NATURAL SUGAR, **0 g** ADDED SUGAR) **570 mg** SODIUM

Mediterranean Snapper
with Extra Virgin Salsa Verde

SERVES: 4   PREP TIME: 15 MINUTES   COOK TIME: 10 MINUTES

Snapper is great for those who are resistant to trying seafood or looking to dip their toes into the Mediterranean water. It doesn't have a typical fishy taste, and the texture is light and flaky. And it's an eco-friendly pick that's lower in contaminants than some other popular options. If you're feeling adventurous, have your fishmonger clean a whole snapper and throw it on the grill or broil it in the oven. Then top the protein-packed, lean fish with a scrumptious salsa verde, and it becomes an exciting entrée featuring an explosion of flavors. You can also use the salsa verde as a topper for seared scallops, roast chicken, lean steak, or even baked potatoes.

SALSA VERDE
makes 1 cup

1 medium shallot, finely chopped

2 cloves garlic, minced

3 tablespoons red wine vinegar or lemon juice

1 teaspoon kosher salt

¾ cup minced fresh parsley

2 tablespoons minced fresh rosemary

1½ tablespoons minced fresh oregano (or ⅛ teaspoon dried oregano)

6 to 7 tablespoons extra-virgin olive oil

SNAPPER

1½ pounds skin-on red snapper fillets, patted dry

½ teaspoon kosher salt

⅛ teaspoon black pepper

1 FOR THE SALSA VERDE: In a small bowl, combine all of the salsa ingredients and set aside.

2 FOR THE SNAPPER: Mist a large skillet with nonstick olive oil spray and warm over medium heat. Mist both sides of the fish fillets with aditiooil spray and place skin-side down in the skillet. Sprinkle on salt and pepper and cook for about 4 minutes, gently pushing the fillets down with a spatula so the skin comes in full contact with the heated pan and browns evenly. Carefully flip the fish and cook for 4 more minutes, or until the fish is flaky and opaque.

TO SERVE: Transfer the fish to a serving platter and drizzle each fillet with 2 tablespoons of the salsa verde. Serve the remaining salsa on the side.

PER SERVING **280** CALORIES **35 g** PROTEIN **15 g** FAT (**12.5 g** UNSATURATED FAT, **2.5 g** SATURATED FAT) **65 mg** CHOLESTEROL **2 g** CARBS **1 g** FIBER **0 g** SUGAR **580 mg** SODIUM

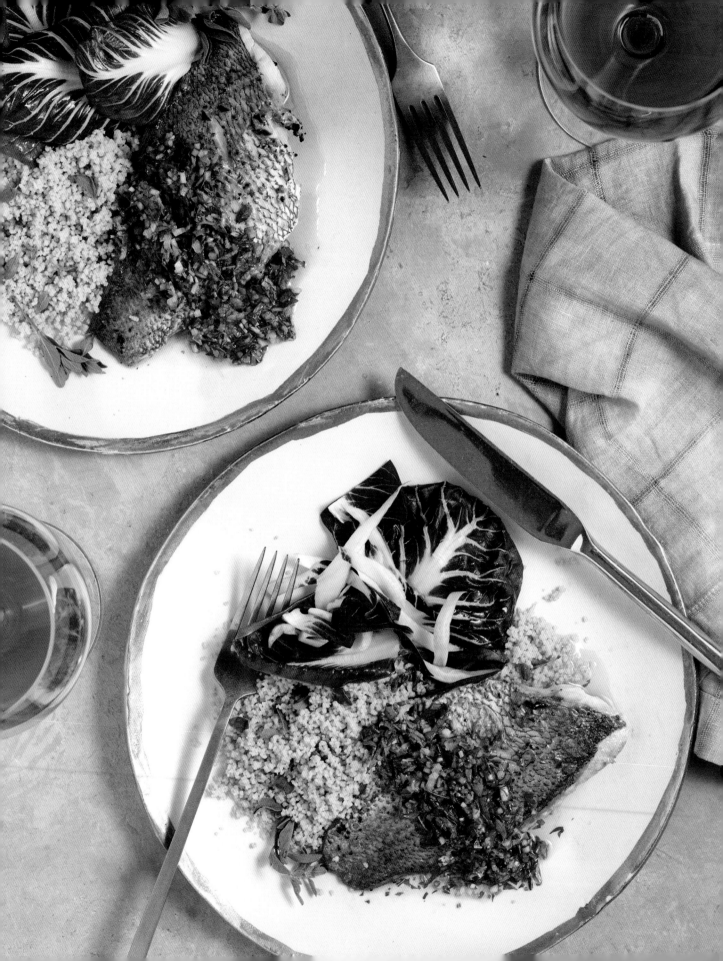

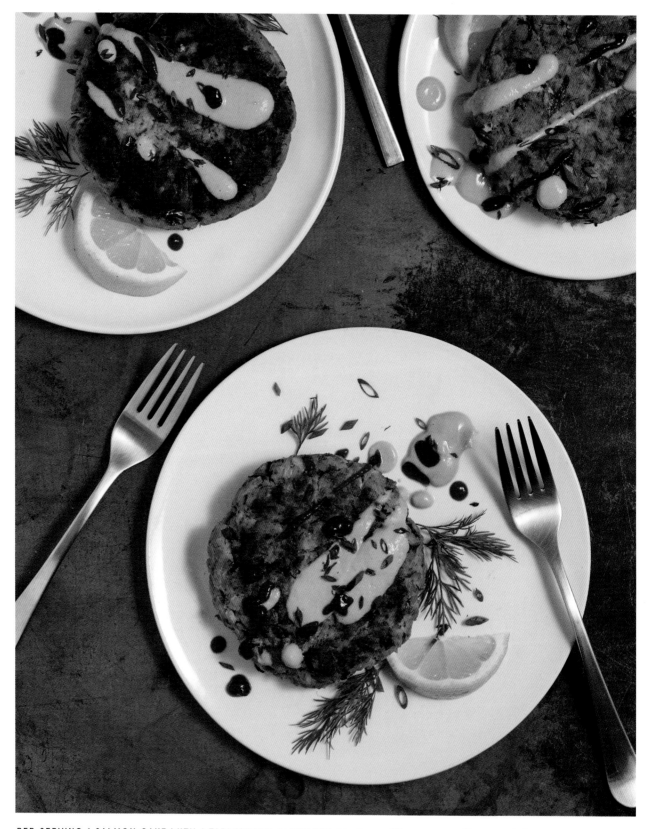

PER SERVING 1 SALMON CAKE WITH 1 TABLESPOON SAUCE **220** CALORIES **27 g** PROTEIN **10 g** FAT (**8.5 g** UNSATURATED FAT, **1.5 g** SATURATED FAT) **80 mg** CHOLESTEROL **5 g** CARBS **2 g** FIBER **1 g** SUGAR (**1 g** NATURAL SUGAR, 0 g ADDED SUGAR) **380 mg** SODIUM

Alaskan Salmon Cakes with Lemon Avocado Sauce

SERVES: 8   PREP TIME: 20 MINUTES   COOK TIME: 25 MINUTES

These salmon cakes are a real treat for supper (or a leftover lunch). They're so tasty and packed with nutrition: That's because salmon is loaded with protein and omega-3 fatty acids, and it's also one of the most vitamin D–rich foods out there. The ground flaxseeds may be mini, but they're mighty. In this recipe, they do double duty: They chip in extra omega-3 fats and allow me to cut back on bread crumbs, as they act as a binding agent. The Lemon Avocado Sauce is super creamy and dairy-free—you can also use it to elevate chicken, veggies, and so much more.

SALMON CAKES

- 2 pounds fresh salmon fillets, skin on, pin bones removed
- ¾ teaspoon kosher salt, divided
- ¼ teaspoon black pepper
- ⅓ cup finely diced red, orange, or yellow bell pepper
- 2 scallions, finely minced
- 2 tablespoons finely chopped fresh herbs (such as parsley, cilantro, or dill)
- 1 large egg, beaten
- 1 teaspoon lemon zest
- 1 teaspoon hot sauce, or more to taste (optional)
- 1½ tablespoons ground flaxseeds
- 6 tablespoons panko breadcrumbs (preferably whole grain)

AVOCADO SAUCE
makes about ¾ cup

- 1 medium avocado
- ½ cup roughly chopped fresh cilantro
- 1 to 2 scallions, roughly chopped
- 2 tablespoons lemon juice
- 1 tablespoon chopped jalapeño (optional)
- ½ teaspoon ground cumin
- ½ teaspoon kosher salt, or more to taste
- Ground black pepper

1 FOR THE SALMON CAKES: Preheat the oven to 400°F. Mist a baking sheet with nonstick oil spray.

2 Place the salmon on the baking sheet skin-side down, liberally mist the tops with oil spray, and sprinkle with salt and pepper. Roast for 15 minutes, or until just cooked through and the fish looks light pink inside without any translucency. Set aside to cool completely.

3 Lift the salmon from the skin (discard or enjoy it), flaking the flesh into a large bowl. (Save the baking sheet, as you'll be using it again.) Add the bell pepper, scallions, herbs, egg, lemon zest, and hot sauce, if using. Gently mix with a spatula or your hands. Sprinkle in the ground flaxseeds and breadcrumbs and stir to combine. Shape into 8 patties, place on a plate, and cover. Refrigerate for 10 minutes to firm.

4 Liberally mist a skillet with olive oil spray and warm over medium-high heat. Working in two batches, add the salmon cakes to the skillet and cook for 1 to 2 minutes on each side, until golden brown. Mist the skillet with additional oil spray as needed. Place the patties back on the baking sheet (mist the baking sheet with oil spray before adding the patties) and bake for 6 to 8 minutes, until they start to sizzle.

5 FOR THE SAUCE: In a food processor or blender, combine all of the sauce ingredients and process until smooth. Add 1 to 2 tablespoons of water if it is too thick. Serve the salmon cakes with the sauce on top or on the side.

Shrimp and Spinach Scampi with Spaghetti Squash

SERVES: 4   PREP TIME: 10 MINUTES   COOK TIME: 35 MINUTES

Welcome to scampi scrumptiousness. In this dish—an Italian classic with an American spin—a lean protein and a low-carb pasta alternative pair up to create a saucy and flavorful masterpiece. Spaghetti squash, which twirls up just like spaghetti, plays a starring role. To make cutting the raw squash easier, I recommend microwaving it for about three minutes to soften it up a bit before slicing. This also cuts down on roasting time . . . double bonus. If you're looking to trim your saturated fat intake, you can swap the butter for heart-healthy soft tub spread (make sure the spread contains no trans fats or hydrogenated oils).

1 large spaghetti squash

½ teaspoon kosher salt, divided

Ground black pepper

2 tablespoons butter, divided

2 tablespoons olive oil

1 medium shallot, minced

3 to 4 cloves garlic, minced

¼ teaspoon red pepper flakes, or more to taste

1½ cups grape tomatoes, halved

1 teaspoon fresh thyme

1 teaspoon lemon zest

1 pound raw shrimp, peeled and deveined, tail off

¼ to ⅓ cup white wine or reduced-sodium broth

2 tablespoons lemon juice

4 cups baby spinach

1 tablespoon finely chopped fresh parsley

1 Preheat the oven to 400°F. Mist a baking sheet with nonstick oil spray and set aside.

2 Microwave the spaghetti squash for 3 to 4 minutes. Let cool slightly. Then cut the squash in half lengthwise and scoop out and discard the seeds. Place the squash on the prepared baking sheet cut-side up. Liberally mist each half with olive oil spray and season with ¼ teaspoon of the salt and black pepper to taste. Flip the squash halves over and roast for about 30 minutes. Allow to cool, then, using a fork, gently shred the squash flesh into spaghetti-like strands.

3 While the squash is cooking, melt 1 tablespoon of the butter and warm the oil in a large, deep skillet over medium heat. Add the shallot, garlic, and red pepper flakes. Cook for 1 to 2 minutes, stirring constantly, until the shallot starts to soften. Add the tomatoes and season with the remaining ¼ teaspoon salt and black pepper to taste. Cook for 2 minutes, or until the tomatoes start to release their juices.

4 Add the thyme and lemon zest and cook for another 1 to 2 minutes, until fragrant. Add the shrimp and cook for 3 minutes, or until almost cooked through. Add the wine or broth and lemon juice and scrape any bits and pieces from the bottom of the pan.

5 Add the spinach and toss until it wilts. Add the cooked spaghetti squash strands, the remaining 1 tablespoon butter, and 1½ teaspoons of the parsley and toss gently to combine everything. Season with extra salt and red pepper flakes, if desired. Transfer to serving plates and garnish with the remaining 1½ teaspoons parsley.

PER SERVING 270 CALORIES 19 g PROTEIN 14 g FAT (9 g UNSATURATED FAT, 5 g SATURATED FAT) 160 mg CHOLESTEROL 22 g CARBS 5 g FIBER 6 g SUGAR (6 g NATURAL SUGAR, 0 g ADDED SUGAR) 980 mg SODIUM

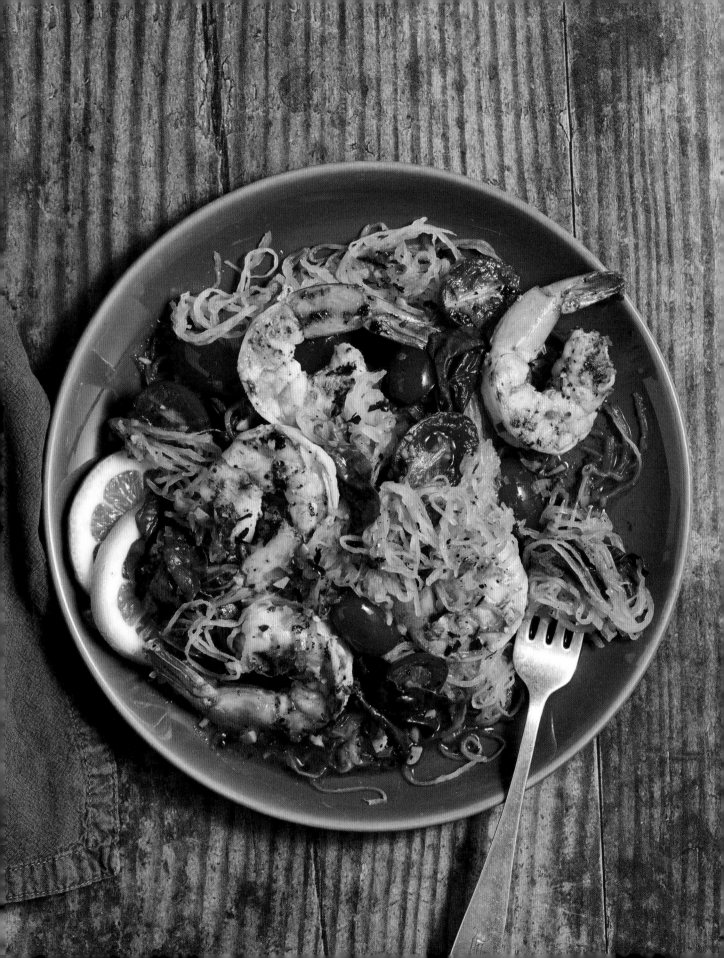

Vegetarian and Vegan Entrées

Roasted Veggies with
Cashew Mac and Cheese Sauce 219

The Incredible Vegan Tacos 220

Eggplant Parmesan Meatballs 222

Roasted Bell Peppers
Stuffed with Quinoa-Mushroom Pilaf 225

Black Lentils with
Coconut Citrus Slaw 226

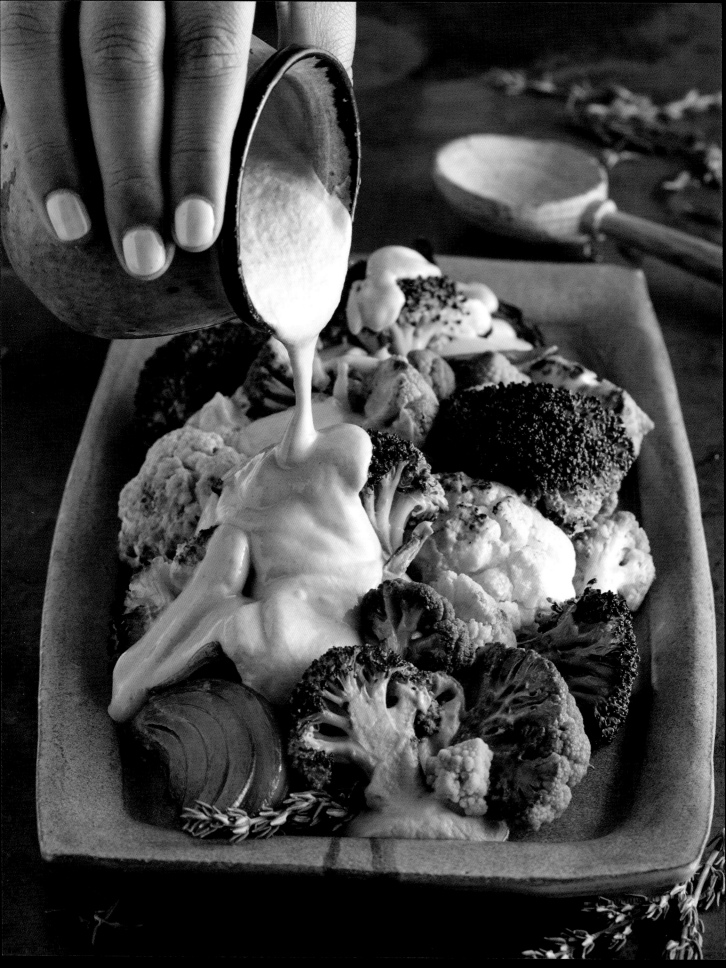

Roasted Veggies with Cashew Mac and Cheese Sauce

SERVES: 7   PREP TIME: 25 MINUTES   COOK TIME: 30 MINUTES

This is not your mama's mac and cheese! This vegan version relies on some culinary creativity. Cashews are a versatile ingredient; soak, drain and puree them with liquid and you'll end up with a luxuriously creamy (dairy-free) sauce. I add nutritional yeast for the amazing umami flavor it provides, lemon juice for brightness, and a dash of red pepper flakes for gentle heat. While the recipe calls for canned pumpkin—because it's convenient and readily available—you can feel free to swap in butternut squash puree or even leftover cooked sweet potato. Also, you can toss the delectable sauce with whole grain elbows when you're craving a more traditional mac and cheese meal.

VEGETABLES
makes about 7 cups

- 4 cups cauliflower florets (about 1 medium head)
- 4 cups broccoli florets
- 3 medium carrots, sliced into rounds
- 1 red onion, thinly sliced
- 2 tablespoons olive oil
- ½ teaspoon kosher salt
- ¼ teaspoon black pepper

CHEESE SAUCE
makes 2 cups

- ⅔ cup raw cashews
- ⅔ cup canned pumpkin puree
- 1 clove garlic, chopped
- 2 tablespoons nutritional yeast
- 1½ teaspoons kosher salt
- ½ teaspoon red pepper flakes
- 1 tablespoon lemon juice
- 1 cup plus 2 tablespoons boiling water

1 Set an oven rack to the middle position and preheat the oven to 450°F. Mist 2 baking sheets with nonstick oil spray. Set aside.

2 FOR THE VEGGIES: In a large bowl, toss together the cauliflower, broccoli, carrots, red onion, oil, salt, and black pepper. Arrange in a single layer on the prepared baking sheet and roast for 30 to 35 minutes, tossing halfway through.

3 FOR THE SAUCE: While the veggies are roasting, place the cashews in a small bowl with boiling water. Cover the bowl and let it soak for about 20 minutes. Drain well.

4 In a high-speed blender or food processor, combine the drained cashews, pumpkin puree, garlic, nutritional yeast, salt, red pepper flakes, lemon juice, and 1 cup plus 2 tablespoons boiling water. Blend for about 1 minute, scraping down the sides as needed. If the sauce is too thick, add more boiling water 1 tablespoon at a time until you reach your desired consistency.

TO SERVE: Place the roasted veggies on a platter and drizzle the warm "cream" sauce on top. Garnish with fresh herbs, if desired.

PER SERVING 1 CUP VEGGIES WITH 2 TABLESPOONS SAUCE **150** CALORIES **5 g** PROTEIN **9 g** FAT (**7.5 g** UNSATURATED FAT, **1.5 g** SATURATED FAT) **0 mg** CHOLESTEROL **14 g** CARBS **4 g** FIBER **5 g** SUGAR (**5 g** NATURAL, **0 g** ADDED) **600 mg** SODIUM

The Incredible Vegan Tacos

SERVES: 10 (MAKES ABOUT 20 TACOS)   PREP TIME: 10 MINUTES

COOK TIME: 30 MINUTES

If I had my choice, Tuesdays would occur more than once a week. That's because on Tuesdays, we eat tacos. This combo of lentils and black beans with walnuts creates a hearty-beefy taco experience . . . with serious plant-based health perks. Then there's the DIY taco seasoning blend, which is a cinch to put together. For those following a vegan plan, this is a great option. Note: The recipe makes 5 heaping cups of filling, and it also tastes terrific on salads and sammies.

TACO "MEAT"

1 cup raw walnuts

1 cup dry lentils

2 cups reduced-sodium vegetable broth

1 (14-ounce) can black beans, drained and rinsed

TACO SEASONING
makes 6 tablespoons

2 tablespoons chili powder

1 tablespoon ground cumin

2½ teaspoons kosher salt

2 teaspoons black pepper

1 teaspoon paprika

½ teaspoon garlic powder

½ teaspoon onion powder

½ teaspoon red pepper flakes

½ teaspoon dried oregano

TACOS

20 hard or soft taco shells

Chopped lettuce

Chopped tomatoes

OPTIONAL TOPPERS

Corn, sliced jalapeños, chopped onions, sliced avocado, salsa

1   FOR THE TOASTED WALNUTS: Preheat the oven to 300°F. Spread the walnuts on a baking sheet and toast in the oven for about 10 minutes, until lightly browned. Remove from the oven and set aside.

2   FOR THE TACO SEASONING: In a small bowl, mix all the seasoning ingredients and set aside.

3   FOR THE TACO "MEAT": Combine the lentils and broth in a medium pot and bring to a boil. Reduce the heat to low and simmer for 20 to 30 minutes, until tender. Drain well and transfer to the bowl of a food processor. Add the black beans and walnuts. Gently pulse to combine and slightly break down the mixture, but do not puree it. There should still be lots of texture with pieces of nuts and some whole beans.

4   Liberally coat a large skillet with nonstick oil spray and warm over medium-low heat. Add the lentil-bean-walnut mixture along with ¼ cup of the taco seasoning blend and 2 tablespoons warm water. Gently fold and stir the mixture to incorporate all of the seasonings and warm everything, but be careful not to mash it into a puree (maintain as much texture as possible). Taste and add more taco seasoning, if desired (I typically add 1 to 2 more tablespoons).

5   TO ASSEMBLE: Add ¼ cup filling to each taco shell, along with lettuce, tomatoes, and optional toppings.

PER SERVING 2 TACOS **320** CALORIES **12 g** PROTEIN **16 g** (**14.5 g** UNSATURATED FAT, **1.5 g** SATURATED FAT) **0 mg** CHOLESTEROL **35 g** CARBS **7 g** FIBER **1 g** SUGAR (**1 g** NATURAL SUGAR, **0 g** ADDED SUGAR) **610 mg** SODIUM

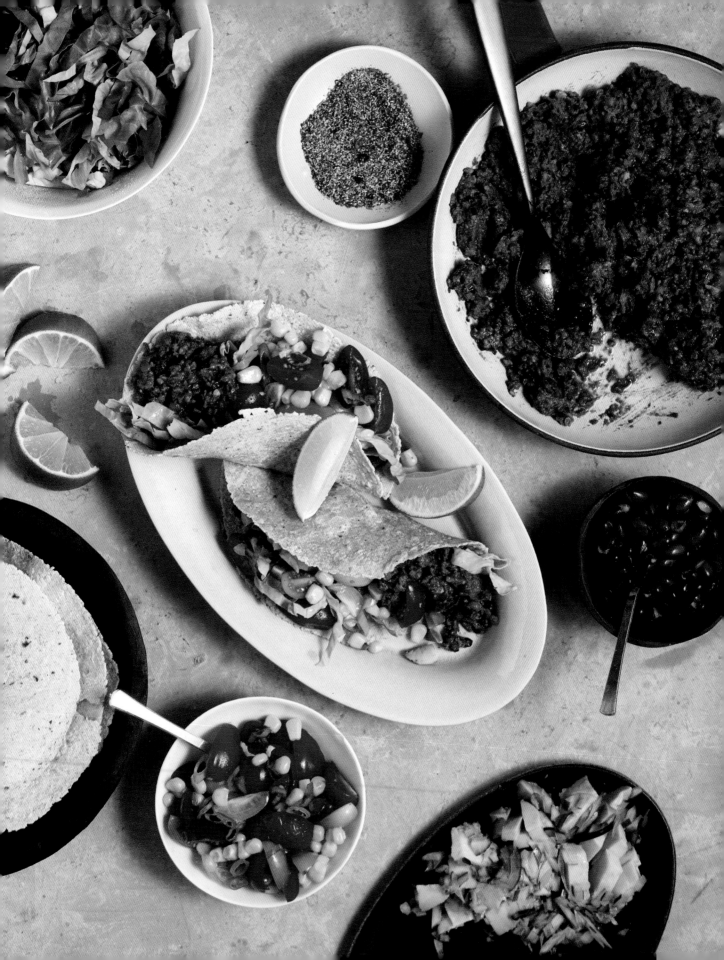

Eggplant Parmesan Meatballs

SERVES: 4   PREP TIME: 40 MINUTES   COOK TIME: 1 HOUR

Meatballs are always a crowd favorite, and so I decided to take the classic for a vegetarian spin. When roasting the eggplant, be sure to follow the instructions for using two baking sheets; this allows adequate space between pieces so the moisture can efficiently evaporate. If you cram them all on one sheet, they may get soggy. The roasting also helps intensify the eggplant flavor and is key for forming the meatballs and creating that meaty consistency. Btw, you can peel the eggplant using an regular old vegetable peeler, and be sure to use a good-quality pecorino or Parmesan for that pop of cheesy flavor in every bite. These meatballs are firm and crisp on the outside but super-moist and delish on the inside. My gang devours them and I'm hoping yours will, too!

MEATBALLS

- 2 large or 3 medium eggplants, peeled and cut into 1½-inch cubes (about 12 cups)
- ½ teaspoon kosher salt, or more to taste
- ⅛ teaspoon black pepper, or more to taste
- ½ teaspoon garlic powder
- ¾ teaspoon dried oregano
- ⅛ teaspoon red pepper flakes, or more to taste
- 1 small onion, diced
- 1 clove garlic, minced
- 2 large egg whites
- ¼ cup grated Pecorino Romano or Parmesan cheese, plus more for serving
- 2 tablespoons minced fresh basil
- 1 tablespoon minced fresh parsley
- 6 tablespoons panko breadcrumbs (preferably whole grain)
- 1 (24-ounce) jar marinara sauce
- ½ cup shredded part-skim mozzarella cheese (optional)

1 FOR THE EGGPLANT: Preheat the oven to 400°F. Line 2 baking sheets with parchment paper.

2 Add the eggplant to a large bowl and generously mist with olive oil spray. Add the salt, black pepper, garlic powder, oregano, and red pepper flakes into the bowl and toss with the eggplant to evenly distribute. Spread the eggplant out on the prepared baking sheets, mist with additional olive oil spray, and sprinkle on leftover seasonings from the bowl. Roast for 20 to 25 minutes, until the eggplant is browned on the edges and soft throughout. Remove from the oven and set aside to cool. Reserve the large bowl and one of the baking sheets to use for the meatballs.

3 FOR THE MEATBALLS: Mist a large saucepan with olive oil spray and warm over medium-high heat. Add the onion and garlic and cook, stirring occasionally, for 5 to 7 minutes. Transfer to the bowl you mixed the eggplant in and allow to cool slightly. Add the roasted eggplant, egg whites, Pecorino or Parmesan cheese, the basil, parsley, and panko to the bowl and mix with a spatula or your hands to break up the eggplant and combine all the ingredients. Using a ¼-cup measure, portion 16 piles of the mixture on your prepared baking sheet. Using your hands, pick up each portion and press to compact them into smooth, round meatball shapes. Generously mist the tops with oil spray and bake for about 20 minutes, until evenly browned. (Before removing from the oven, gently lift one meatball to ensure the bottom is browned.)

4 Spread about 1 cup of marinara sauce on the bottom of a 9 by 13-inch baking dish. Add the meatballs, top with the remaining sauce, and sprinkle with extra cheese, if desired. Cook for 6 to 8 minutes, until the cheese is melted.

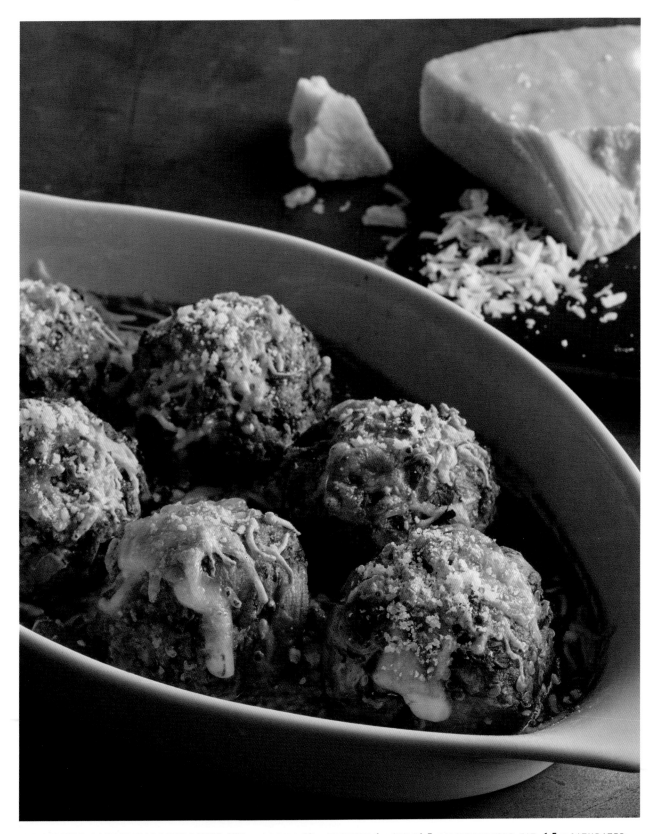

PER SERVING 4 MEATBALLS WITH SAUCE **220** CALORIES **10 g** PROTEIN **6 g** FAT (**4.5 g** UNSATURATED FAT, **1.5 g** SATURATED FAT) **5 M** CHOLESTEROL **38 g** CARBS **12 g** FIBER **18 g** SUGAR **800 mg** SODIUM

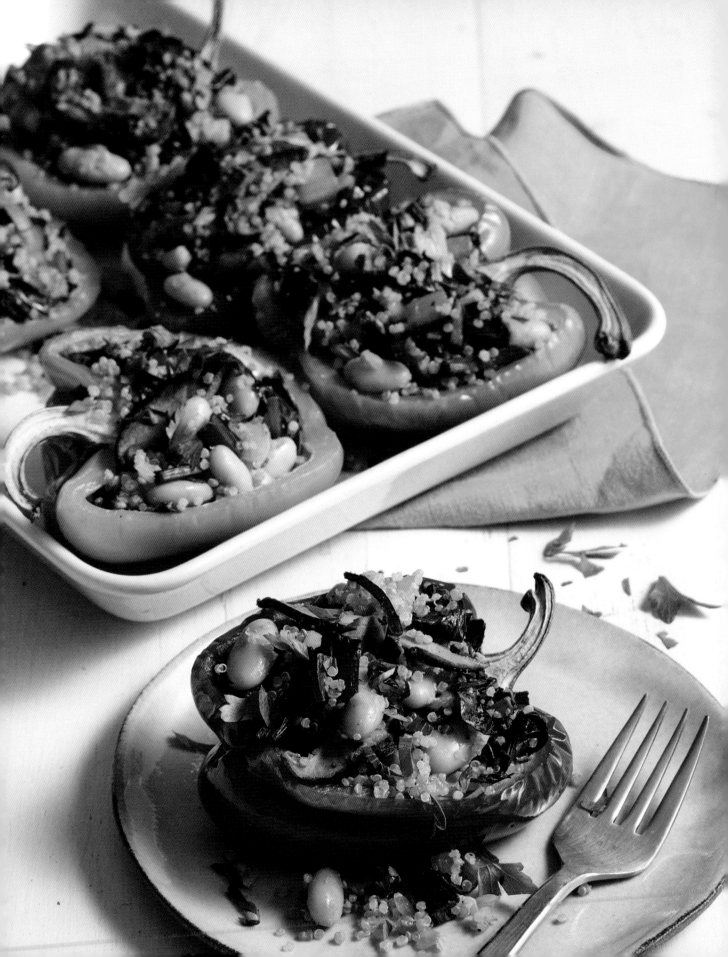

Roasted Bell Peppers
Stuffed with Quinoa-Mushroom Pilaf

MAKES: TK HALVES   PREP TIME: 15 MINUTES   COOK TIME: 50 MINUTES

This dish is beautiful—but peppers aren't just a pretty face. One pepper delivers more than twice your daily needs for vitamin C. However, if you're not a fan of peppers or want to save yourself some time, make the nutrient-packed filling as a standalone. I do it often, and it makes a super-delicious side or entrée. And hey, as the saying goes, "it's what's inside that counts!"

3 medium red, yellow, or orange bell peppers

2 teaspoons olive oil

¾ cup dry quinoa

1¾ cups reduced-sodium vegetable broth, divided

2 to 3 fresh thyme sprigs

1 teaspoon kosher salt, divided

½ teaspoon ground black pepper, divided

8 ounces mushrooms, sliced

1 small onion, chopped

2 cloves garlic, minced

¼ teaspoon red pepper flakes

1 bunch rainbow or Swiss chard (about 6 cups), stems and leaves separated, finely chopped

1 (15.5-ounce) can white beans, rinsed and drained

2 tablespoons nutritional yeast

Fresh parsley for garnish

1 Preheat the oven to 400°F. Mist a baking sheet with olive oil spray. Set aside.

2 Slice the bell peppers in half lengthwise and remove the seeds and membrane. Place the pepper halves on the baking sheet cut-side up and liberally mist with olive oil spray. Roast for 18 to 20 minutes, until tender. Remove from the oven, leaving the peppers on the baking sheet, and set aside.

3 While the bell peppers are in the oven, warm the oil in a medium saucepan over high heat. Add the quinoa, stir to coat it in the oil, and toast for about 30 seconds. Add 1½ cups of the broth and the thyme sprigs and bring to a boil. Cover, reduce the heat to low, and simmer for 15 minutes, or until the quinoa has puffed and the broth has absorbed. Remove the thyme sprigs and season with ½ teaspoon of the salt and ¼ teaspoon black pepper.

4 While the quinoa is simmering, liberally mist a large skillet with oil spray and warm over medium heat. Add the mushrooms and cook for 5 to 7 minutes, until golden brown. Transfer the mushrooms to a plate and set aside. Reapply oil spray to the skillet, add the onion, and cook for about 5 minutes. Add the garlic and red pepper flakes and cook for 1 more minute, stirring constantly (mist with more oil spray if the pan becomes dry). Add the chard stems (reserving the leaves) and white beans and cook for 3 minutes, or until the chard stems start to soften. Add the chard leaves and cook, stirring, until the leaves wilt down. Fold in the cooked quinoa, cooked mushrooms, and nutritional yeast, add the reserved ¼ cup broth, and season with the remaining ½ teaspoon salt and ¼ teaspoon black pepper, plus additional if needed.

5 Fill each pepper half with about ¾ cup of the quinoa stuffing, lightly packing the stuffing down to make sure it does not fall out. Place the peppers back in the oven for about 5 minutes, until everything is heated through. Garnish with parsley.

PER SERVING 1 BELL PEPPER HALF **190** CALORIES **9 g** PROTEIN **4 g** FAT (**4 g** UNSATURATED FAT, **0 g** UNSATURATED FAT) **0 mg** CHOLESTEROL **31 g** CARBS **7 g** FIBER **5 g** SUGAR **300 mg** SODIUM

Black Lentils with Coconut Citrus Slaw

SERVES: 6   PREP TIME: 10 MINUTES   COOK TIME: 30 MINUTES

Pack up and head to the tropics with this delicious, island-inspired dish that reinvents classic rice and beans. In addition to whole grain rice, I use black lentils (also called beluga lentils, because they resemble their namesake beluga caviar) which are exploding with nutrition. Just one cup of cooked lentils contains nearly 16 grams of fiber—more than half the daily recommended amount—and 18 grams of protein. They're an inexpensive canvas to soak up a number of flavors, and they'll keep you feeling full for hours on end. I always have multiple bags stashed in my pantry and countless ideas for enjoying them.

RICE

3 to 6 cups cooked brown rice, wild rice, or quinoa

BLACK LENTILS

3 cloves garlic, minced

1 yellow onion, finely diced

1 medium carrot, finely diced

2 stalks celery, finely diced

½ teaspoon kosher salt

2 cups dry black lentils (also called beluga; can substitute French green lentils)

1 tablespoon tomato paste

1½ teaspoon dried thyme

1 teaspoon ground cumin

2 cups reduced-sodium vegetable broth

COCONUT CITRUS SLAW
makes about 2½ cups

1 cup unsweetened coconut shreds or flakes

1 cup shredded red/purple cabbage

1 small red onion, finely chopped

2 tablespoons minced jalapeño

2 tablespoons lime juice

1 teaspoon orange zest (optional)

2 tablespoons orange juice

¼ to ½ cup chopped fresh cilantro

½ teaspoon kosher salt

1 FOR THE LENTILS: Liberally mist a medium saucepan with nonstick oil spray and warm over medium-high heat. Add the garlic and cook for about 1 minute, stirring constantly. Add the onion, carrot, celery, and salt and cook for about 5 minutes, stirring occasionally, until the veggies begin to soften. Add more oil spray if the pan becomes dry.

2 Add the lentils, tomato paste, thyme, and cumin and stir to combine. Add the broth, bring to a boil, then reduce the heat to low, cover, and simmer for 20 to 30 minutes, until the lentils are tender but retain their shape.

3 FOR THE COCONUT SLAW: In a medium bowl, combine all of the slaw ingredients and let sit for a few minutes so the flavors can mingle. Season with extra salt, if desired.

TO SERVE: Spoon the lentils over the rice or quinoa and top with the coconut citrus slaw. Garnish with your choice of toppers like sliced avocado, cilantro, and lime juice.

PER SERVING ½ CUP RICE OR QUINOA, 1 CUP LENTILS, PLUS ½ CUP COCONUT SLAW **450** CALORIES **21 g** PROTEIN **9 g** FAT (**3 g** UNSATURATED FAT, **6 g** SATURATED FAT) **0 mg** CHOLESTEROL **74 g** CARBS **17 g** FIBER **5 g** SUGAR (**5 g** NATURAL SUGAR, **0 g** ADDED SUGAR) **400 mg** SODIUM

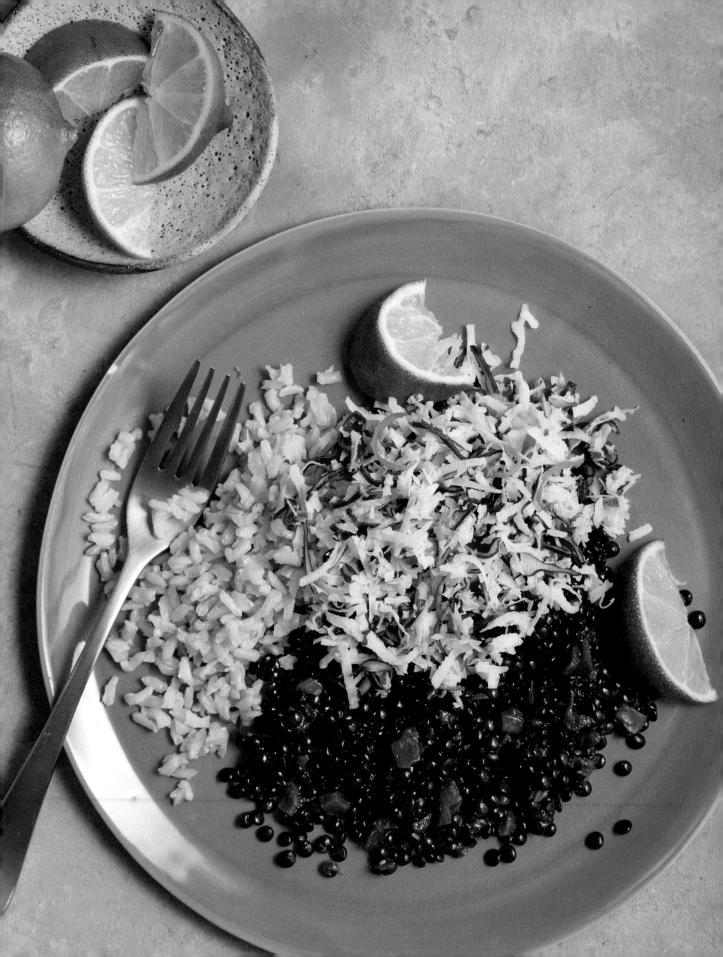

Sweet and Savory Treats

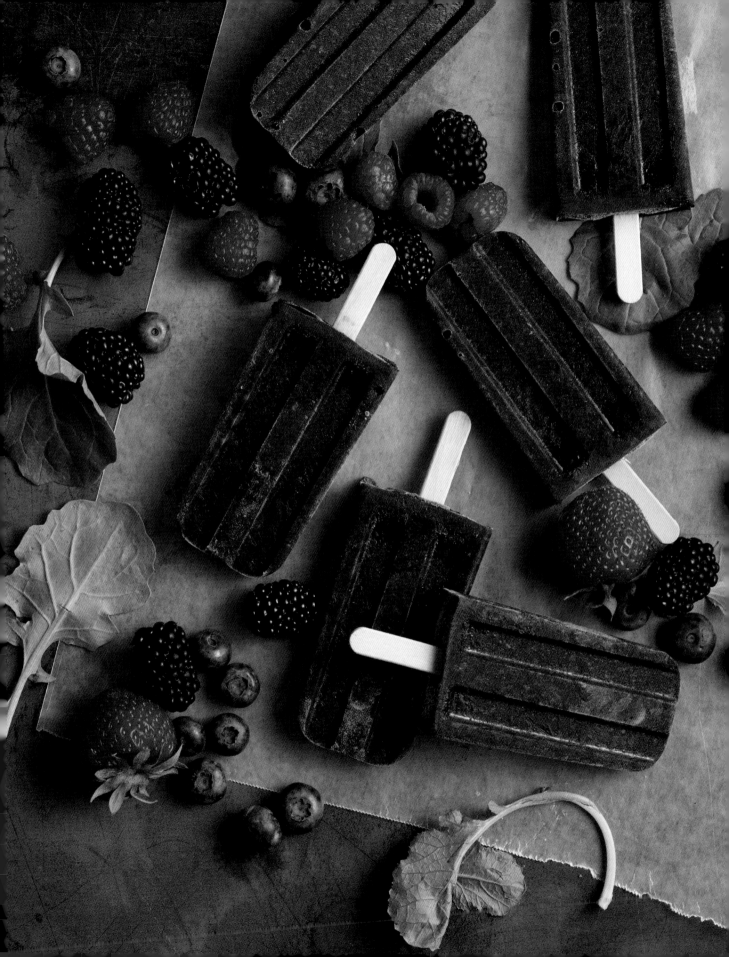

Superfood Ice Pops

MAKES: 9 ICE POPS   PREP TIME: 5 MINUTES,
PLUS AT LEAST 4 HOURS IN THE FREEZER

Store-bought ice pops are often loaded with sugar, colorings, and other junky ingredients. But these are a sweet surprise: They're jam-packed with good-for-you magic, including fiber-rich berries and kale; potassium-packed banana; heart-healthy flaxseeds, plus one special superfood ingredient that I have to take a minute to brag about: matcha. This powder is made from ground-up green tea leaves and is even more antioxidant-rich (ten times to be exact) than other types of green tea. That's because you end up consuming the entire leaf rather than just the brewed water, while the leaves (or tea bag) are discarded.

All these outstanding ingredients and perks for just 40 calories a pop. My nieces and nephews go crazy for them—and I'm excited for you to give them a try!

2 cups fresh or frozen mixed berries

1 cup almond milk (or any milk of choice)

1 fresh or frozen ripe banana

1 cup loosely packed fresh kale or baby spinach leaves

1 tablespoon lime juice

2 to 3 teaspoons honey

1 tablespoon ground flaxseeds

1 teaspoon matcha powder

1 In a blender, combine all the ingredients and blend until smooth. Pour the mixture into ice pop molds and freeze until the pops are firm and solid, at least 4 hours.

PER 1 POP **40** CALORIES **1 g** PROTEIN **1 g** FAT (**1 g** UNSATURATED FAT, **0 g** SATURATED FAT) **0 mg** CHOLESTEROL **8 g** CARBS **1 g** FIBER **5 g** SUGAR (**4 g** NATURAL SUGAR, **1 g** ADDED SUGAR) **20 mg** SODIUM

Soft Baked Almond Butter– Chocolate Chip Cookies

MAKES: ABOUT 40 SMALL COOKIES   PREP TIME: 5 MINUTES   COOK TIME: 15 MINUTES

In the mood for something sweet and special? Say hello to your new favorite cookie fix. These treats—warm and irresistible straight from the oven—deliver on both taste and nutrition. Instead of flour, I rely on canned chickpeas, a legume rich in folate and tryptophan, a nutrient that the body uses to make serotonin, a feel-good chemical. You may be skeptical; my family and *TODAY* show pals were, too. But the soft and chewy texture won them over. Almond butter also plays a starring role, bringing protein, fiber, and heart-healthy fat to the (dessert) table. If you have nut allergies in the house, swap in soy or sunflower seed butter.

Plus, they're a snap to make: Everything gets tossed into the food processor. And instead of having to clean another bowl, I just remove the blade after the batter is smooth and mix in the chips by hand. Then I place the cookies, one at a time, on the prepped baking sheet. Easy as . . . cookies! They're best served warm, but they do freeze well, too. Each scrumptious gem is filled with goodness, so go ahead and enjoy one . . . or two . . . or three with a glass of milk or a soothing cup of flavorful tea.

1 (15-ounce) can chickpeas, drained and rinsed

1 cup creamy almond butter*

1 large egg, beaten

½ cup honey

1 teaspoon baking soda

2 teaspoons vanilla extract

1 tablespoon vegetable oil (or melted butter)

½ to ¾ cup semisweet or dark chocolate chips

* *For nut allergies, swap in sunflower seed butter or soy nut butter.*

1 Preheat the oven to 350°F. Mist a large baking sheet (or 2 standard baking sheets) with nonstick oil spray or line with parchment paper and set aside.

2 Toss all the ingredients except the chocolate chips into a food processor and pulse until the chickpeas are pureed and everything is well combined. Do not overmix. Turn off the motor, remove the blade, and mix in the chocolate chips by hand. Place 1 heaping tablespoon of batter per cookie on the prepared baking sheet(s). (I like to mist my spoon periodically with oil spray so the batter slides off more easily.) You may choose to sprinkle a few extra decorative chocolate chips on top. Bake for about 15 minutes. They're extra delicious served soft and warm right out of the oven.

PER COOKIE **70** CALORIES **2 g** PROTEIN **4.5 g** FAT (**4 g** UNSATURATED FAT, **0.5 g** SATURATED FAT) **5 mg** CHOLESTEROL **8 g** CARBS **1 g** FIBER **5 g** SUGAR (**1 g** NATURAL SUGAR, **4 g** ADDED SUGAR) **35 mg** SODIUM

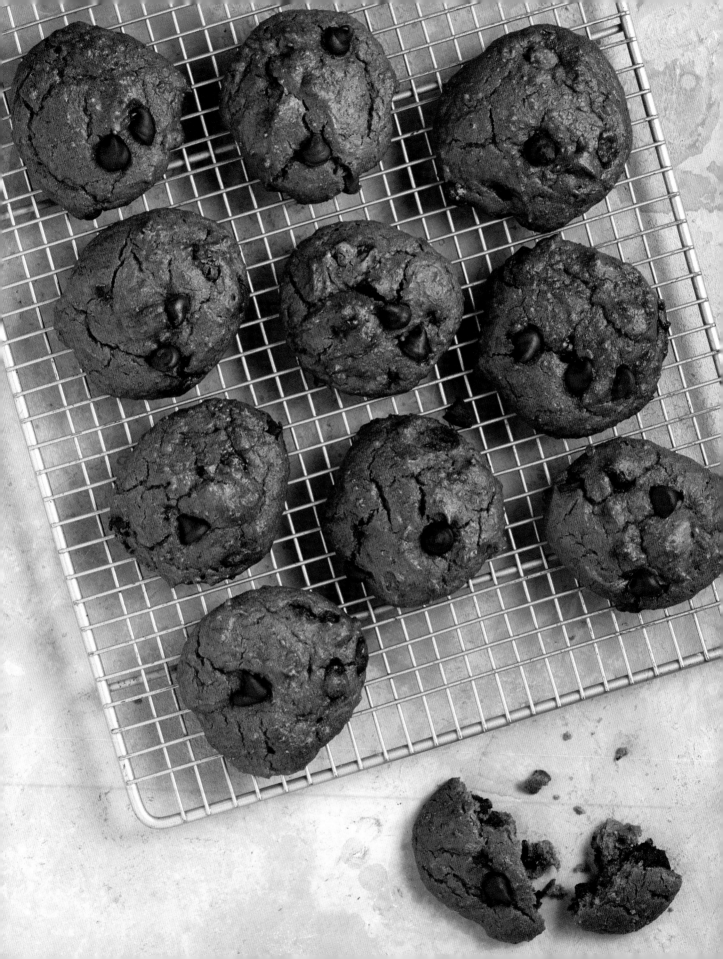

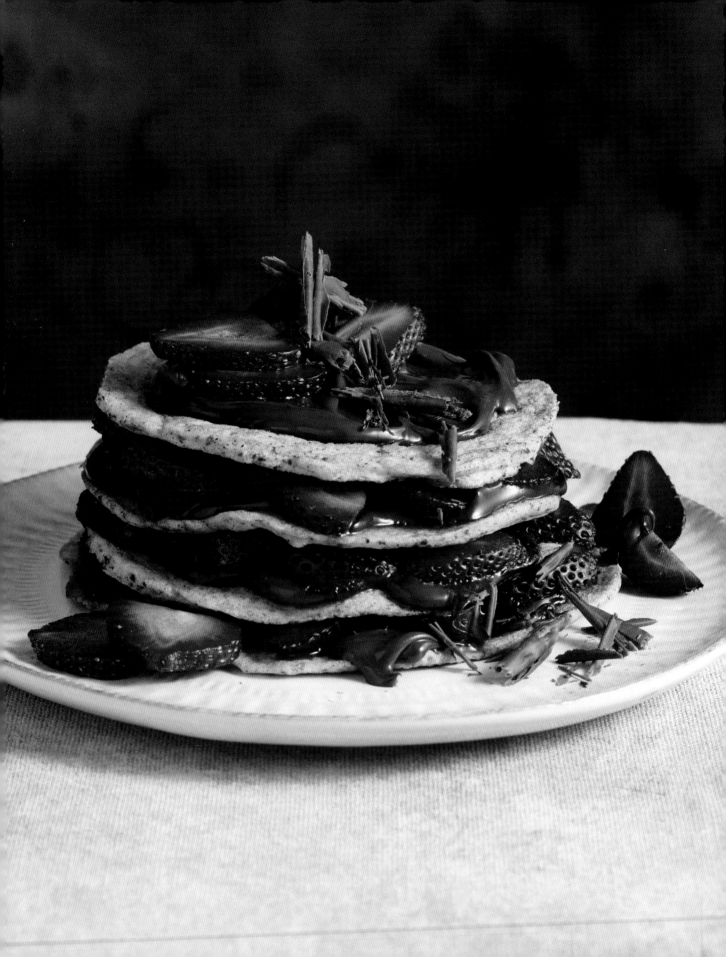

Layered Chocolate Crepe Cake

SERVES: 4   PREP TIME: 10 MINUTES   COOK TIME: 10 MINUTES

This is obscenely rich and indulgent. One layer after another of creamy chocolate and sweet strawberries results in dessert heaven. The first time I tested out this cake recipe, Ian and I devoured it. Then Ian commented "Hmmm, I think you should test this again . . . tomorrow." Success! I like to think of the spread as my lightened-up version of Nutella.

CREPES

4 large egg whites

2 tablespoons ground flaxseeds

2 tablespoons tapioca flour or arrowroot

2 tablespoons blanched almond flour

¼ teaspoon kosher salt

CHOCOLATE SPREAD AND BERRIES

¾ cup powdered peanut butter

¼ cup cocoa powder

3 tablespoons sugar

Pinch of kosher salt

1 cup strawberries, sliced

1 **FOR THE CREPES:** In a small bowl, combine the egg whites and flaxseeds and whisk with a fork. Set aside for 5 minutes to allow the mixture to gel.

2 In a separate small bowl, combine the tapioca flour, almond flour, and salt. Whisk the flour mixture into the gelled egg mixture. It will be lumpy at first, but keep whisking until it's smooth, about 1 minute total.

3 Mist an 8-inch pan with nonstick oil spray and warm over medium heat. Add about ¼ cup of the crepe batter to the pan and smooth out the top using a spatula or the back of a spoon until it reaches about 5 inches in diameter. Cook for 1 to 2 minutes per side. Repeat until all of the batter is used up and you have 4 crepes.

4 **FOR THE SPREAD:** In a small bowl, mix the peanut powder, cocoa powder, sugar, and salt. Add 5 tablespoons water and mix for about 30 seconds to create a velvety smooth paste. If it's too thick, add more water very sparingly, just 1 teaspoon at a time.

5 **TO ASSEMBLE:** Spread each crepe with 2 tablespoons of the chocolate spread (you'll have some left over) and top with the strawberries. Carefully place one crepe on top of the other to build four layers. Garnish with shaved chocolate, if desired.

PER SERVING 150 CALORIES 10 g PROTEIN 5 g FAT (5 g UNSATURATED FAT, 0 g SATURATED FAT) 0 mg CHOLESTEROL 19 g CARBS 5 g FIBER 8 g SUGAR (3 NATURAL SUGAR, 5 g ADDED SUGAR) 260 mg SODIUM

Super Bark
(Nutty Traditional, Super Seed with Sea Salt, Tropical Superfood)

MAKES: ABOUT 24 PIECES EACH   PREP TIME: 10 MINUTES FOR EACH, PLUS 20 MINUTES IN THE REFRIGERATOR

Chocolate lovers, rejoice! Here you have three different variations of dark chocolaty bark to satisfy every kind of sweet tooth. Version one is chock-full of chunky goodness, as many mix-ins as chocolate, so you'll get plenty of crunchy action in every bite. The second version is a Hawaiian escape with a mouthwatering combo of sweet, chewy pineapple, buttery, crunchy macadamia nuts, and creamy, tropical coconut. In the last, super-seed version, I usually use white seeds so you get a result that looks like nonpareils or Sno-Caps. (Full disclosure: This was one of my favorite movie theater treats from back in the day before I was a nutritionist, lol.) How do you choose? No need to decide . . . enjoy all of them!

TEMPERED DARK CHOCOLATE

2 cups dark chocolate chips, ideally at least 60% cocoa

1 In a medium bowl, melt 1⅓ cups of the chocolate chips in the microwave by heating for 15 to 30 seconds at a time, stirring in between, until the chocolate is smooth and velvety. Then stir in the remaining ⅔ cup chocolate chips until they're completely melted and blended in. If they don't melt completely from stirring, microwave for another 5 seconds at a time until fully melted. Use this tempered base for the following three variations; it helped to maintain a glossy finish and keeps the chocolate firm and snappy.

RECIPE FOR THREE DELICIOUS VARIATIONS CONTINUES ON PAGE 238

TRADITIONAL NUTTY SUPERFOOD BAR PER SERVING 1 PIECE **170** CALORIES **4 g** PROTEIN **13.5 g** FAT (**9 g** UNSATURATED FAT, **4.5 g** SATURATED FAT) **0 mg** CHOLESTEROL **10 g** CARBS **1 g** FIBER **7 g** SUGAR (**7** NATURAL SUGAR, **<1 g** ADDED SUGAR) **60 mg** SODIUM

SUPER SEED BARK WITH SEA SALT PER SERVING 1 PIECE **100** CALORIES **2 g** PROTEIN **6 g** FAT (**2.5 g** UNSATURATED FAT, **3.5 g** SATURATED FAT) **0 mg** CHOLESTEROL **8 g** CARBS **1 g** FIBER **6 g** SUGAR (**6** NATURAL SUGAR, **<1 g** ADDED SUGAR) **60 mg** SODIUM

TROPICAL SUPERFOOD BARK PER SERVING 1 PIECE **140** CALORIES **1 g** PROTEIN **9 g** FAT (**4 g** UNSATURATED FAT, **5 g** SATURATED FAT) **0 mg** CHOLESTEROL **14 g** CARBS **1 g** FIBER **11 g** SUGAR (**11** NATURAL SUGAR, **<1 g** ADDED SUGAR) **60 mg** SODIUM

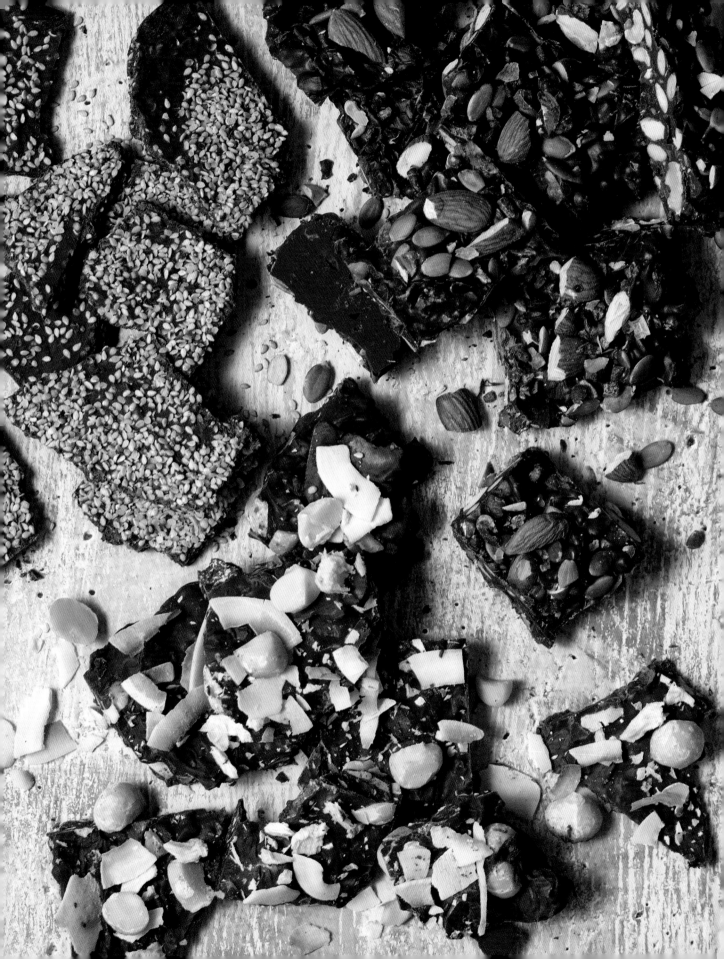

TRADITIONAL NUTTY SUPERFOOD BARK

2 cups tempered dark chocolate (see recipe)

1 cup toasted almonds, roughly chopped*

¾ cup toasted walnuts, roughly chopped*

¾ cup toasted pumpkin seeds, roughly chopped*

2 tablespoons cocoa nibs

¾ teaspoon kosher salt

* *If using raw nuts or seeds, spread them out on a baking sheet and toast in the oven at 350°F for about 10 minutes. Allow them to cool before chopping.*

1 Line a baking sheet with parchment paper and set aside.

2 In a small bowl, combine the nuts and seeds. Set aside 2 tablespoons.

3 Mix the nut-seed mixture and salt into the melted chocolate. Spread the mixture evenly onto the prepared baking sheet, then sprinkle the reserved nut-seed mixture and the cocoa nibs over the top. Use a rubber spatula or your fingers to gently press the toppings into the chocolate so they stick. Place the bark in the fridge for about 20 minutes, until completely cooled and set. Cut or break it into 24 pieces.

SUPER SEED BARK WITH SEA SALT

2 cups tempered dark chocolate (see recipe)

¼ cup hemp seeds (also called hemp hearts)

½ cup sesame seeds

¾ teaspoon flaked sea salt (fleur de sel) or kosher salt

1 Line a baking sheet with parchment paper and set aside.

2 In a small bowl, combine the hemp seeds and sesame seeds. Set aside 1 tablespoon of the mixture.

3 Add the seed mixture into the melted chocolate. Spread the mixture evenly onto the prepared baking sheet, then sprinkle the reserved seeds and the salt over the top. Use a rubber spatula or your fingers to gently press the toppings into the chocolate so they stick. Place the bark in the fridge for 20 minutes, or until completely cooled and set. Cut or break it into 24 pieces.

TROPICAL SUPERFOOD BARK

2 cups tempered dark chocolate (see recipe)

¾ cup unsalted macadamia nuts, chopped

¾ cup unsweetened coconut flakes, roughly chopped

¾ cup chopped unsweetened dried or freeze-dried pineapple

¾ teaspoon flaked sea salt (fleur de sel) or kosher salt

1 Line a baking sheet with parchment paper and set aside.

2 In a small bowl, combine the macadamia nuts, coconut flakes, and pineapple. Set aside 2 tablespoons of the mixture.

3 Add the macadamia-fruit mixture into the melted chocolate. Spread the mixture evenly onto the prepared baking sheet, then sprinkle the reserved nut-fruit mixture and salt on top. Use a rubber spatula or your fingers to gently press the toppings into the chocolate so they stick. Place the bark in the fridge for about 20 minutes, until it's completely cooled and set. Cut or break it into 24 pieces.

Rosemary-Spiced Walnuts

MAKES: 2 CUPS   PREP TIME: 2 MINUTES   COOK TIME: 8 MINUTES

Five ingredients–including salt and pepper—is all it takes to create a savory snack that's loaded with delicious crunch and plant-based omega-3 fats. In fact, walnuts are the only nut that provides these heart-healthy fats in significant amounts. Toasting them brings out their rich and slightly buttery flavor, elevating every satisfying bite.

If you're looking for a great app to bring to a party or you want to impress your sweetie on date night, this is *the* recipe. Or you can make a big stash and enjoy a handful or two whenever you're looking for a snack. I often store mine in the freezer; they're extra-crispy and will keep fresh for months.

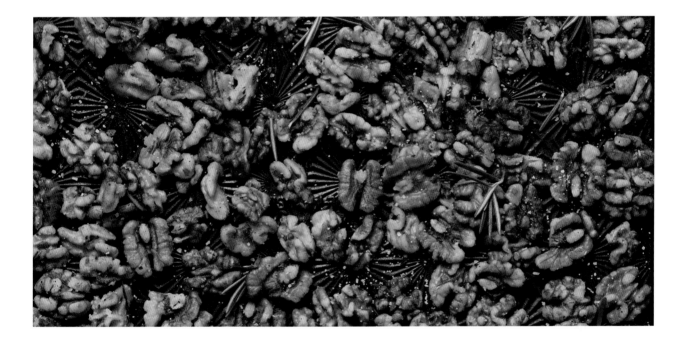

2 cups raw walnuts

1 tablespoon olive oil

2 teaspoons finely chopped fresh rosemary

¼ to ½ teaspoon kosher salt

¼ teaspoon black pepper

1 Preheat the oven to 400°F.

2 Place the walnuts in a medium bowl and toss with the oil, rosemary, salt, and pepper to fully coat.

3 Transfer to a baking sheet and spread the nuts out in a single layer. Bake for 8 minutes. Remove from the oven and let slightly cool before serving.

PER SERVING ¼ CUP **180** CALORIES **4 g** PROTEIN **18 g** FAT (**16 g** UNSATURATED FAT, **2 g** SATURATED FAT) **0 mg** CHOLESTEROL **4 g** CARBS **2 g** FIBER **0 g** SUGAR **60 mg** SODIUM

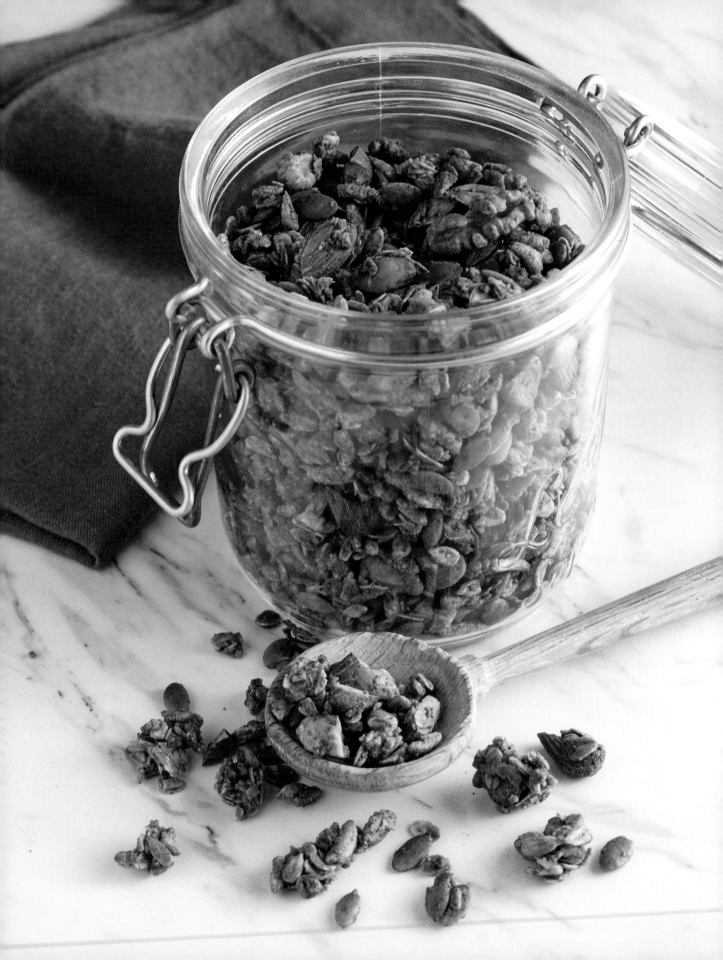

Crispy Turmeric Granola

MAKES: ABOUT 9 CUPS

PREP TIME: 5 MINUTES   COOK TIME: 25 MINUTES

Turmeric helps to ease aches and pain, thanks to its active ingredient, curcumin. I'm always looking for interesting ways to incorporate the power ingredient into my cooking. But truth be told, not everyone is a fan of its pungent flavor and bright yellow color (which has ruined more manicures than I care to admit, haha). However, it's not overpowering in this crunchy granola recipe, so don't let it scare you, or your kiddos, off. In fact, you can't even really detect the taste. This satisfying snack is totally kid- and family-friendly—whip it up and watch it disappear.

Feel free to adjust the seed ratio based on what you have on hand or like best. And if you prefer a bolder spice experience, add 2 teaspoons of garam masala or curry powder.

1 cup raw almonds, chopped

½ cup raw walnuts, chopped

¾ cup raw pumpkin seeds, chopped

¼ cup raw sunflower seeds, chopped

2 cups uncooked old-fashioned oats

2 cups crispy brown rice cereal

⅔ cup honey

2 large egg whites

2 tablespoons ground turmeric

2 teaspoons ground cinnamon

1 teaspoon kosher salt

1 Preheat the oven to 325°F and line 2 baking sheets (or 1 very large sheet) with parchment paper. Lightly mist the parchment paper with nonstick oil spray. Set aside.

2 In a large bowl, combine the almonds, walnuts, pumpkin seeds, sunflower seeds, oats, and brown rice cereal.

3 Mist the bottom of a small bowl with oil spray, then add the honey, egg whites, turmeric, cinnamon, and salt. Stir until everything is well combined. Be sure to blend all of the spices into the honey by mashing any visible clumps with the back of a spoon or spatula until you have a smooth consistency. Pour the honey blend into the nut-oat mixture and stir until everything is well coated.

4 Add the granola mixture to the prepared sheet(s) and spread out in an even layer. Bake for 25 to 30 minutes, stirring the granola and rotating the pans halfway through. Remove from the oven and allow the granola to cool completely. As the granola cools, it will become super crunchy. Store in an airtight container for up to 1 month.

PER SERVING ½ CUP **180** CALORIES **5 g** PROTEIN **9 g** FAT (**8 g** UNSATURATED FAT, **1 g** SATURATED FAT) **0 mg** CHOLESTEROL **22 g** CARBS **3 g** FIBER **11 g** SUGAR (**1 g** NATURAL SUGAR, **10 g** ADDED SUGAR) **135 mg** SODIUM

Sweet Ricotta Cream with Mixed Berries

SERVES: 1   PREP TIME: 4 MINUTES

This is a dessert with benefits: The ricotta provides protein and bone-building calcium. The berries (your choice: You can stick with one favorite or opt for a mix) add fiber, memory-boosting antioxidants, and a beautiful combo of colors. I love tossing this together when I'm craving something sweet and satisfying but don't feel like fussing with a formal recipe. It requires just four simple ingredients, a bowl, and a spoon. It hits the spot every time.

½ cup part-skim ricotta cheese

1 teaspoon vanilla extract

1 teaspoon honey

½ to 1 cup fresh berries

1 In a small bowl, mix together the ricotta, vanilla, and honey until thoroughly combined. Top with the fresh berries.

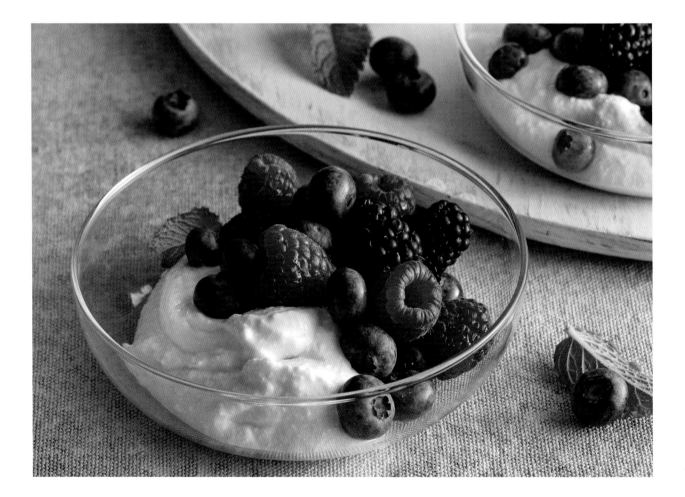

PER SERVING **270** CALORIES **15 g** PROTEIN **10 g** FAT (**4 g** UNSATURATED FAT, **6 g** SATURATED FAT) **40 mg** CHOLESTEROL **30 g** CARBS **3 g** FIBER **16 g** SUGAR (**11 g** NATURAL SUGAR, **5 g** ADDED SUGAR) **125 mg** SODIUM

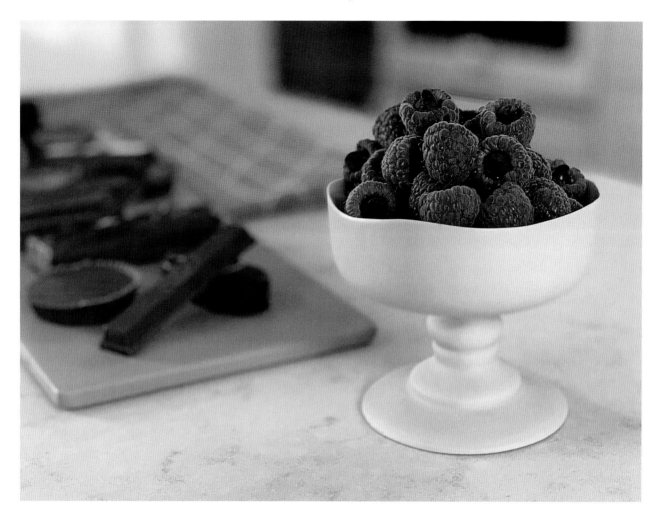

Dark Chocolate–Stuffed Raspberries

SERVES: 1   PREP TIME: 5 MINUTES

You can enjoy 7 of these rich, candy-like berries for just 25 calories. At that number, you can feel free to go back for seconds (and even thirds!). They're great as a stand-alone dessert or snack or you can use them to garnish ice cream, cupcakes, or even fruit salad. Who wouldn't be delighted to scoop one of these up? They're a true treat. Not to mention, this is the easiest recipe in the whole book!

7 raspberries

7 semisweet or dark chocolate chips

1 Stuff each raspberry with 1 chocolate chip. Enjoy chilled or at room temperature.

PER SERVING **25** CALORIES **0 g** PROTEIN **1 g** FAT (**0.5 g** UNSATURATED FAT, **0.5 g** SATURATED FAT) **0 mg** CHOLESTEROL **4 g** CARBS **1 g** FIBER **2 g** SUGAR (**0 g** NATURAL SUGAR, **2 g** ADDED SUGAR) **0 mg** SODIUM

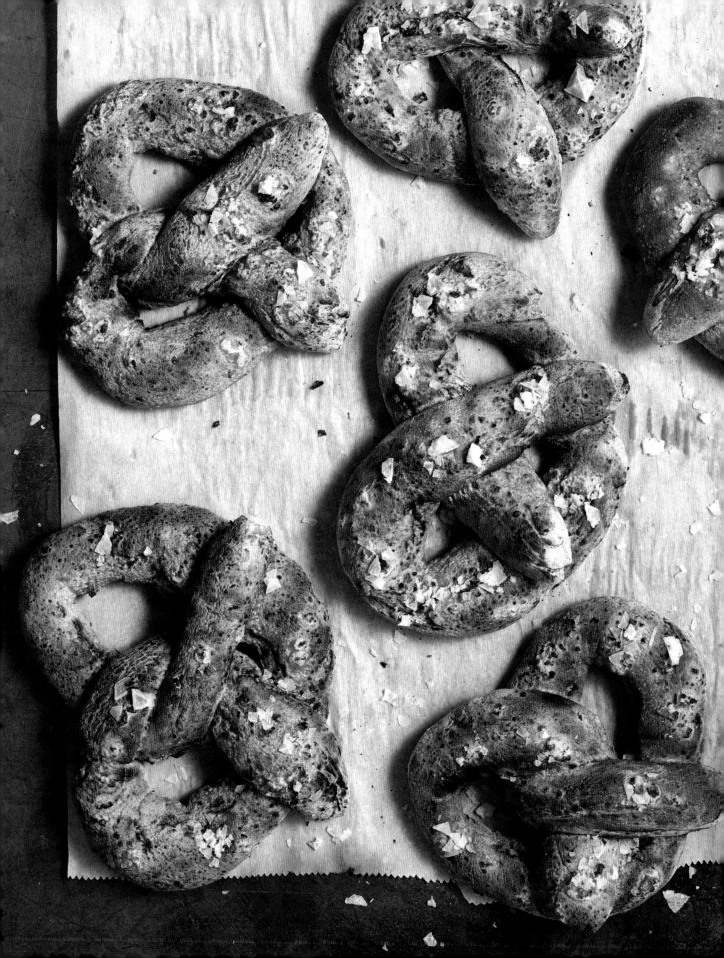

Soft and Doughy Protein Pretzels

MAKES: 8 PRETZELS   PREP TIME: 5 MINUTES   COOK TIME: 20 MINUTES

Remember those doughy pretzels as big as your face that you couldn't wait to enjoy at ball games or carnivals? They sure are delicious, but they're loaded with starchy carbs . . . and not much else. Instead, whip up your own version at home using just a few basic—and wholesome—ingredients. Thanks to the Greek yogurt and whole wheat flour (the same dough as my bagel bites, page 37), each one delivers 10 grams of protein and 4 grams of fiber.

P.S.: I like to dip mine in spicy mustard or warm marinara sauce. They're ridiculously tasty and freeze well, too!

2 cups whole wheat flour

1 tablespoon baking powder

1 teaspoon kosher salt

2 cups nonfat plain Greek yogurt

1 large egg, beaten

OPTIONAL TOPPERS

Coarse sea salt or kosher salt for the pretzel tops, spicy brown mustard and warm marinara sauce for dipping

1   Preheat the oven to 350°F. Line a baking sheet with parchment paper and set aside.

2   In a large bowl, combine the flour, baking powder, and kosher salt. Add the yogurt and mix until all the flour is incorporated to make a batter. Knead the dough with clean hands until it's dry and elastic (this will take about 1 minute). Divide into 8 balls.

3   One at a time, form each ball into one long rope (if it breaks, just squish it back together). If the batter is sticky, add some flour to your hands. (If it still feels too sticky to roll, incorporate a dash of additional flour into the dough.) Lay each rope on the parchment paper and form it into a pretzel shape.

4   Brush the egg wash over the tops and generously sprinkle on the coarse salt, if desired. Bake for about 20 minutes. Serve the pretzels with a side of mustard or marinara sauce for dipping, if desired.

PER SERVING 1 PRETZEL **140** CALORIES **10 g** PROTEIN **1 g** FAT (**1 g** UNSATURATED FAT, **0 g** SATURATED FAT) **12 mg** CHOLESTEROL **24 g** CARBS **4 g** FIBER **2 g** SUGAR (**2 g** NATURAL SUGAR, **0 g** ADDED SUGAR) **280 mg** SODIUM

Chocolate Sunflower Butter Cups

MAKES: 24 MINI CUPS   PREP TIME: 5 MINUTES,
PLUS AT LEAST 1 HOUR IN THE FREEZER   COOK TIME: 2 MINUTES

A 5-minute dessert that includes chocolate? I'm in! I came up with these tasty treats while experimenting with leftover sunflower butter—my niece, Becca, is allergic to nuts, and I wanted to make her something yummy. Sunflower seed butter is a great alternative for people with nut allergies because it features the same rich creaminess as peanut butter, but, of course, it's nut-free. And the nutrition profile is so similar to nuts: The little seed is loaded with heart-healthy fats, fiber, and folate, one of the B vitamins needed to convert carbohydrates into energy. I keep a stash of these dreamy cups in the freezer and reach for one when a craving strikes.

1 ripe banana

¼ cup creamy sunflower seed butter

½ teaspoon vanilla extract

1½ cups semisweet or dark chocolate chips

Sunflower seeds for garnish

1   In a small bowl, combine the banana, sunflower seed butter, and vanilla. Mash everything together until there are no lumps and set aside.

2   Prepare a 24-compartment mini-muffin tin by misting the individual compartments with nonstick oil spray (this will help the chocolate cups pop out easily when they're ready). This recipe works best *without* muffin liners.

3   TO MELT AND TEMPER THE CHOCOLATE: Place 1 cup of the chocolate chips in a bowl and microwave for 15 to 30 seconds at a time, stirring in between, until the chocolate is smooth and velvety. Stir in the remaining ½ cup chocolate chips until they're all melted and blended. If they haven't all melted, microwave for another 5 seconds at a time and stir.

4   TO ASSEMBLE: Add 1 generous teaspoon of melted chocolate to the bottom of each muffin compartment. Spread out the chocolate with your fingers to cover the bottom. Next, add a layer of sunflower butter filling on top (you'll be using about 1 generous teaspoon per cup) and, again, spread the second layer out with your fingers. Finally, add the remaining melted chocolate on top, using your fingers to level it out. Garnish with a few sunflower seeds. (It's a messy process; don't worry if they don't appear perfect. They'll turn out looking and tasting amazing.)

5   Place the muffin tin in the freezer to firm up for at least 1 hour or overnight. When you're ready to eat them, carefully pop them out of the muffin tins, using the tip of a knife.

NOTE: Keep in the freezer until right before you're ready to serve, as the middle layer starts to soften up rather quickly. Or transfer them from the muffin tin directly to a storage bag or container and stash in the freezer for future treats. They'll last in the freezer for months.

PER 1 MINI CUP **70** CALORIES **1 g** PROTEIN **4 g** FAT (**2 g** UNSATURATED FAT, **2 g** SATURATED FAT) **0 mg** CHOLESTEROL **1 g** FIBER **6 g** SUGAR (**0.5 g** NATURAL SUGAR, **5.5 g** ADDED SUGAR) **5 mg** SODIUM

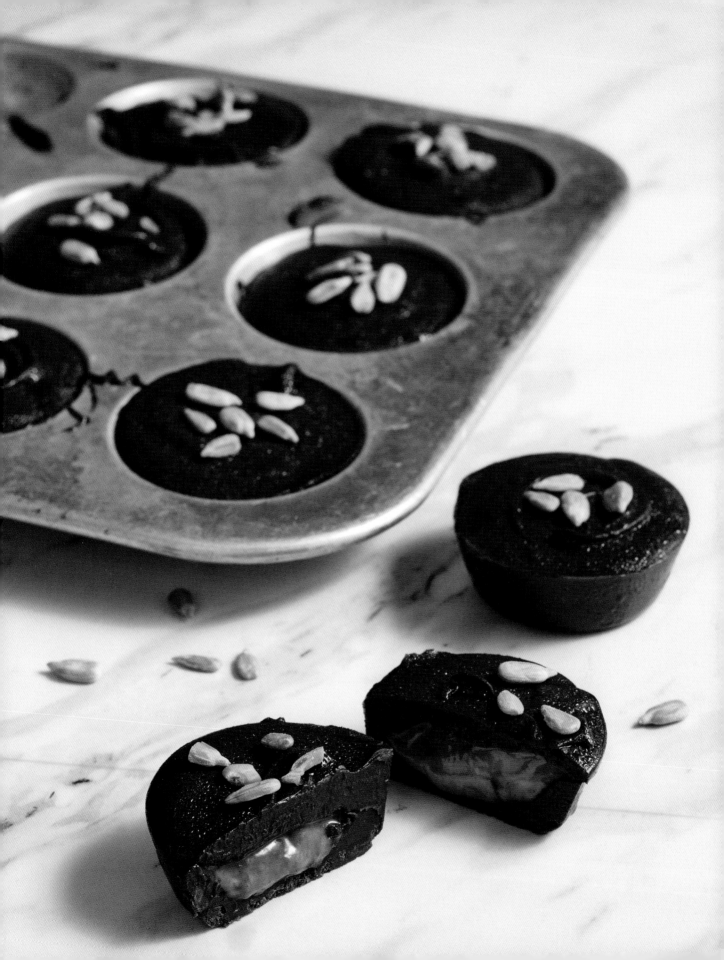

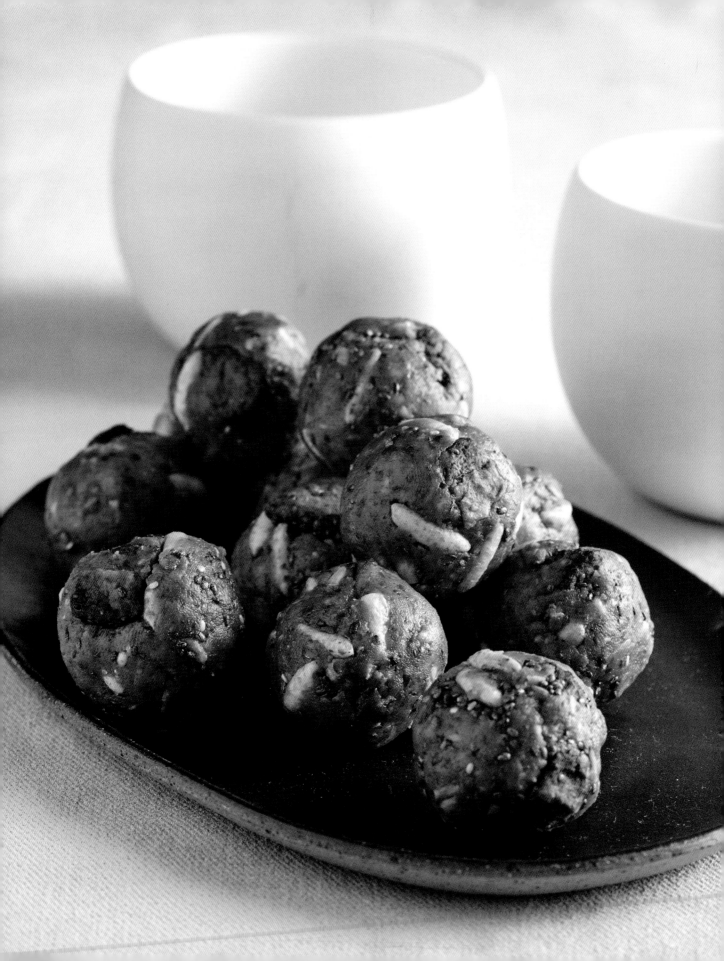

PB & Strawberry Energy Bites

MAKES: 60 BITES   PREP TIME: 5 MINUTES

There's so much to love about these little balls of goodness. For one, they require no baking. Just whirl the ingredients in a food processor and press them together with your fingers. These are great for an afternoon snack or a pre-workout nibble. I also have to mention that the recipe makes a lot (about 60 small bites, or you can make 30 jumbo ping pong-sized balls), so you can store leftovers in the freezer for future snacks or healthy treats. I actually prefer these slightly frozen. I love that you'll find (count 'em) seven superfoods—protein-rich nut butter, sweet dates, fiber-filled oats and brown rice, antioxidant-packed berries, and omega-3-filled flax and chia—in such a small package.

1 packed cup pitted dried dates*

1 cup plus 1 tablespoon creamy peanut butter, divided

1 tablespoon honey

2 tablespoons coconut oil, divided

½ cup uncooked old-fashioned oats

3 tablespoons ground flaxseeds

2 tablespoons chia seeds

½ cup crispy brown rice cereal

1 cup freeze-dried strawberries, crushed into smaller pieces

*   *If your dates are a bit dried out, soak them in 1 cup boiling water for 1 to 2 minutes to soften them up, then drain well before using.*

1. In the bowl of a food processor, combine the dates and 1 cup of the peanut butter and process to form a paste, 1½ to 2 minutes, scraping down the bowl halfway through to ensure everything gets incorporated. Add the honey and 1 tablespoon of the oil and process until smooth. Add the oats, flaxseeds, and chia seeds and pulse until the oats have broken down into smaller pieces and they're mixed into the paste, another 2 minutes or so. Transfer the mixture to a large bowl. Using your hands, mix in the crispy rice cereal and crushed freeze-dried strawberries.

2. In a small microwave-safe bowl, heat the remaining 1 tablespoon coconut oil and 1 tablespoon peanut butter for about 20 seconds to create a liquid. Whisk them together, then add to the bowl with the batter and blend everything using your hands. The mixture will be crumbly but should come together easily when squeezed with your fingers. Form the mixture into 60 (1-inch) balls, pressing and molding to form each bite. Store your bites in a sealed container in the freezer for up to 2 months.

PER BITE **50** CALORIES **1 g** PROTEIN **3 g** FAT (**2 g** UNSATURATED FAT, **1 g** SATURATED FAT) **0 mg** CHOLESTEROL **5 g** CARBS **1 g** FIBER **2 g** SUGAR (**1 g** NATURAL SUGAR, **1 g** ADDED SUGAR) **20 mg** SODIUM

Pumpkin Pie Ice Cream

SERVES: 6   PREP TIME: 5 MINUTES, PLUS AT LEAST 3 HOURS IN THE FREEZER

I'm using the fall superstar to create a dairy-free frozen treat. The perks: You don't need a special ice cream maker to whip it up; you can use a standard blender or food processor. And you can use up any ripe bananas you may have lying around, which means you're not only reducing food waste but also getting a double punch of potassium (pumpkin also contains the nutrient), which helps with blood pressure, bloating, and cramping. Also, pretty fantastic to enjoy an ice cream with 4 grams of fiber.

4 ripe bananas

1 (15-ounce) can pumpkin puree (about 1½ cups)

¼ cup maple syrup

1 tablespoon pumpkin pie spice

¼ teaspoon ground cinnamon

¼ teaspoon kosher salt

1 Peel the bananas and freeze for at least 3 hours.

2 Break the frozen bananas into large pieces and place in the bowl of a food processor or high-speed blender. Add the remaining ingredients and process until completely smooth with no frozen chunks remaining. If the bananas are too hard to blend, add a splash of milk to help them along.

Enjoy immediately as soft serve ice cream. Or, to firm it up, divide among small serving bowls, cover, and freeze for at least 30 minutes before serving. Let it sit on the counter for a few minutes to soften before digging in. Garnish with chopped toasted pecans, if desired.

PER SERVING ½ CUP **120** CALORIES **1 g** PROTEIN **0 g** FAT **0 mg** CHOLESTEROL **37 g** CARBS **4 g** FIBER **19 g** SUGAR (**11 g** NATURAL SUGAR, **8 g** ADDED SUGAR) **85 mg** SODIUM *ADD 50 CALORIES FOR THE PECANS.

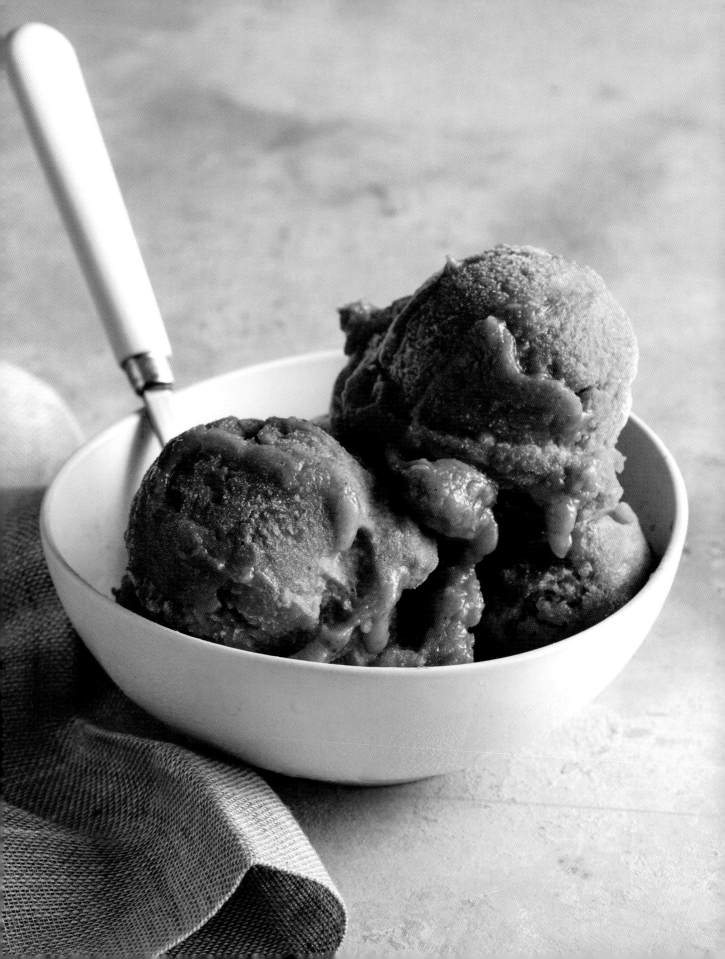

Fudgy Lentil Brownies

MAKES: 12 BROWNIES   PREP TIME: 10 MINUTES   COOK TIME: 40 MINUTES

I enjoy sneaking surprise ingredients into indulgent desserts. Take these fudgy lentil brownies. I use them as an opportunity to show lentils some long-overdue love. The fiber-rich pulses are taking over the plant-based food scene because they're tasty, easy to prepare, budget-friendly, and loaded with the good stuff. Couple them with three more power foods—cocoa powder, rolled oats, and almond butter—and you have a chocolaty treat that boasts 5 grams of protein and 4 grams of fiber.

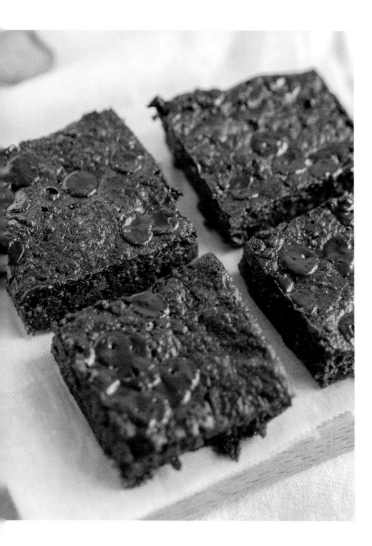

½ cup dry light brown lentils

1 cup uncooked old-fashioned oats

¼ cup cocoa powder

1½ teaspoons baking powder

½ teaspoon baking soda

¼ teaspoon kosher salt

½ cup natural applesauce

1 large egg

¼ cup almond butter

2 teaspoons vanilla extract

⅓ cup honey

1¼ cups semisweet or dark chocolate chips

1 Preheat the oven to 350°F. Mist an 8-inch-square baking dish with nonstick oil spray. Set aside.

2 In a small saucepan, combine the lentils and 1 cup water. Bring to a boil over medium-high heat, then reduce the heat, cover, and simmer for 15 to 20 minutes, until the lentils are tender and most of the liquid is gone.

3 In a food processor, combine the oats, cocoa powder, baking powder, baking soda, and salt. Pulse until a fine powder forms. Add the cooked lentils (and any liquid remaining in the pan), the applesauce, egg, almond butter, vanilla, and honey and process until a smooth batter forms. Using a spoon, fold in at least 1 cup of the chocolate chips.

4 Pour the batter into the prepared baking dish and spread evenly with a spatula. Sprinkle the remaining ¼ cup chocolate chips over the top. Bake for about 25 minutes. Let cool for at least 10 minutes before cutting and serving.

PER SERVING 1 BROWNIE **210** CALORIES **5 g** PROTEIN **9 g** FAT (**5.5 g** UNSATURATED FAT, **3.5 g** SATURATED FAT) **15 mg** CHOLESTEROL **31 g** CARBS **4 g** FIBER **12 g** SUGAR (**2 g** NATURAL SUGAR, **10 g** ADDED SUGAR) **115 mg** SODIUM

Dark Chocolate Turtles

MAKES: ABOUT 28 TURTLES   PREP TIME: 15 MINUTES   COOK TIME: 2 MINUTES

Teenage Mutant Ninja Turtles (sometimes known as TMNT) were huge when my kids were younger. I made my own edible TMNTs—*Totally Mouthwatering Nutty Turtles*—that are sure to be as big a hit with your little ones (oh, and adults, too!). Unlike traditional turtles, which are made with milk chocolate and sugary caramel, these mini masterpieces contain ingredients you can feel good about. Even better, your friends and family won't even suspect the smart swaps. First, I trade the milk chocolate for dark, which contains more health-boosting flavanols. Instead of candy caramel, I rely on dates, which provide the same gooey caramel-like chew with the added benefit of fiber. No swaps needed on antioxidant-rich pecans, another signature turtle ingredients. Bonus: These chocolate goodies freeze perfectly so you can stash a batch for future cravings.

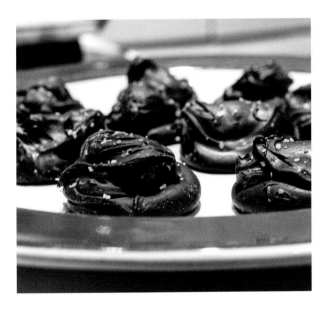

2 cups dark chocolate chips (at least 60% cocoa), divided

⅓ cup (28 pieces) toasted pecan halves*

¾ cup pitted dried dates, cut in half lengthwise

¾ teaspoon flaked sea salt (fleur de sel) or kosher salt

* *To toast raw pecans, spread them on a baking sheet and place in an oven set at 350°F for 5 to 6 minutes. Remove and let cool.*

1   Line 2 baking sheets with parchment paper. Set aside.

2   **TO TEMPER THE CHOCOLATE:** In a medium bowl, add 1⅓ cups of the chocolate chips and microwave for 15 to 30 seconds at a time, stirring in between, until the chocolate is smooth and velvety. Stir in the reserved ⅔ cup chocolate chips until they're completely melted. (If they don't fully melt, microwave for another 10 seconds and stir.)

3   **TO ASSEMBLE:** Place a 1-teaspoon-size dollop of the melted chocolate on one of the prepared baking sheets. Place a pecan half on top and gently press down to slightly flatten out the chocolate underneath. Add a date half on top of the pecan, then add another teaspoon of the melted chocolate. Top the "turtle" with a small pinch of salt. Repeat this process, using up all of the chocolate, pecan halves and date halves to make a full batch of turtles. If the melted chocolate starts to harden before you're done prepping, pop it back in the microwave for another 5 to 10 seconds and stir. Place the turtles in the fridge for at least 10 minutes, or until they harden and firm.

PER TURTLE **90** CALORIES **1 g** PROTEIN **5 g** FAT (**2 g** UNSATURATED FAT, **3 g** SATURATED FAT) **0 mg** CHOLESTEROL **9 g** CARBS **0 g** FIBER **7 g** SUGARS (**7 g** NATURAL SUGAR, **0 g** ADDED SUGAR) **50 mg** SODIUM

Oatmeal Cookie Walnut Butter

MAKES: ABOUT 1 CUP   PREP TIME: 15 MINUTES

This. Spread. Is. Addictive. It has similar nutrition stats as straight nut butter with the added benefits of walnuts and whole grain oats. Plus, you'll appreciate the sweet deliciousness of vanilla, cinnamon, and honey. Just toss all ingredients into a blender or food processor, puree, and dig in.

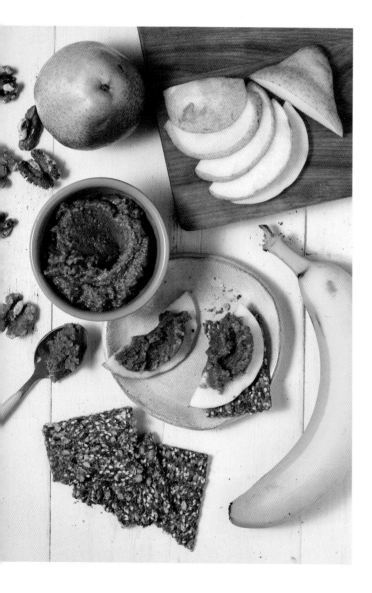

2 cups raw walnuts

¼ cup uncooked old-fashioned oats

1 tablespoon plus 1 teaspoon honey

1 teaspoon vanilla extract

½ teaspoon ground cinnamon

¼ teaspoon kosher salt or sea salt

1   Combine all the ingredients in the bowl of a food processor or high-speed blender and process for about 10 minutes, until the batter is thick and creamy. Stop every few minutes to scrape down the sides and loosen up the contents underneath the blades. While the batter may look like its done after just a few minutes, try to continue processing for the full 10 minutes, as this will create a creamier nut butter.

TO SERVE: Spread on sliced apples, pears, and bananas, or use as a topper for whole grain waffles, toast, and crackers. This will keep in an airtight container in the fridge for up to 6 weeks. (If it becomes crumbly in the fridge, microwave for about 20 seconds before eating to restore its creaminess.)

PER SERVING 2 TABLESPOONS **180** CALORIES **4 g** PROTEIN **15 g** FAT (**13.5 g** UNSATURATED FAT, **1.5 g** SATURATED FAT) **0 mg** CHOLESTEROL **7 g** CARBS **2 g** FIBER **3 g** SUGAR (**1 g** NATURAL SUGAR, **2 g** ADDED SUGAR) **45 mg** SODIUM

Peanut Butter–Stuffed Strawberries

SERVES: 1   PREP TIME: 5 MINUTES

Powdered peanut butter is a fantastic way to enjoy PB goodness with far fewer calories. It's made from peanuts that are defatted and then ground into a fine powder. When you're ready to enjoy, all you have to do is add water and mix until it's creamy.

Don't get me wrong, I think peanuts—and natural nut butters—are fabulous. They offer heart-healthy fats and a whole lot of goodness, but the powdered version works really well in some recipes, including this one. There are several different brands of PB powder; you can find it in the peanut butter section of the grocery store.

In this strawberry spin, I hollow out fiber-rich berries and then pipe the peanut butter in. They make a fun snack, dessert, or even energizing breakfast. A serving (8 to 10 filled berries) delivers an impressive 10 g fiber and 21 g protein. They're *berry* good!

8 to 10 strawberries

½ cup peanut butter powder, prepared with water according to the package directions

1 tablespoon chia seeds (optional)

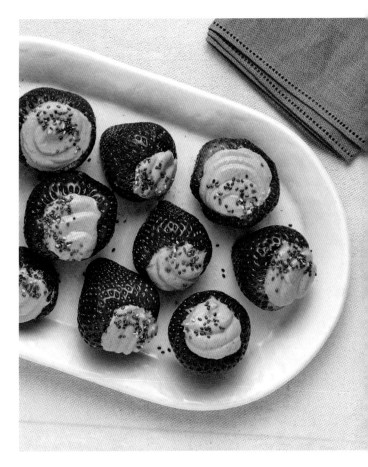

1   Slightly hollow out the strawberries to create just enough space for the peanut butter. (If you'd like the strawberries to stand up straight, slice a tiny piece off the bottom to create a flat base.)

2   Place the peanut butter in a zip-top bag and cut one *tiny* hole in the corner of the bag. Pipe the peanut butter into the strawberries. Sprinkle the chia seeds on top, if desired.

PER SERVING 240 CALORIES 21 g PROTEIN 6 g FAT (6 g UNSATURATED FAT, 0 g SATURATED FAT) 0 mg CHOLESTEROL 34 g CARBS 10 g FIBER 14 g SUGAR (14 g NATURAL SUGAR, 0 g ADDED SUGAR) 380 mg SODIUM

Salted Caramel Chia Pudding

SERVES: 4   PREP TIME: 5 MINUTES, PLUS AT LEAST 2 HOURS IN THE REFRIGERATOR

It's pudding time! I love this rich dessert—it's a no-bake, vegan pudding that contains 11 grams of fiber (yes, you read that correctly). One of the key ingredients is chia seeds. These "nutrition sprinkles" are flavor-neutral and help add thickness to recipes, giving this decadent dessert a rich and luxurious consistency. They absorb the liquid while it sits in the fridge; the longer the mixture chills, the more pudding-like it becomes. The taste sort of reminds me of a creamy tapioca pudding with a little crunch. And gelling is not all these super seeds do—they also contribute fiber, protein, and plant-based omega-3s. Another power ingredient is dates, which lend a sweet caramel flavor along with offering up potassium, magnesium, and fiber.

If you prefer a less sweet dessert, skip the added maple syrup. But if you do decide to use it, note that it tacks on only 3 grams of added sugar, and in my opinion, it's totally worth it. Craving chocolate? Simply toss in a tablespoon of cocoa powder to the blender, or you can wait until your pudding is firm from the fridge and mix 1 to 2 teaspoons into each single serving. Caramel or chocolate . . . it's a tough decision.

Heaping ½ cup pitted dried dates

1½ cups unsweetened almond milk (or other milk of choice)

1 teaspoon vanilla extract

½ teaspoon maple extract or maple flavor

1 tablespoon maple syrup

½ teaspoon kosher salt or sea salt

6 tablespoons chia seeds

1 Combine the dates, milk, vanilla, maple extract or flavor, maple syrup, and salt in a high-speed blender and pulse until the dates are completely broken down and the mixture is smooth, 1½ to 2 minutes. Add the chia seeds and pulse again to blend everything together.

2 Transfer the mixture into a bowl or container (it's okay if there are some small date pieces). Cover and chill in the fridge for at least 2 hours or overnight. Do not skip the chilling time, as it enables the chia seeds to thicken and turn the mixture into pudding.

Serve in pretty parfait glasses or ramekins and garnish with optional toasted coconut, chopped dates, or shaved dark chocolate.

PER SERVING ½ CUP **190** CALORIES **6 g** PROTEIN **9 g** FAT (**8 g** UNSATURATED FAT, **1 g** SATURATED FAT) **0 mg** CHOLESTEROL **28 g** CARBS **11 g** FIBER **14 g** SUGAR (**11 g** NATURAL SUGAR, **3 g** ADDED SUGAR) **380 mg** SODIUM

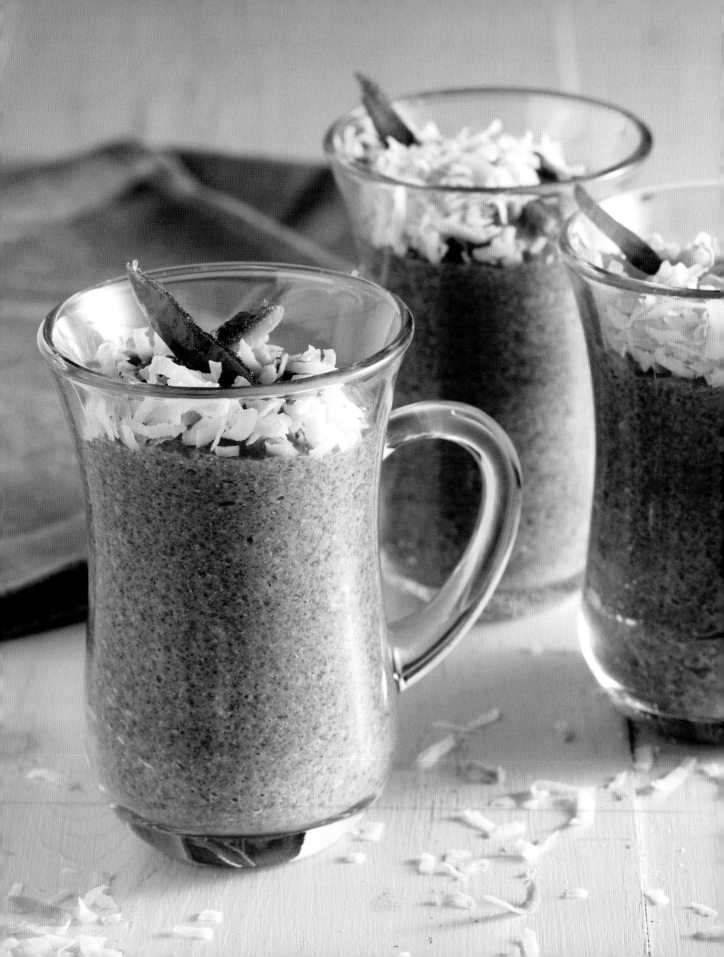

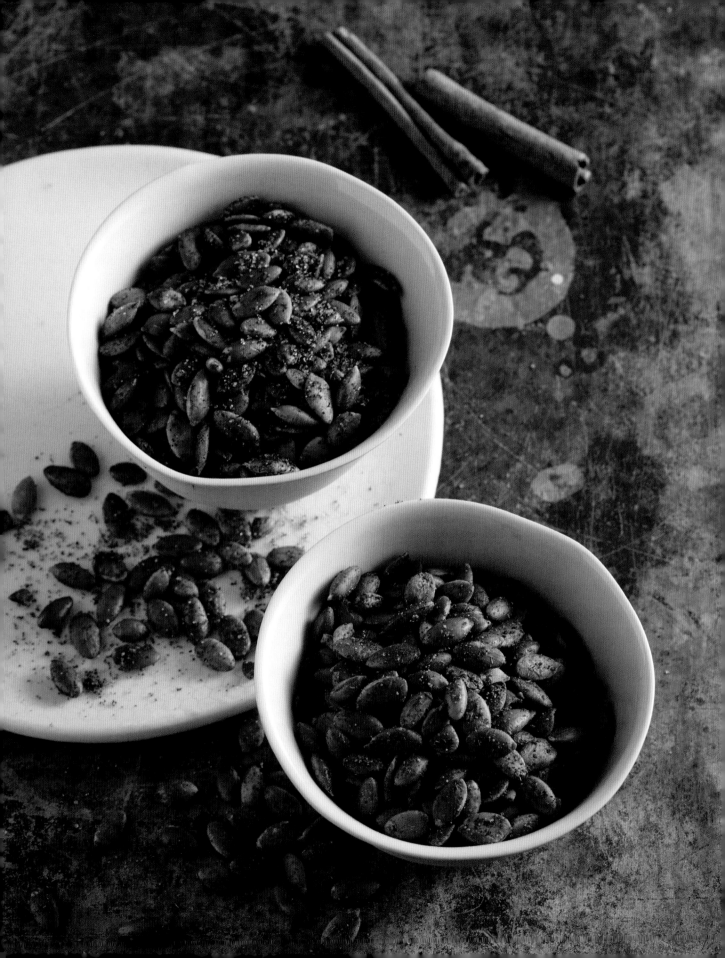

Roasted Pepitas
(Cinnamon-Sugar and Cumin-Cayenne)

SERVES: 4   PREP TIME: 2 MINUTES   COOK TIME: 10 MINUTES

Pepitas are nutritious and delicious shell-less pumpkin seeds. They come packaged with magnesium (helpful for headache sufferers) and zinc (an immune-booster) as well as protein and fiber (useful for managing blood sugar, appetite, and mood). And they're the star ingredient in these two easy-breezy recipes, Cinnamon-Sugar and Cumin-Cayenne Roasted Pepitas. Make a batch and enjoy them right out of your hand, or on yogurt and oatmeal, in salads, pancakes, muffins, and cookies—you can even use these flavorful gems to garnish creamy soups, stews, and chili!

CINNAMON-SUGAR PEPITAS

1 cup raw pepitas

1 teaspoon olive oil

1½ teaspoons ground cinnamon

1 tablespoon sugar

¼ teaspoon kosher salt

1 Preheat the oven to 325°F. Line a baking sheet with parchment paper and set aside.

2 In a small bowl, combine the pepitas and oil and toss with a spoon to coat. Add the cinnamon, sugar, and salt and mix to combine. Lay the mixture out on the prepared baking sheet in a single layer and roast for about 10 minutes. If you'd like them a bit toastier and crunchier, remove from the oven, shake the seeds around, then put back in the oven for another 2 to 4 minutes. Watch closely so they don't burn. Let cool and enjoy.

PER SERVING ¼ CUP **200** CALORIES **9 g** PROTEIN **15 g** FAT (**11.5 g** UNSATURATED FAT, **3.5 g** SATURATED FAT) **0 mg** CHOLESTEROL **8 g** CARBS **4 g** FIBER **4 g** SUGAR (**1 g** NATURAL SUGAR, **3 g** ADDED SUGAR) **125 mg** SODIUM

CUMIN-CAYENNE PEPITAS

1 cup raw pepitas

1 teaspoon olive oil

1 teaspoon kosher salt

½ teaspoon garlic powder

½ teaspoon ground cumin

¼ teaspoon chili powder

¼ teaspoon ground cayenne

1 Preheat the oven to 325°F. Line a baking sheet with parchment paper and set aside.

2 In a small bowl, combine the pepitas and oil and toss with a spoon to coat. Add the salt, garlic powder, cumin, chili powder, and cayenne and mix to combine. Lay the mixture out on the prepared baking sheet in a single layer and roast for 10 minutes. If you'd like them a bit toastier and crunchier, remove from the oven, shake the seeds around, then put back in the oven for another 2 to 4 minutes. Watch closely so they don't burn. Let cool and enjoy.

PER SERVING ¼ CUP **190** CALORIES **9 g** PROTEIN **15 g** FAT (**11.5 g** UNSATURATED FAT, **3.5 g** SATURATED FAT) **0 mg** CHOLESTEROL **5 g** CARBS **3 g** FIBER **1 g** SUGAR (**1 g** NATURAL SUGAR, **0 g** ADDED SUGAR) **490 mg** SODIUM

PB Coconut Cookie Dough Dip

MAKES: 1 HEAPING CUP   PREP TIME: 5 MINUTES

I wasn't sure what to call this addictive recipe—it tastes like a sweet, rich peanut butter–coconut cookie dough, but it has a thinner dip-like consistency, so I landed on cookie dough dip.

Pro tip: Mist your measuring cup with nonstick oil spray before adding your PB (same with the tablespoon for the honey) so they slide out more easily. You'll totally flip for this dip!

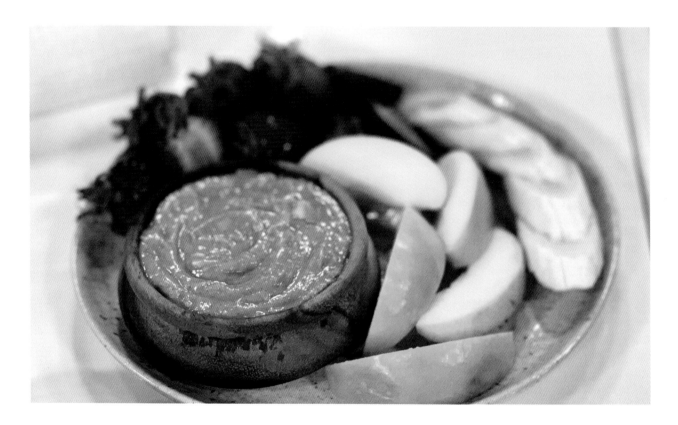

½ cup creamy peanut butter

½ cup unsweetened vanilla almond milk

1 tablespoon honey

1 teaspoon ground cinnamon

1 teaspoon vanilla extract

Pinch sea salt

½ cup unsweetened coconut flakes

Apple slices, strawberries, or banana slices for serving

1 Combine the peanut butter, almond milk, honey, cinnamon, vanilla, and salt in a blender or food processor. Pulse until smooth, 1 to 2 minutes, scraping down the sides as necessary to incorporate all the ingredients. Add the coconut and pulse until well combined. (For a thinner, smoother consistency, add an additional 1 to 2 tablespoons almond milk with the coconut flakes.) Serve with fruit for dipping. Store in a sealed container in the fridge for up to 3 weeks.

PER SERVING 2 TABLESPOONS **140** CALORIES **4 g** PROTEIN **11 g** FAT (**7.5 g** UNSATURATED FAT, **3.5 g** SATURATED FAT) **0 mg** CHOLESTEROL **7 g** CARBS **2 g** FIBER **3 g** SUGAR (**1 g** NATURAL SUGAR, **2 g** ADDED SUGAR) **70 mg** SODIUM

Gooey Apple Pie Filling with Toasty Pecans

SERVES: 2   PREP TIME: 5 MINUTES   COOK TIME: 2 MINUTES

This dessert features a thick, gooey apple-pie-filling-like consistency and is packed with warm, indulgent apple-cinnamon flavor. I mix in rolled oats and leave the skin on the apples for extra fiber. The recipe comes together lickety-split and thickens up quickly, so it's best served warm and freshly made right before you're ready to dig in. It's a fuss-free dessert that delivers the classic feel-good flavors of apple pie for a fraction of the calories, sugar, fat, and prep time. Apple pie perfection.

1 unpeeled apple, cored and finely diced

¼ cup old-fashioned oats

1 tablespoon maple syrup

½ teaspoon ground cinnamon, plus more for garnish

1 tablespoon arrowroot*

¼ teaspoon vanilla extract

2 to 4 tablespoons toasted pecan halves

Aerated whipped topping for serving

*   *If you can't find arrowroot, swap in cornstarch.*

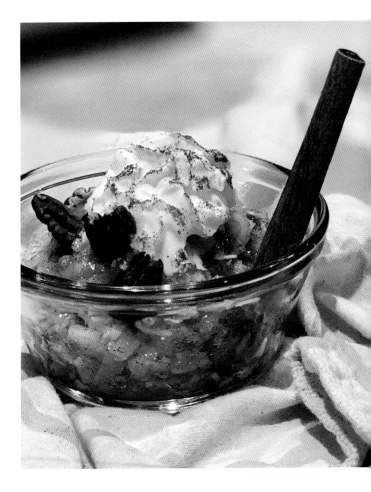

1 Mix the apple, oats, maple syrup, and cinnamon in a medium microwave-safe bowl. In a small bowl, dissolve the arrowroot in ¼ cup cold water until smooth and no lumps remain. Add the arrowroot mixture to the bowl with the chopped apples and mix until everything is well combined. Microwave for 1 minute, remove the bowl, add the vanilla, and mix well. Microwave for another minute and mix again. The mixture should be thick and gooey. Add the toasted pecans and divide the mixture between 2 ramekins.

Serve with an optional squirt of whipped topping and sprinkling of cinnamon.

PER SERVING **140** CALORIES **1 g** PROTEIN **5 g** FAT (**4.5 g** UNSATURATED FAT, **0.5 g** SATURATED FAT) **5 mg** CHOLESTEROL **25 g** CARBS **3 g** FIBER **16 g** SUGAR (**10 g** NATURAL SUGAR, **6 g** ADDED SUGAR) **0 mg** SODIUM

Smoothies, Slushies, Beneficial Bevvies, and Grown-up Cocktails

Longevity Smoothie

Superfoods: berries, banana, kale, nuts, seeds, green tea

SERVES: 1   PREP TIME: 5 MINUTES

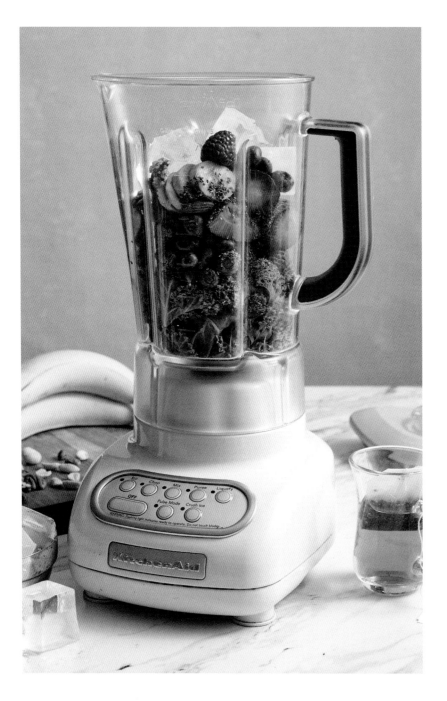

2 cups fresh or frozen mixed berries (any type)

½ to 1 ripe banana

1 cup loosely packed kale or spinach leaves

6 nuts (1 almond + 1 peanut + 1 macadamia + 1 pecan + 1 walnut + 1 pistachio)*

1 teaspoon chia seeds or ground flaxseeds

½ cup green tea, chilled

3 to 5 ice cubes (optional)

* *You may substitute any nuts you have on hand.*

Place all the ingredients in a blender and puree until smooth. Pour into a glass and enjoy.

PER SERVING ABOUT 2 CUPS **230** CALORIES **6 g** PROTEIN **8 g** (**7 g** UNSATURATED FAT), **1 g** SATURATED FAT, **0 mg** CHOLESTEROL **42 g** CARBS **14 g** FIBER **23 g** SUGAR (**23 g** NATURAL SUGAR, **0 g** ADDED SUGAR) **25 mg** SODIUM

Mint Chocolate Shamrock Shake

Superfoods: cocoa powder, bananas

SERVES: 2   PREP TIME: 5 MINUTES

2 ripe bananas, peeled and frozen

¼ cup cocoa powder

½ to ¾ cup almond milk (or milk of choice)

1 drop mint extract (it's very strong)

½ teaspoon vanilla extract

½ cup ice cubes

OPTIONAL TOPPERS

Aerated whipped topping, mint leaves, cocoa powder

Break the frozen bananas into large pieces. Combine all the ingredients in a blender and puree until smooth and frothy. Add a splash of extra milk if you have trouble blending. Pour into glasses and garnish with optional toppings.

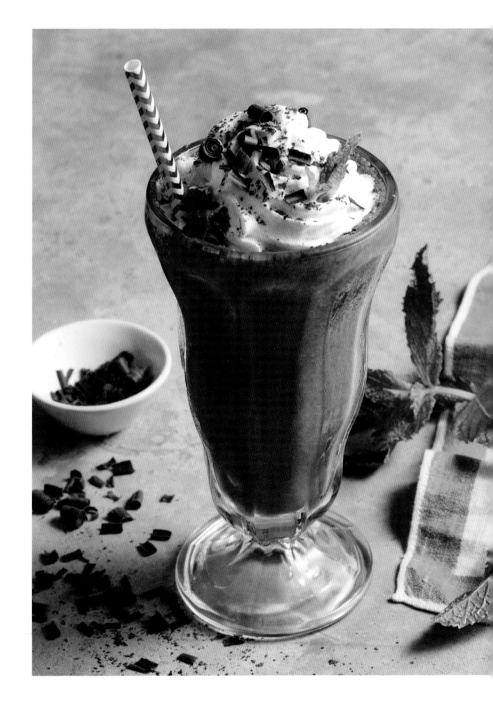

PER SERVING 1 HEAPING CUP **120** CALORIES **3 g** PROTEIN **2 g** TOTAL FAT (**2 g** UNSATURATED FAT, **0 g** SATURATED FAT) **0 mg** CHOLESTEROL **30 g** CARBS **7 g** FIBER **12 g** SUGAR (**12 g** NATURAL SUGAR, **0 g** ADDED SUGAR) **50 mg** SODIUM

Sweet Cherry Slushy

Superfoods: cherries, pineapple

SERVES: 2   PREP TIME: 2 MINUTES

2 cups frozen pitted sweet cherries

½ cup frozen pineapple chunks

1 cup cherry–flavored sparkling water

1 cup ice cubes

Combine all the ingredients in a blender and process until thick and slushy. Add additional sparkling water or ice as needed to achieve your desired slushy consistency. Pour into glasses and serve.

Blueberry Raspberry Slushy

Superfoods: blueberries, raspberries

SERVES: 2   PREP TIME: 2 MINUTES

1½ cups fresh or frozen blueberries

1½ cups fresh or frozen raspberries

1 (12-ounce) can berry-flavored sparkling water

Place all the ingredients in a blender and process until thick and slushy. Pour into glasses and garnish with a few floating berries if desired.

PER SERVING ABOUT 1½ CUPS **110** CALORIES **1 g** PROTEIN **0 g** FAT **0 mg** CHOLESTEROL **28 g** CARBS **4 g** FIBER **19 g** SUGAR (**19 g** NATURAL SUGAR, **0 g** ADDED SUGAR) **0 mg** SODIUM

PER SERVING 1½ CUPS **110** CALORIES **2 g** PROTEIN **1 g** FAT (**1 g** UNSATURATED FAT, **0 g** SATURATED FAT) **0 mg** CHOLESTEROL **27 g** CARBS **9 g** FIBER **15 g** SUGAR (**15 g** NATURAL SUGAR, **0 g** ADDED SUGAR) **0 mg** SODIUM

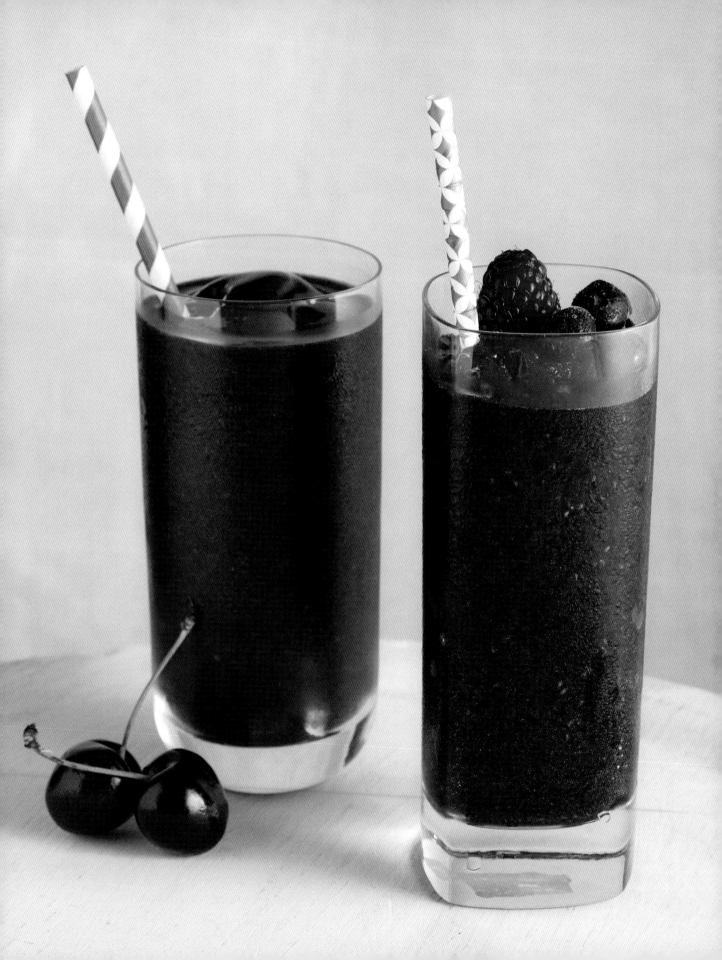

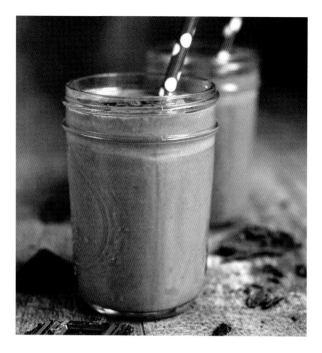

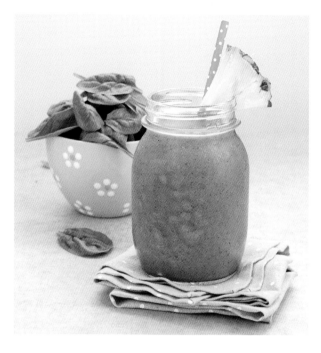

Mocha-mazing Smoothie

Superfoods: coffee, banana, spinach, flaxseeds, almond butter, cocoa powder

SERVES: 2   PREP TIME: 5 MINUTES

1 cup brewed coffee, chilled or at room temperature

1 ripe banana, peeled and frozen

1 cup loosely packed baby spinach

2 tablespoons ground flaxseeds

2 tablespoons almond butter

1 tablespoon cocoa powder

½ cup unsweetened almond milk (or milk of choice)

½ cup ice cubes

Honey or sugar (optional)

Break the frozen banana into a few large pieces. Combine all the ingredients in a blender and puree until thick and frothy. Pour into glasses and enjoy.

PER SERVING 1¼ CUPS **200** CALORIES **7 g** PROTEIN **12 g** FAT (**11 g** UNSATURATED FAT, **1 g** SATURATED FAT) **0 mg** CHOLESTEROL **19 g** CARBS **7 g** FIBER **7 g** SUGAR (**7 g** NATURAL SUGAR, **0 g** ADDED SUGAR) **75 mg** SODIUM

Super Green Smoothie

Superfoods: dates, strawberries, pineapple, kale, almond butter, chia seeds

SERVES: 2   PREP TIME: 5 MINUTES

1 cup unsweetened almond milk

1 cup frozen strawberries

1 cup frozen pineapple chunks

4 to 5 pitted dried dates

1 cup spinach or kale leaves

1 tablespoon almond butter

2 to 3 teaspoons chia seeds or ground flaxseeds

1 teaspoon vanilla extract

3 to 5 ice cubes

Combine all the ingredients in a blender and puree until smooth and frothy. Pour into glasses and enjoy.

PER SERVING 1¼ CUPS **220** CALORIES **5 g** PROTEIN **8 g** FAT (**7.5 g** UNSATURATED FAT, **0.5 g** SATURATED FAT) **0 mg** CHOLESTEROL **36 g** CARBS **7 g** FIBER **22 g** SUGAR (**22 g** NATURAL SUGAR, **0 g** ADDED SUGAR) **130 mg** SODIUM

Salted Caramel Milkshake

Superfoods: dates, pineapple, almond butter

SERVES: 2   PREP TIME: 5 MINUTES

Caramel hard candy, crushed into very small pieces

1 cup unsweetened vanilla almond milk

½ cup pitted dried dates

Heaping ½ cup frozen pineapple chunks

1 to 2 tablespoons almond butter

1 teaspoon vanilla extract

¼ teaspoon maple extract or maple flavor

Heaping ½ cup ice cubes

2 pinches of sea salt (optional)

Dip the rims of 2 tall glasses in water, then into the crushed caramel candy to line them.

In a blender, combine the milk and dates and process until well combined and there are virtually no date bits and pieces visible. Add the pineapple, almond butter, vanilla, maple extract or flavor, and ice cubes. Blend on medium speed just until the ice cubes are pureed and the beverage is thick and frothy. Pour into the candy-rimmed glasses, add a pinch of sea salt to each, if desired.

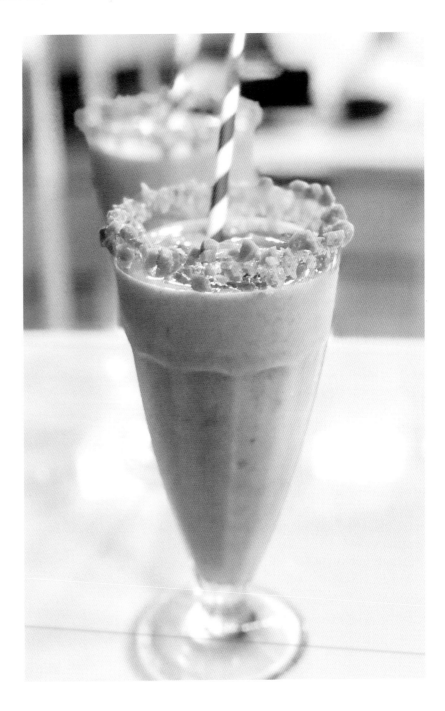

PER SERVING **180** CALORIES **4 g** PROTEIN **6 g** TOTAL FAT (**5.5 g** UNSATURATED FAT, **0.5** SATURATED FAT) **0 mg** CHOLESTEROL **31 g** CARBS **4 g** FIBER **22 g** SUGAR (**22 g** NATURAL SUGAR, **0 g** ADDED SUGAR) **150 mg** SODIUM

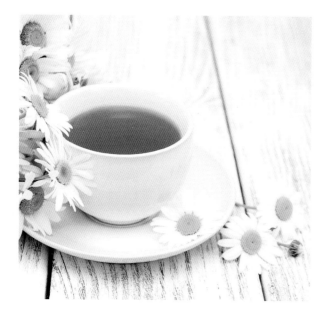

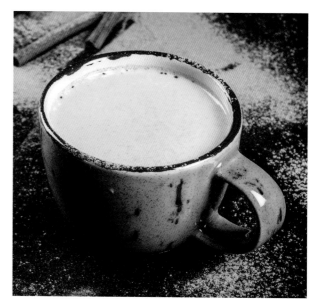

Turmeric-Ginger Tea

Superfoods: turmeric, ginger, cinnamon

SERVES: 2   PREP TIME: 5 MINUTES
COOK TIME: 10 MINUTES

1 (1-inch) piece fresh
   ginger root, thinly sliced

1 (2-inch) piece fresh
   turmeric root, thinly
   sliced

1 cinnamon stick

Honey (optional)

In a small saucepan, combine 2 cups water, the ginger, turmeric, and cinnamon. Stir to combine, cover, and bring to a boil over medium heat. Reduce the heat to low and simmer for 10 minutes. Strain the tea through a fine-mesh strainer into mugs, stir in some honey, if desired.

PER SERVING 1 CUP **0** CALORIES **0 g** PROTEIN **0 g** FAT **0 mg** CHOLESTEROL **1 g** CARBS **0 g** FIBER **0 g** SUGAR **10 mg** SODIUM

Golden Turmeric Milk

Superfoods: turmeric, cinnamon, almond

SERVES: 1   PREP TIME: 3 MINUTES
COOK TIME: 5 MINUTES

½ cup canned lite
   coconut milk*

½ cup unsweetened
   almond milk

1 teaspoon ground
   turmeric

1 to 2 teaspoons honey

¼ teaspoon ground
   cinnamon

⅛ teaspoon ground black
   pepper

Pinch of ground ginger
   (optional)

*   Or mix ¼ cup full-fat
    coconut milk with
    ¼ cup water to create
    lite coconut milk.

In a small saucepan, whisk together the coconut milk, almond milk, turmeric, honey, cinnamon, black pepper, and ginger, if using, and bring to a boil over medium heat. Reduce the heat to low and simmer for about 5 minutes. Pour into a mug and enjoy.

PER SERVING **110** CALORIES **0 g** PROTEIN **8 g** FAT (**7 g** SATURATED FAT, **1 g** UNSATURATED FAT) **0 mg** CHOLESTEROL **10 g** CARBS **1 g** FIBER **5 g** SUGAR (**0 g** NATURAL SUGAR, **5 g** ADDED SUGAR) **25 mg** SODIUM

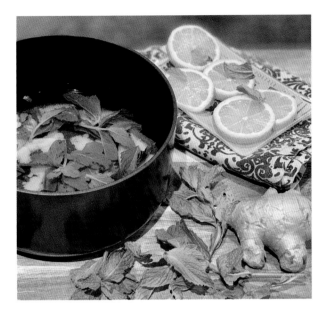

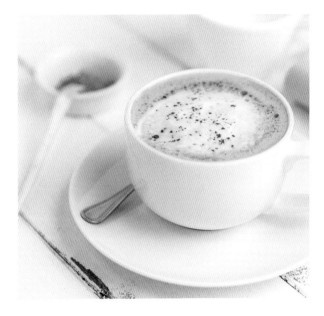

Infusion Mint Tea

Superfoods: mint, ginger, lemon

SERVES: 2 PREP TIME: 3 MINUTES
COOK TIME: 3 MINUTES

⅔ cup fresh mint leaves

1 (2-inch) piece fresh
  ginger root, thinly
  sliced

6 strips lemon zest
  (from 1 lemon)

1 teaspoon honey
  (optional)

In a small saucepan, bring 2 cups water to a boil. Turn off the heat, add the mint, ginger, lemon zest, and honey, if desired. Cover and steep for 3 minutes (or longer for stronger-flavored tea). Remove the mint, ginger, and lemon zest and pour into mugs.

PER SERVING 5 CALORIES 0 g PROTEIN 0 g FAT 0 mg CHO-LESTEROL 1 g CARBS 1 g FIBER 0 g SUGAR 10 mg SODIUM

Matcha Latte

Superfood: matcha

SERVES: 1 PREP TIME: 3 MINUTES

½ cup boiling water

½ cup canned lite
  coconut milk*

1 teaspoon matcha powder

½ teaspoon vanilla extract

1 teaspoon honey, or more
  to taste

* To trim calories and
   saturated fat, swap in
   almond milk or low-fat
   cow's milk.

Add the boiling water, coconut milk, matcha, vanilla, and honey to a small blender and process for about 1 minute, until the ingredients are well combined and frothy. Serve immediately, or microwave for 30 to 60 seconds to get it piping hot.

PER SERVING 1 CUP, WITH COCONUT MILK 110 CAL-ORIES 2 g PROTEIN 6 g FAT (1.5 g UNSATURATED FAT, 4.5 g SATURATED FAT) 0 mg CHOLESTEROL 12 g CARBS 1 g FIBER 9 g SUGAR (4 g NATURAL SUGAR, 5 g ADDED SUGAR) 45 mg SODIUM

PER SERVING 1 CUP, WITH ALMOND MILK 50 CALORIES 3 g PROTEIN 1.5 g FAT (1.5 g UNSATURATED FAT, 0 g SATURAT-ED FAT) 0 mg CHOLESTEROL 7 g CARBS 1 g FIBER 6 g SUGAR (1 g NATURAL SUGAR, 5 g ADDED SUGAR) 95 mg SODIUM

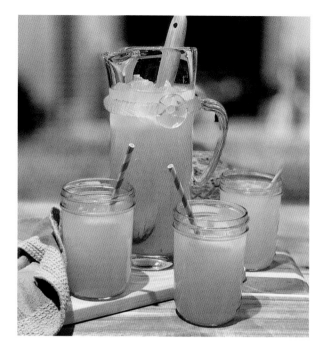

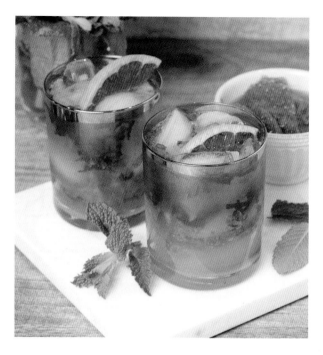

Golden Pineapple Kombucha Mocktail

Superfoods: turmeric, ginger, kombucha

SERVES: ABOUT 8
PREP TIME: 3 MINUTES

2 cups turmeric-ginger tea, at room temperature or chilled (recipe on page 270)

2 cups pineapple juice

4 cups kombucha (plain or ginger-flavored) or sparkling water (plain or pineapple-flavored)

Fill a pitcher with ice and add the turmeric-ginger tea, pineapple juice, and kombucha or sparkling water. Give it a stir.

PER SERVING 1 CUP MADE WITH KOMBUCHA **45** CALORIES **0 g** PROTEIN **0 g** FAT **0 mg** CHOLESTEROL **11 g** CARBS **0 g** FIBER **9 g** SUGAR **10 mg** SODIUM

PER SERVING 1 CUP MADE WITH SPARKLING WATER **30** CALORIES **0 g** PROTEIN **0 g** FAT **0 mg** CHOLESTEROL **8 g** CARBS **0 g** FIBER **8 g** SUGAR **10 mg** SODIUM

Pink Grapefruit Mojito Mocktail

Superfoods: pink grapefruit, lime, mint

SERVES: 1   PREP TIME: 5 MINUTES

8 fresh mint leaves

½ pink grapefruit, sectioned, skin and flesh removed

1 tablespoon lime juice

½ cup crushed ice

½ to ¾ cup grapefruit-flavored sparkling water

Combine the mint leaves, grapefruit sections, and lime juice in a glass. Use the back of a spoon or a muddler to gently crush the ingredients. You'll need just about 4 or 5 turns, until you start to smell a minty scent. Stir in the crushed ice and sparkling water.

PER SERVING **45** CALORIES **1 g** PROTEIN **0 g** FAT **0 mg** CHOLESTEROL **12 g** CARBS **2 g** CARBS **2 g** FIBER **9 g** SUGAR (**9 g** NATURAL SUGAR, **0 g** ADDED SUGAR) **0 mg** SODIUM

Tropical Piña Colada

Superfood: pineapple

SERVES: 2   PREP TIME: 5 MINUTES

1½ cups frozen pineapple chunks

¾ cup canned lite coconut milk*

3 to 5 ice cubes

1½ ounces rum

1 to 2 drops coconut extract

2 tablespoons unsweetened shredded coconut (optional)

2 wedges fresh pineapple (optional)

*   *Or mix ¼ cup full-fat coconut milk with ¼ cup water to create lite coconut milk.*

In a blender, combine all the ingredients and process until smooth and creamy. Pour into glasses and garnish each with an optional pineapple wedge.

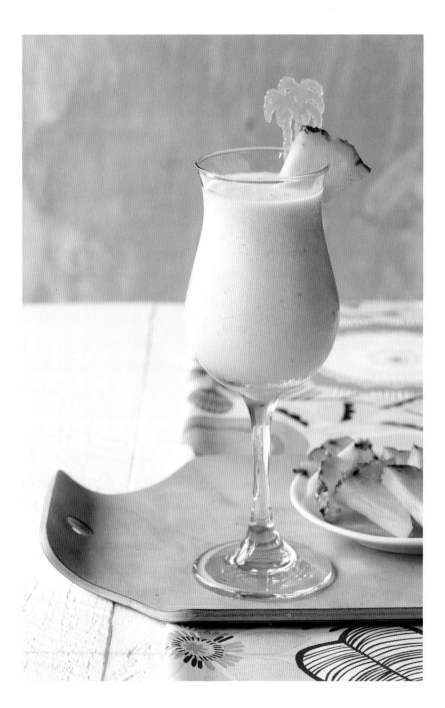

PER SERVING **160** CALORIES **2 g** PROTEIN **5 g** FAT (**0.5 g** UNSATURATED FAT, **4.5** SATURATED FAT) **16 g** CARBS **2 g** FIBER **12 g** SUGAR (**12 g** NATURAL SUGAR, **0 g** ADDED SUGAR) **20 mg** SODIUM

Blackberry Margarita

Superfoods: blackberries, lime

SERVES: 1   PREP TIME: 5 MINUTES

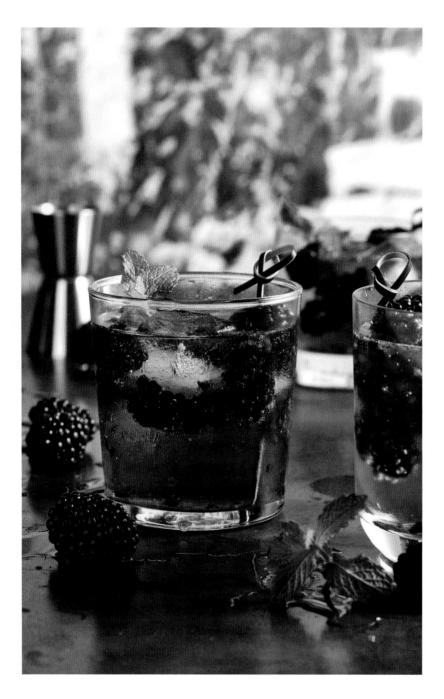

¾ cup fresh blackberries, divided

1 to 2 teaspoons honey

1 tablespoon lime juice

1 ounce tequila

½ cup ice cubes

¼ cup sparkling wine or champagne

In a glass, lightly muddle ½ cup of the blackberries with the honey and lime juice using a wooden spoon. Add the tequila, ice cubes, and the remaining ¼ cup blackberries (leave them whole) and gently stir. Top with the sparkling wine or champagne. For an extra-special touch, line your glass rims with salt or sugar before making your cocktails.

PER SERVING **190** CALORIES **2 g** PROTEIN **0.5 g** FAT (**0.5 g** UNSATURATED FAT, **0 g** SATURATED FAT) **0 mg** CHOLESTEROL **19 g** CARBS **5 g** FIBER **12 g** SUGAR (**6 g** NATURAL SUGAR, **6 g** ADDED SUGAR) **0 mg** SODIUM

Matcha Moscow Mule

Superfoods: ginger, lime, matcha

SERVES: 1   PREP TIME: 2 MINUTES

1 ounce vodka

1 ounce pineapple juice*

1 teaspoon grated fresh ginger root

2 tablespoons lime juice

½ teaspoon matcha powder

Ice cubes

¼ cup club soda or sparkling water

*   *You can swap 1 teaspoon honey
    for the pineapple juice.*

In a glass, combine the vodka,
pineapple juice, ginger, lime
juice, and matcha and mix until
well combined. Add ice cubes,
top it off with the club soda or
sparkling water.

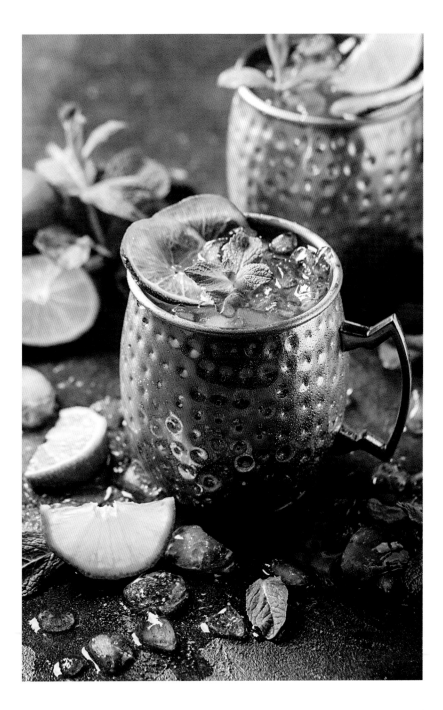

PER SERVING **90** CALORIES **1 g** PROTEIN **0 g** FAT **0 mg** CHOLESTEROL **7 g** CARBS **0 g** FIBER **4 g** SUGAR (**4 g** NATURAL SUGAR,
0 g ADDED SUGAR) **0 mg** SODIUM

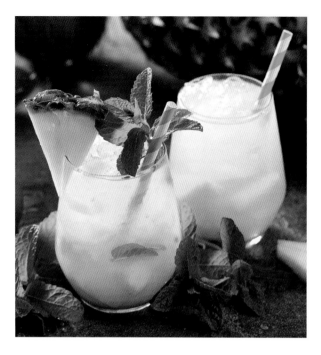

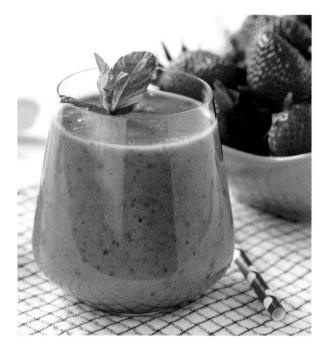

Piña Colada on the Rocks

Superfood: kiwi

SERVES: 1   PREP TIME: 2 MINUTES

3 kiwi, peeled

¼ cup canned lite coconut milk

¼ cup pineapple juice

¼ cup coconut or lime-flavored sparkling water

1 ounce rum

Puree kiwi in a blender, pour into an ice cube tray and freeze. (1 kiwi makes about 2 cubes.)

In a cocktail glass, combine the coconut milk, pineapple juice, sparkling water, rum, and ice cubes and mix well. Add a few "kiwi cubes" to your glass.

PER SERVING **140** CALORIES **0 g** PROTEIN **4 g** FAT (**0.5 g** UNSATURATED FAT, **3.5 g** SATURATED FAT) **0 mg** CHOLESTEROL **8 g** CARBS **0 g** FIBER **7 g** SUGAR (**7 g** NATURAL SUGAR, **0 g** ADDED SUGAR) **15 mg** SODIUM

Strawberry Daiquiri

Superfood: strawberries

SERVES: 2   PREP TIME: 5 MINUTES

2 cups sliced fresh strawberries

1 to 2 teaspoons sugar

2 cups sliced frozen strawberries

1½ ounces rum

3 to 5 ice cubes

In a small bowl, mix the strawberries and sugar to macerate. Cover and refrigerate for 20 to 30 minutes, until the strawberries begin to sweeten and release their natural juices.

Put the fresh strawberry-sugar mixture into a blender, add the frozen strawberries, rum, and ice cubes, and process until smooth and frothy. Pour into glasses and enjoy.

PER SERVING 1 CUP **160** CALORIES **2 g** PROTEIN **1 g** FAT (**1 g** UNSATURATED FAT, **0 g** SATURATED FAT) **0 mg** CHOLESTEROL **27 g** CARBS **7 g** FIBER **18 g** SUGAR (**16 g** NATURAL SUGAR, **2 g** ADDED SUGAR) **0 mg** SODIUM

Pomegranate Sangria

Superfoods: orange, apple, strawberries, pomegranate

MAKES: 12 CUPS   PREP TIME: 10 MINUTES, PLUS AT LEAST 6 HOURS IN THE REFRIGERATOR

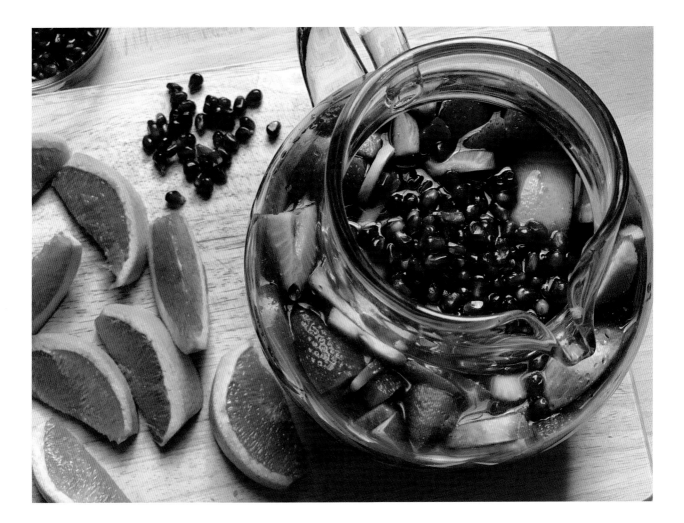

1 orange, sliced

1 red apple, sliced

3 cups strawberries, sliced

½ cup pomegranate seeds, plus more for garnish (optional)

1 (750-ml) bottle red table wine (like Pinot Noir)

1 cup pomegranate juice

½ to 1 cup chilled sparkling water, plain or pomegranate-flavored

Place the orange, apple, strawberries, and pomegranate seeds in a large pitcher. Add the wine and pomegranate juice. Refrigerate for at least 6 hours or overnight (so the fruit has time to incorporate all the delicious juice and wine flavor). When you're ready to serve, pour into glasses and top each glass off with a splash of sparkling water and a sprinkling of pomegranate seeds, if desired. Stir and enjoy.

PER SERVING 1 CUP **90** CALORIES **1 g** PROTEIN **0 g** FAT **0 mg** CHOLESTEROL **12 g** CARBS **2 g** FIBER **8 g** SUGAR (**8 g** NATURAL SUGAR, **0 g** ADDED SUGAR) **5 mg** SODIUM

Miami Vice

Superfoods: pineapple, strawberries

SERVES: 4   PREP TIME: 10 MINUTES

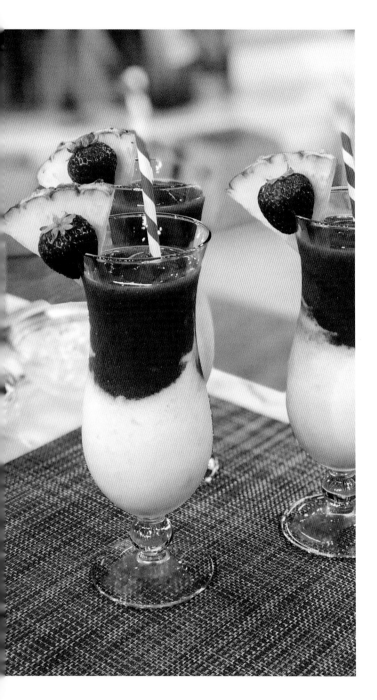

PIÑA COLADA

1½ cups frozen pineapple chunks

¾ cup canned lite coconut milk*

1½ ounces rum

1 to 2 drops coconut extract or natural flavor

2 tablespoons unsweetened shredded coconut

3 to 5 ice cubes

STRAWBERRY DAIQUIRI

2 cups sliced fresh strawberries

1 to 2 teaspoons sugar

2 cups sliced frozen strawberries

1 ounce rum

3 to 5 ice cubes (add more for an icier consistency)

FOR THE PIÑA COLADA: Add all the ingredients to a blender and process until smooth and creamy.

FOR THE STRAWBERRY DAIQUIRI: In small bowl, mix the fresh strawberries and sugar. Cover and refrigerate for 20 to 30 minutes, until the strawberries begin to release their natural juices. Then place them in a blender with the frozen strawberries, rum, and ice cubes and process until smooth and frothy.

TO ASSEMBLE: Pour ½ cup of the piña colada into each glass, followed by ½ cup of the strawberry daiquiri. Garnish with pineapple wedges and strawberries on the rim, if desired.

* FOR MIAMI VICE ICE POPS: Fill ice pop molds halfway with the piña colada mixture and stash in the freezer for about 1 hour to set. Then, add the strawberry daiquiri mixture on top. Place back in the freezer for at least 5 to 6 hours or overnight. 55 calories each.

PER SERVING 130 CALORIES 2 g PROTEIN 3 g FAT (0.5 g UNSATURATED FAT, 2.5 g SATURATED FAT) 0 mg CHOLESTEROL 17 g CARBS 3 g FIBER 12 g SUGAR (11 g NATURAL SUGAR, 1 g ADDED SUGAR) 10 mg SODIUM

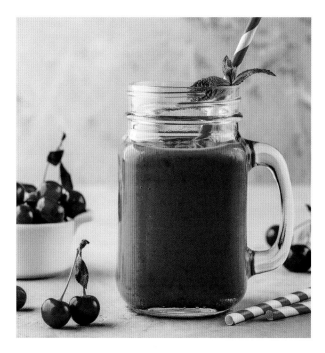

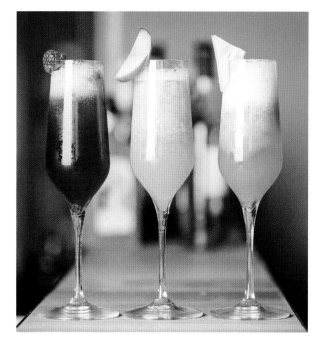

Fruit-Infused Frosé

Superfoods: cherries, pineapple

SERVES: 2   PREP TIME: 3 MINUTES

2 cups frozen sweet pitted cherries

½ cup frozen pineapple chunks

¾ to 1 cup rosé wine

3 to 5 ice cubes (optional)

In a blender, combine all the ingredients and blend until smooth. Pour into glasses and enjoy.

Fruity Champagne Sparkler

Superfoods: orange, cranberry, tart cherry, or pink grapefruit

SERVES: 1   PREP TIME: 2 MINUTES

3 ounces sparkling wine or champagne

1 ounce fruit juice of choice (orange, cranberry, tart cherry, pink grapefruit, etc.)

1 to 2 slices of fresh fruit

Pour the sparkling wine into a champagne flute. Top it off with your preferred fruit juice and a slice of corresponding fruit.

PER SERVING 190 CALORIES 2 g PROTEIN 0 g FAT 0 mg CHOLESTEROL 31 g CARBS 4 g FIBER 24 g SUGAR (24 g NATURAL SUGAR, 0 g ADDED SUGAR) 0 mg SODIUM

PER SERVING 90 CALORIES 0 g PROTEIN 0 g FAT 0 mg CHOLESTEROL 6 g CARBS 0 g FIBER 3 g SUGAR (3 g NATURAL SUGAR, 0 g ADDED SUGAR) 0 mg SODIUM

Acknowledgments

Feeling gratitude and not expressing it is like wrapping a present and not giving it.
—William Arthur Ward

I am super grateful to so many amazing people who made this book possible, and I am thrilled to give them the gift of my eternal thanks.

My entire work life is only possible because of the continuous support and unparalleled expertise of my outstanding editorial director, Donna Fennessy. Donna works meticulously with precision and grace to cover every detail, whether it involves an article, research report, or, in this case, a full-fledged book. Her unyielding dedication over the past year has transformed 150 recipes into a delicious and important resource that will help countless people live healthier and longer lives. Donna is quite literally the wizard behind my health curtain. I am equally grateful to her amazing family:—her husband, Jack, and three beautiful children, Lucy, Allie, and Jack—for so generously sharing their incredible wife and mom with me.

And I'm indebted to my lead nutritionist, Rebecca Jay Forman, RDN. She is invaluable because she brings a confident, calm, and insightful approach to everything she does. Whether she's helping me test recipes, analyze math, vet through research, or keep any one of hundreds of balls in the air at any point in time, I couldn't imagine doing this without her. She is a beloved employee and cherished friend.

Deepest gratitude to Leslie Orlandini, Jessie Levin, and Amanda Heckert, three gifted and innovative chefs who helped create recipes and test them over and over again.

Thanks also to Ryan Nord, Jane Dystel, and Miriam Goderich, for always being my biggest cheerleaders and ardent supporters. Major thanks to Jami Kandel, who has been with me almost from the beginning in helping to spread my message.

To my entire NBC *TODAY* family, who allow me the chance to share my creations and tasty tidbits with their audience day in and day out. I'm so grateful to be part of their brilliant team in our mission to help millions of people live their best lives.

To Abrams Books, in particular Holly Dolce, for approving this fun and informative idea and for being my beyond-outstanding and crackerjack editor, along with Lisa Silverman. A million thanks to Lucy Schaeffer for the seriously drool-worthy photography. And to Leslie Orlandini for being a magician extraordinaire at food styling. Also, to Ryan Lui and Andrea

Patton for having an impeccable eye for props, and to Danielle Terry and Kelly O'Neil for making me cover-worthy—no easy task. And to Robin Maizes, Nathan Congleton, and Tara Rochford for their stunning additions. Also to Reed Alexander for his wizardry with words.

And special thanks to Jordan Solomon and Katie Maloney for their unending support and sage advice. And to Hedda Boege, Tia Cannon, Julia Chatzky, Olivia Gutherz, Ali McGowan, and Danielle Ziegelstein for their contributions to this book.

One giant hug to my large and loving family (including Debra, Steve, Ben, Noah, Becca, Chloe, Jenny, Casey, Rosie, Pam, Dan, Charlie, Cooper, Granger, Elena, Glenn, Trey, Billie, Levi, Mabel, Mia, Jason, Annabelle, Zachary, Bailey, Harley, Alee, Nancy, Camron, Pam, Kaheo, Jason, Madeline, Marci, Rob, Pamela, Brandon, Scarlett, Dave, Beth, and Stewie) for always being willing to gather and taste test—*recipe after recipe*—until each is perfect. I know it has involved loosening the belt buckle on more than one occasion! I truly appreciate you all.

To my mom and dad, Ellen and Artie Schloss; my other mom and dad, Carol and Vic Bauer; my husband, Ian; my three kids, Jesse, Cole, and Ayden Jane; and my favorite fur-baby, Gatsby . . . you are my superfuel, my superjoy, my super-everything.

Metric Conversions

Below is a list of conversions from imperial/U.S. measurements to metric measurements (by weight) for some commonly used ingredients. Note: Use volume (not weight) equivalents for nut butters, including tahini; oils that are liquid at room temperature; milks, sour cream, and yogurt; syrups and honey; and jams, preserves, and purees.

Ingredient	¼ cup	⅓ cup	½ cup	⅔ cup	¾ cup	1 cup
almond flour	30 g	35 g	60 g	75 g	85 g	115 g
arrowroot flour	30 g	45 g	65 g	85 g	95 g	130 g
baking powder	50 g	65 g	100 g	130 g	145 g	195 g
baking soda	45 g	60 g	90 g	120 g	135 g	180 g
basil, fresh chopped	10 g	15 g	20 g	25 g	30 g	40 g
blueberries	35 g	50 g	75 g	95 g	110 g	145 g
breadcrumbs, panko	20 g	25 g	40 g	55 g	60 g	80 g
butter	55 g	75 g	115 g	150 g	170 g	225 g
cashews, halves or pieces	40 g	45 g	65 g	85 g	100 g	130 g
chia seeds, black or white	40 g	55 g	80 g	110 g	120 g	165 g
chickpea flour	25 g	30 g	45 g	60 g	70 g	90 g
chocolate chips, dark, semisweet, or milk	45 g	60 g	85 g	115 g	130 g	175 g
cilantro, fresh chopped	10 g	15 g	20 g	25 g	30 g	40 g
cheese, shredded	30 g	40 g	55 g	75 g	85 g	115 g
feta cheese, crumbled	40 g	50 g	75 g	100 g	115 g	150 g
goat cheese	30 g	40 g	55 g	75 g	85 g	115 g
cocoa powder	25 g	30 g	50 g	65 g	70 g	95 g
cream cheese	60 g	75 g	115 g	155 g	175 g	230 g
dates, pitted, whole	30 g	40 g	65 g	85 g	95 g	125 g
dill, chopped	13 g	17 g	25 g	35 g	40 g	50 g
flax seeds, ground	35 g	45 g	65 g	85 g	100 g	130 g
whole wheat flour (and white whole wheat flour)	30 g	40 g	65 g	80 g	95 g	125 g
lentils	50 g	65 g	95 g	130 g	145 g	190 g
oats, rolled (old-fashioned)	20 g	30 g	45 g	60 g	65 g	90 g
onions, chopped	35/30 g	40/35 g	65/55 g	85/75 g	95/85 g	125/110 g
Parmesan (or similar) cheese, grated	25 g	30 g	50 g	65 g	70 g	100 g
parsley, fresh chopped	13 g	17 g	25 g	35 g	40 g	50 g
peppers, chile (jalapeño, etc.), chopped	40 g	50 g	75 g	100 g	115 g	150 g
pumpkin seeds (pepitas)	15 g	20 g	30 g	40 g	50 g	65 g
quinoa (uncooked)	45 g	55 g	85 g	115 g	130 g	170 g
ricotta (whole or part skim)	60 g	80 g	125 g	165 g	185 g	245 g
sesame seeds, white or yellow	40 g	50 g	75 g	100 g	115 g	150 g
spinach (fresh), chopped	8 g	10 g	15 g	20 g	23 g	30 g
spinach (frozen), chopped	40 g	50 g	80 g	105 g	115 g	155 g
sugar (granulated)	50 g	65 g	100 g	135 g	150 g	200 g
walnuts, chopped or pieces	30 g	40 g	60 g	80 g	90 g	120 g

Index